State Standard of the People's Republic of China

The Location of Acupoints

Approved by the State Administration of Traditional Chinese Medicine
Compiled by the Institute of Acupuncture and Moxibustion of the China Academy of Traditional Chinese Medicine

FOREIGN LANGUAGES PRESS BEIJING

First Edition 1990

ISBN 0-8351-2749-4
ISBN 7-119-01368-8

Published by Foreign Languages Press
24 Baiwanzhuang Road, Beijing 100037, China

Printed by Printing House of the Chinese Academy of Sciences

Distributed by China International Book Trading Corporation
21 Chegongzhuang Xilu, Beijing 100044, China
P.O. Box 399, Beijing, China

Printed in the People's Republic of China

Publication Note

This standard, put forward by the State Administration of Traditional Chinese Medicine, specifies the methods for the location of points and the standard locations of 361 regular points and 48 extra points. It will facilitate the teaching, research and clinical practice of acupuncture, as well as academic information exchange on a global scale.

The researchers for this standard are Deng Liangyue, Li Ding, Chen Keqin, Wang Deshen, Gao Xizhu, Yan Zhenguo, Li Ruiwu, Gu Li, Zhao Xin, Huang Longxiang and Liu Weihong.

The experts and administrative personnel who have appraised and approved the text are Chen Youbang, Lu Zhijun, Wang Xuetai, Chen Shaowu, He Puren, Cheng Xinnong, Yang Jiasan, Zhao Erkang, Huang Xianming, Wei Jia, Wang Fuxiong, Ma Jixing, Shi Xuemin, Liu Quanjun, Yang Jiebin, He Shuhuai, Geng Enguang, Lu Jingshan, Zhang Shaozhen, Qiu Shuhua, Zhang Jianzhong, Han Yuqing, Li Dazong, Zhang Yizhi, Jia Weicheng, Liu Weidong, Zhang Ruixiang, Sha Fengtong and Zhao Lu.

The English text of this standard was prepared by Du Wei, Chen Yan, Chen Zhengrong, Hong Tao, Jin Zhigao, Li Ruiwu, Lin Huanyin, Luo Mingfu, Wang Huizhu, Xue Kuiyang, Yan Zhenguo, Zhang Jianhua and Yu Min; and edited by Wang Tai, Ou Ming, Zhang Kai, Fang Tingyu, Li Yanwen and Huang Guoqi.

The Institute of Acupuncture and Moxibustion of the China Academy of Traditional Chinese Medicine shall be responsible for the explanation of this standard.

CONTENTS

PART ONE

1. The Basis and Methods for the Location of Points

1. 1 The Basis for the Location of Points

The standard locations of the points of the 14 meridians and a part of the extra points are presented in this State Standard on a thorough study of the classical literature of traditional Chinese medicine and the monographs of acupuncture and moxibustion through the ages, such as *The Yellow Emperor's Canon of Internal Medicine* (*Huangdi Neijing*), *The Classic of Sphygmology* (*Mai Jing*), *A-B Classic of Acupuncture and Moxibustion* (*Zhen Jiu Jia Yi Jing*), *Illustrated Manual of Points for Acupuncture and Moxibustion on a Bronze Statue with Acupoints* (*Tong Ren Shu Xue Zhen Jiu Tu Jing*), and the newly published textbooks of the medical colleges and universities and the international acupunture training centres, and also based on the deep-going analysis and discussion of the clinical experience and the achievements of modern scientific researches.

The basic theories of traditional Chinese medicine, the theory of meridians and collaterals, and the principles for localization of points are taken as the guidance to determine the standard locations of points. The descriptions of the portions of the human body in traditional Chinese medicine are not always the same as those in modern anatomy. The palmar (flexor) side of the upper limbs is named the "medial side," where the three yin meridians of the hand are distributed, while the dorsal (extensor) side is known as the "lateral side," where the three yang meridians of the hand are distributed. The side of the lower limbs facing the sagittal plane of the body is called the "medial side," where the three yin meridians of the foot are distributed, while the sides where the three yang meridians of the foot are distributed are the "lateral side" and the "posterior side."

The transitional border between the palm and the dorsum of the hand and between the sole and the dorsum of the foot is called the "red and white skin junction"; the eminence of the metacarpophalangeal and metatarsophalangeal joints (including the part covered with joint capsule) is named "Benjie" in traditional Chinese medicine, the part distal to that is known as "anterior to Benjie," and the part proximal to that as "posterior to Benjie." In the upper limbs, the radial side of the thumb is termed as the "anterior side," and the ulnar side of the little finger as the "posterior side."

The anterior and posterior midlines on the head and trunk of the body are the places where the Ren (Conception Vessel) and Du (Governor Vessel) meridians are distributed, which are taken as the landmarks for locating the bilateral three yin and three yang meridians.

1. 2 The Methods for the Location of Points

There are three methods for locating points, surface anatomical landmarks, bone proportional measurement and finger measurement. They should be used in combination, but the first one is the fundamental and the other two the supplemental ones.

1. 2. 1 Surface Anatomical Landmarks

This is a method to determine the location of points on the basis of anatomical landmarks on the body surface, which are divided into the fixed and movable landmarks.

The fixed landmarks include the prominences and depressions formed by the joints and muscles, the configuration of the five sense organs, hairline, fingernails and toenails, nipples and umbilicus. For instance, Yanglingquan (GB 34) is in the depression anterior and inferior to the head of the fibula; Binao (LI 14) is at the end of the insertion of the deltoid muscle; Cuanzhu (BL 2) is at the medial end of the eyebrow; Yintang (EX-HN3) is midway between the eyebrows; and Danzhong (RN 17) is at the midpoint between the two nipples.

The movable landmarks refer to the clefts, depressions, wrinkles or prominences appearing on the joints, muscles, tendons and skin during motion. For example, Tinggong (SI 19) is between the tragus and mandibular joint, where a depression is formed when the mouth is slightly open; Quchi (LI 11) is in the depression at the lateral end of the cubital crease when the elbow is flexed.

The major anatomical landmarks on the human body surface are listed as follows:

On the head are:

1) the midpoint of the anterior hairline;

2) the midpoint of the posterior hairline;

3) the corner of the forehead (at the corner of the anterior hairline); and

4) the mastoid process.

On the face are:

1) Yintang (EX-HN3) (at the midpoint between the eyebrows); and

2) the pupil (in the erect sitting position and looking straight forward), or the centre of the eye (at the midpoint of the line between the inner and outer canthi).

On the neck is:

1) the laryngeal protuberance.

On the chest are:

1) the suprasternal fossa (in the depression above the suprasternal notch);

2) the midpoint of sternoxyphoid symphysis (at the conjunction of the sternum and xyphoid process); and

3) the nipple (the centre of the nipple).

On the abdomen are:

1) the umbilicus (Shenque, RN 8) (the centre of the umbilicus);

2) the upper border of the pubic symphysis at the crossing point of the upper border of the pubic symphysis and the anterior midline); and

3) the anterior superior iliac spine.

On the lateral side of the chest and abdomen are:

1) the apex of the axilla (the highest point of the axillary fossa); and

2) the free end of the 11th rib.

On the back, low back and sacrum are:

1) the spinous process of the 7th cervical vertebra;

2) the spinous processes from the 1st to the 12th thoracic vertebrae and from the 1st to the 5th lumbar vertebrae, the median sacral crest and the coccyx;

3) the medial and the scapular spine (on the medial border of the scapula);

4) the acromial angle; and

5) the posterior superior iliac spine.

On the upper limbs are:

1) anterior axillary fold (the anterior end of the axillary crease);

2) the posterior axillary fold (the posterior end of the axillary crease);

3) the cubital crease;

4) the tip of the elbow (olecranon); and

5) the dorsal and palmar creases of the wrist (the styloid crease between the distal ends of the styloid processes of the ulna and radius).

On the lower limbs are:

1) the greater trochanter of the femur;

2) the medial epicondyle of the femur;

3) the medial epicondyle of the tibia;

4) the inferior gluteal crease (the border between the buttocks and thigh);

5) Dubi (ST 35) (in the centre of the depression lateral to the patella ligament);

6) the popliteal crease;

7) the tip of the medial malleolus; and

8) the tip of the lateral malleolus.

1. 2. 2 Bone Proportional Measurement

In this method the joints are taken as the main landmarks to measure the length and width of various portions of the human body. The proportional measurement of various portions of the human body defined in the *Miraculous Pivot* (*Ling Shu*) is taken as the basis for the location of points in combination with the modified methods introduced by the acupuncturists through the ages. The length between two joints is divided into several equal portions, each portion as one *cun* and 10 portions as one *chi*. The main bone proportional measurements are listed in the following table.

Table of Bone Proportional Measurement (Figs. 1, 2 & 3)

Position	Origin and end points	Portion (*cun*)	Method of measurement	Remarks
Head and face	From the midpoint of the anterior hairline to the midpoint of the posterior hairline	12	Longitudinal measurement	Used for measuring the longitudinal distance of the points on the head
	From Yintang (EX-HN3) to the midpoint of the anterior hairline	3	Longitudinal measurement	Used for measuring the longitudinal distance of the points on the anterior and posterior hairline and the head
	From the point below the spinous process of the 7th cervical vertebra (Dazhui, DU 14) to the midpoint of the posterior hairline	3	Longitudinal measurement	

	From Yintang (EX-HN3) to the midpoint of the posterior hairline and then to the point below the spinous process of the 7th cervical vertebra (Dazhui, DU 14)	18	Longitudinal measurement	
	Between the corners of the forehead (Touwei, ST 8)	9	Transverse measurement	Used for measuring the transverse distance of the points on the anterior part of the head
	Between the bilateral mastoid processes	9	Transverse measurement	Used for measuring the transverse distance of the points on the posterior part of the head
Chest, abdomen and hypochondrium	From the suprasternal fossa (Tiantu, RN 22) to the midpoint of the sternoxyphoid symphysis	9	Longitudinal measurement	Used for measuring the longitudinal distance of the points of Ren Meridian (Conception Vessel) on the chest
	From the midpoint of the sternoxyphoid symphysis to the centre of the umbilicus	8	Longitudinal measurement	Used for measuring the longitudinal distance of the points on the upper abdomen
	From the centre of the umbilicus to the upper border of the pubic symphysis (Qugu, RN 2)	5	Longitudinal measurement	Used for measuring the longitudinal distance of the points on the lower abdomen
	Between the two nipples	8	Transverse measurement	Used for measuring the transverse distance of the points on the chest and abdomen
	From the apex of the axilla to the free end of the 11th rib (Zhangmen, LR 13)	12	Longitudinal measurement	Used for measuring the longitudinal distance of the points on the hypochondrium
Back and low back	From the medial border of the scapula to the posterior midline	3	Transverse measurement	Used for measuring the transverse distance of the points on the back
	From the acromial angle to the posterior midline	8	Transverse measurement	Used for measuring the transverse distance of the points on the shoulder and back
Upper limbs	From the anterior and posterior axillar folds to the cubital crease	9	Longitudinal measurement	Used for measuring the longitudinal distance of the points on the arm
	From the cubital crease to the			

	dorsal crease of the wrist	12	Longitudinal measurement	Used for measuring the longitudinal distance of the points on the forearm
Lower limbs	From the upper border of the pubic symphysis to the upper border of the medial epicondyle of the femur	18	Longitudinal measurement	Used for measuring the longitudinal distance of the points on the three yin meridians of the foot on the medial side of the lower limbs
	From the lower border of the medial epicondyle of the tibia to the tip of the medial malleolus	13	Longitudinal measurement	
	From the greater trochanter to the popliteal crease	19	Longitudinal measurement	Used for measuring the longitudinal distance of the points on the three yang meridians of the foot on the latero-posterior side of the lower limbs (the distance from the gluteal groove to the popliteal crease is equivalent to 14 *cun*)
	From the politeal crease to the tip of the lateral malleolus	16	Longitudinal measurement	Used for measuring the longitudinal distance of the points on the three yang meridians of the foot on the latero-posterior side of the lower limbs

1. 2. 3 Finger Measurement

This is a method to locate the points by measuring the distance with either the length or width of the patient's finger(s).

1) Middle finger measurement: When the middle finger is flexed, the distance between the radial ends of the two interphalangeal creases of the patient's middle finger is taken as 1 *cun* (Fig. 4).

2) Thumb measurement: The width of the interphalangeal joint of the patient's thumb is taken as 1 *cun* (Fig. 5).

3) Four-finger measurement: When the four fingers (index, middle, ring and little fingers) keep close, their width on the level of the proximal interphalangeal crease of the middle finger is taken as 3 *cun* (Fig. 6).

This method is mainly used for locating the points of the lower limbs. When locating the points, this method should be used in combination with some simple movable landmarks on the basis of the bone proportional measurement.

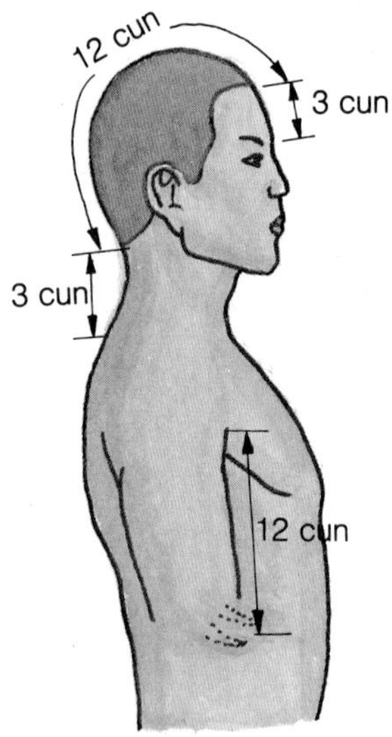

Fig. 1 Longitudinal Measurement of the Head

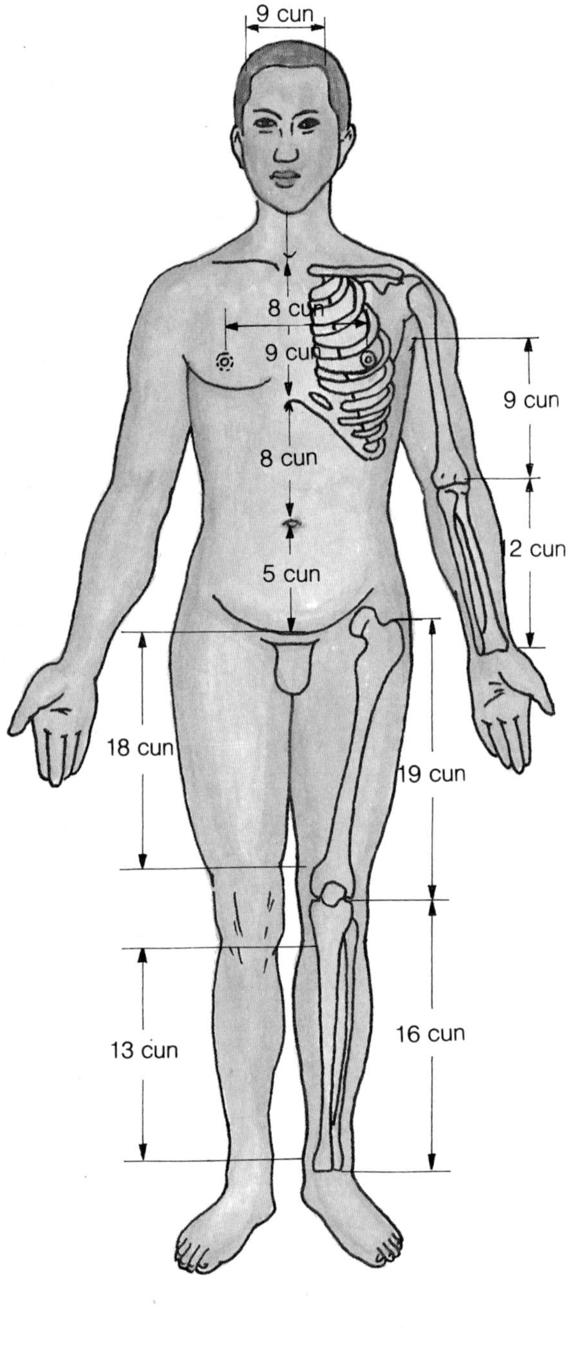

Fig. 2 Bone Proportional Measurement (Front View)

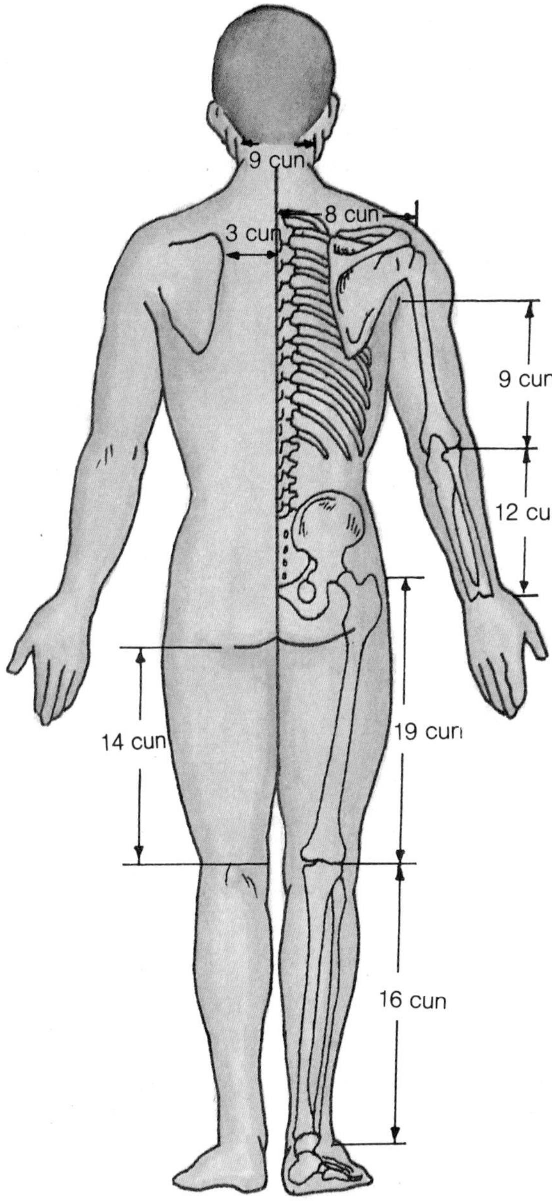

Fig. 3 Bone Proportional Measurement (Back View)

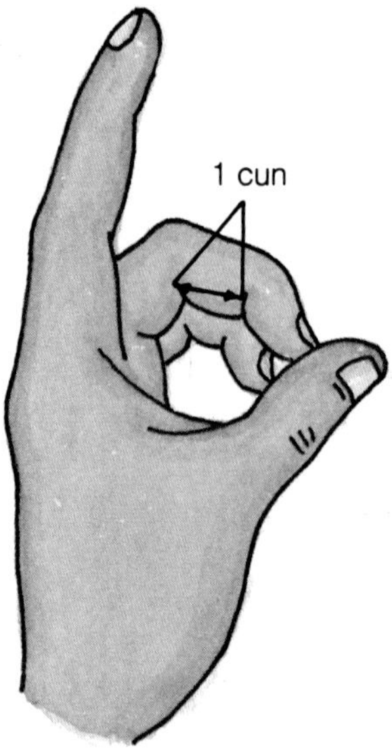

Fig. 4 Middle Finger Measurement

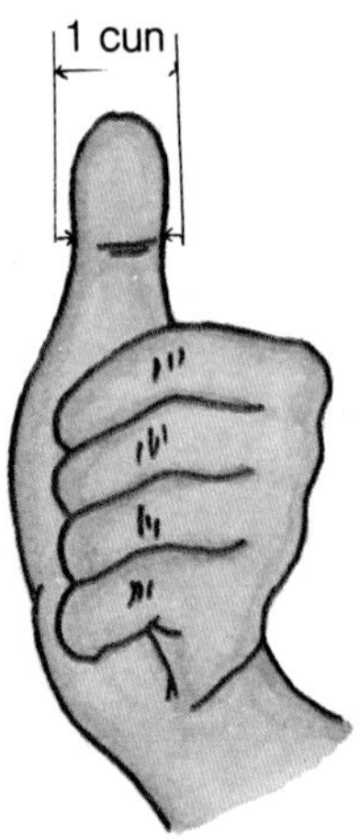

Fig. 5 Thumb Measurement

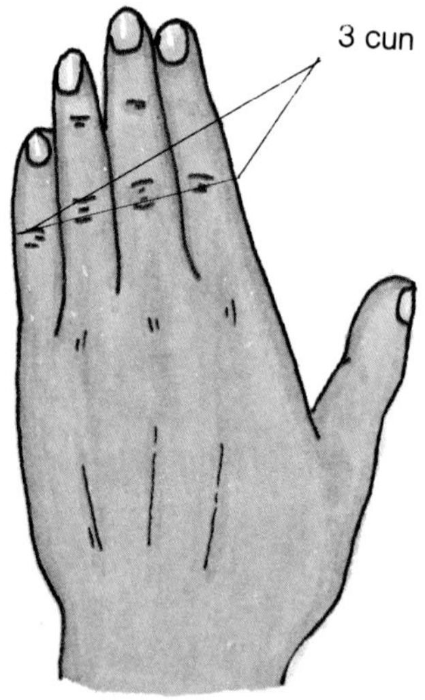

Fig. 6 Four-Finger Measurement

2. Standard Locations of the Points of the 14 Meridians

十四經穴標準定位

Shísì Jīngxué Biāozhŭn Dìngwèi

2. 1 Points of the Lung Meridian of Hand-Taiyin, LU

手太陰肺經穴

Shŏutàiyīn Fèijīng Xué

2. 1. 1 LU 1 Zhōngfŭ 中府

In the superior lateral part of the anterior thoracic wall, 1 *cun* below Yunmen (LU 2), on the level of the 1st intercostal space, 6 *cun* lateral to the anterior midline (Figs. 8 & 11).

2. 1. 2 LU 2 Yúnmén 雲門

In the superior lateral part of the anterior thoracic wall, superior to the coracoid process of the scapula, in the depression of the infraclavicular fossa, 6 *cun* lateral to the anterior midline (Figs. 8 & 12).

2. 1. 3 LU 3 Tiānfŭ 天府

On the medial side of the upper arm and on the radial border of the biceps muscle of the arm, 3 *cun* below the anterior end of the axillary fold (Fig. 11).

2. 1. 4 LU 4 Xiábái 俠白

On the medial side of the upper arm and on the radial border of the biceps muscle of the arm, 4 *cun* below the anterior end of the axillary fold, or 5 *cun* above the cubital crease (Fig. 11).

2. 1. 5 LU 5 Chĭzé 尺澤

In the cubital crease, in the depression of the radial side of the tendon of the biceps muscle of the arm (Figs. 11 & 13).

2. 1. 6 LU 6 Kŏngzuì 孔最

On the radial side of the palmar surface of the forearm, and on the line connecting Chize (LU 5) and Taiyuan (LU 9), 7 *cun* above the cubital crease (Figs. 11 & 13).

2. 1. 7 LU 7 Lièquē 列缺

On the radial side of the forearm, proximal to the styloid process of the radius, 1.5 *cun* above the crease of the wrist, between the brachioradial muscle and the tendon of the long abductor muscle of the thumb (Figs. 11 & 13)

2. 1. 8 LU 8 Jīngqú 經渠

On the radial side of the palmar surface of the forearm, 1 *cun* above the crease of the wrist, in the depression between the styloid process of the radius and radial artery (Figs. 11 & 13).

2. 1. 9 LU 9 Táiyuān 太淵

At the radial end of the crease of the wrist, where the pulsation of the radial artery is palpable (Figs. 11 & 13).

2. 1. 10 LU 10 Yújì 魚際

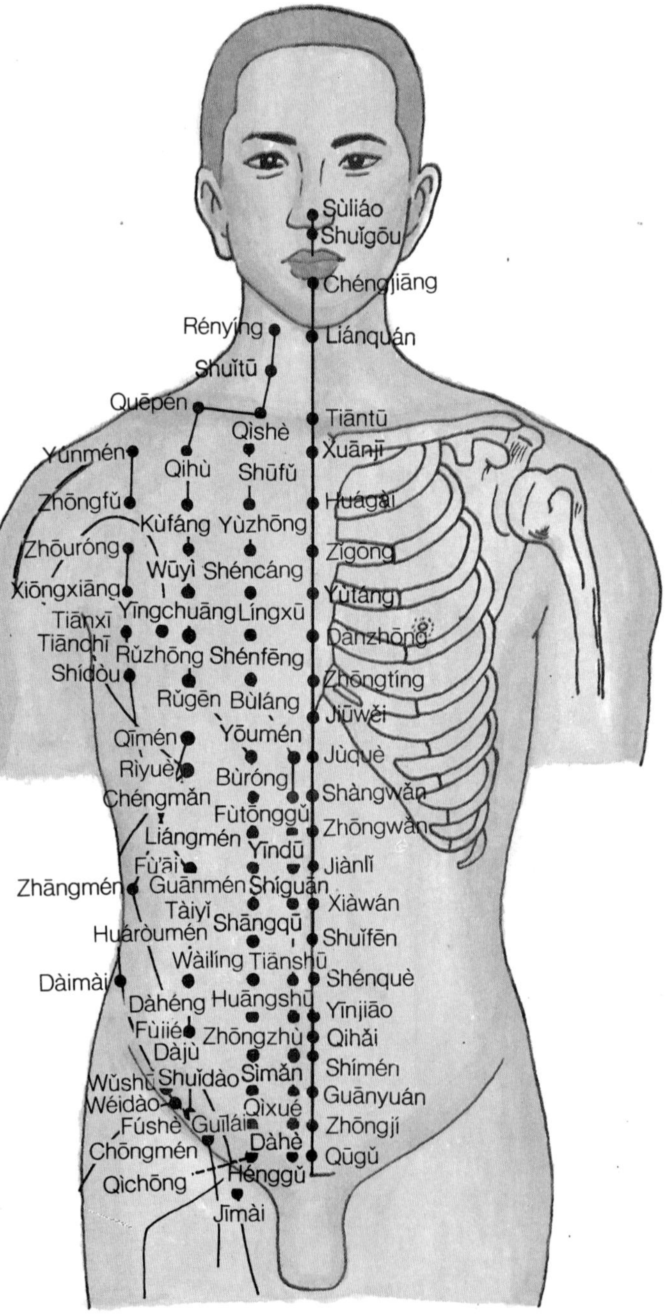

Fig. 8 Points on the Chest and Abdomen

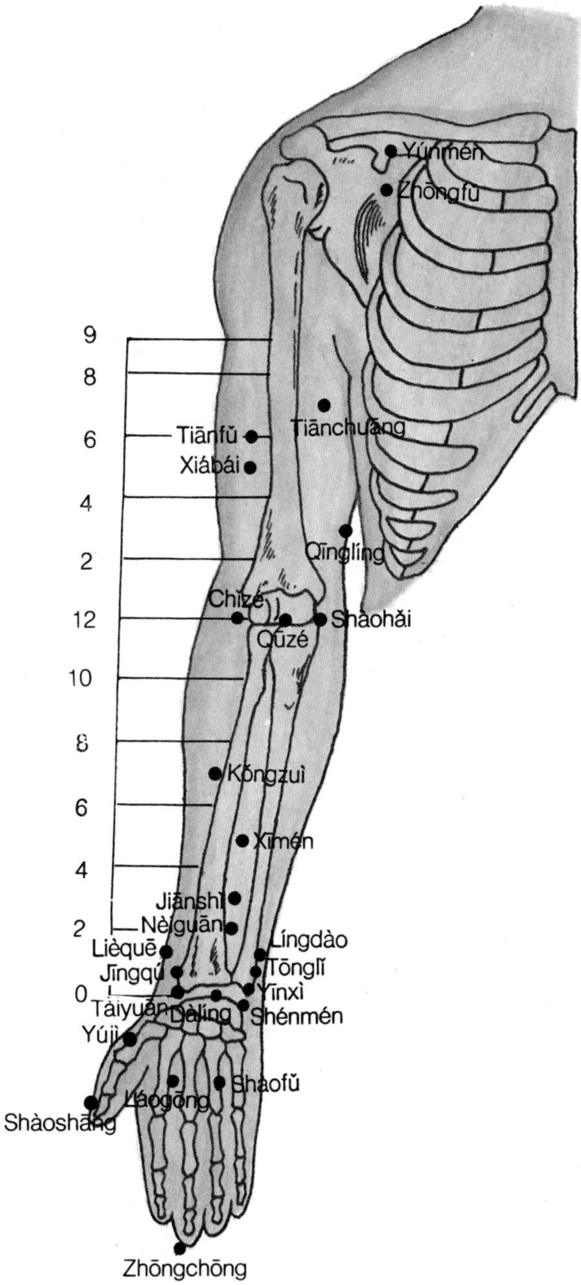

Fig. 11 Points of Three Yin Meridians of the Hand

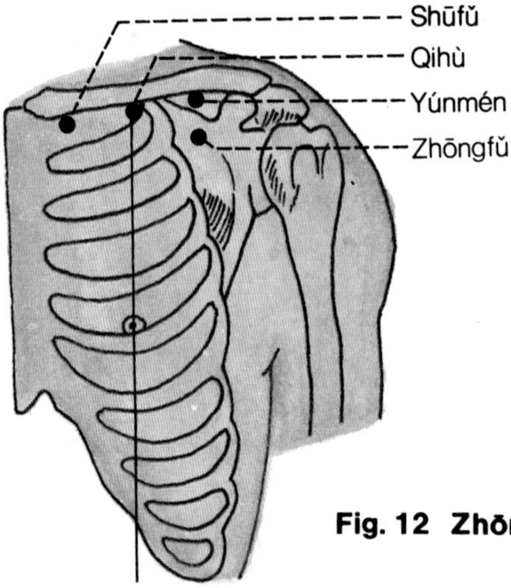

Fig. 12 Zhōngfǔ and Yúnmén Points

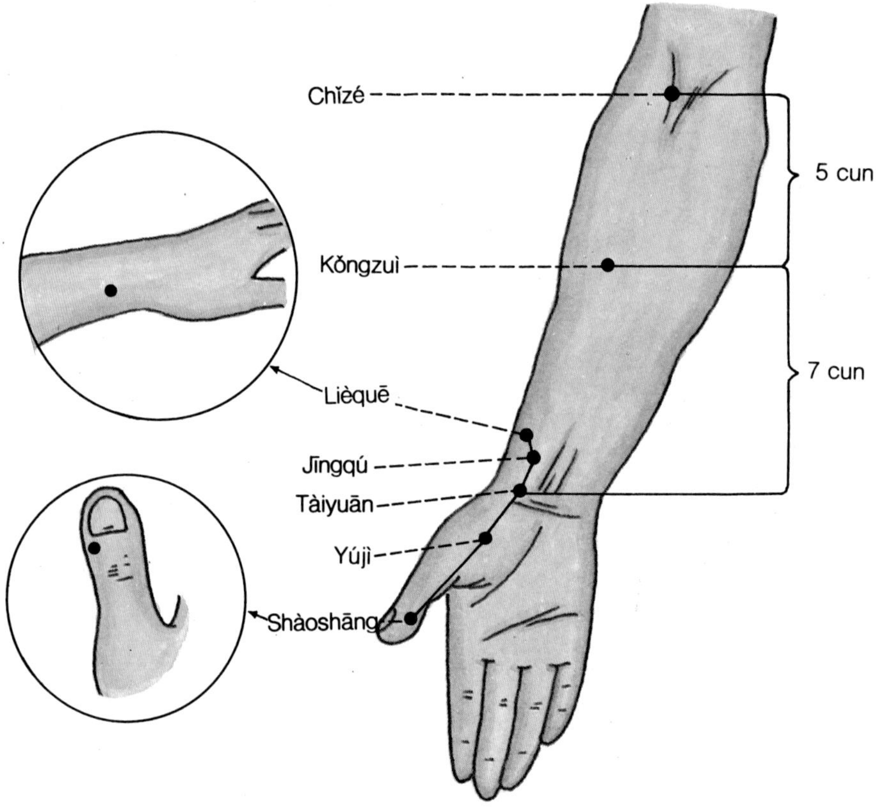

Fig. 13 Points of Lung Meridian (Upper Limbs)

In the depression proximal to the 1st metacarpophalangeal joint, on the radial side of the midpoint of the 1st metacarpal bone, and on the junction of the red and white skin (Figs. 11 & 13).

2. 1. 11 LU 11 Shàoshāng 少商

On the radial side of the distal segment of the thumb, 0.1 *cun* from the corner of the fingernail (Figs. 11 & 13).

2. 2 Points of the Large Intestine Meridian of Hand-Yangming, LI

手陽明大腸經穴

Shǒuyángmíng Dàchángjīng Xué

2. 2. 1 LI 1 Shāngyáng 商陽

On the radial side of the distal segment of the index finger, 0.1 *cun* from the corner of the nail (Figs. 14 & 15).

2. 2. 2 LI 2 Èrjiān 二間

In the depression of the radial side, distal to the 2nd metacarpophalangeal joint when a loose fist is made (Figs. 14 & 15).

2. 2. 3 LI 3 Sānjiān 三間

In the depression of the radial side, proximal to the 2nd metacarpophalangeal joint when a loose fist is made (Figs. 14 & 15).

2. 2. 4 LI 4 Hégǔ 合谷

On the dorsum of the hand, between the 1st and 2nd metacarpal bones, and on the radial side of the midpoint of the 2nd metacarpal bone (Figs. 14 & 15).

2. 2. 5 LI 5 Yángxī 陽谿

At the radial end of the crease of the wrist, in the depression between the tendons of the short extensor and long extensor muscles of the thumb when the thumb is tilted upward (Figs. 14 & 16).

2. 2. 6 LI 6 Piānlì 偏歷

With the elbow slightly flexed, on the radial side of the dorsal surface of the forearm and on the line connecting Yangxi (LI 5) and Quchi (LI 11), 3 *cun* above the crease of the wrist (Fig. 14 & 16).

2. 2. 7 LI 7 Wēnliū 温溜

With the elbow flexed, on the radial side of the dorsal surface of the forearm and on the line connecting Yangxi (LI 5) and Quchi (LI 11), 5 *cun* above the crease of the wrist (Figs. 14 & 16).

2. 2. 8 LI 8 Xiàlián 下廉

On the radial side of the dorsal surface of the forearm and on the line connecting Yangxi (LI 5) and Quchi (LI 11), 4 *cun* below the cubital crease (Figs. 14 & 16).

2. 2. 9 LI 9 Shànglián 上廉

On the radial side of the dorsal surface of the forearm and on the line connecting Yangxi (LI 5) and Quchi (LI 11), 3 *cun* below the cubital crease (Figs. 14 & 16).

2. 2. 10 LI 10 Shǒusānlǐ 手三裏

On the radial side of the dorsal surface of the forearm and on the line connecting Yangxi

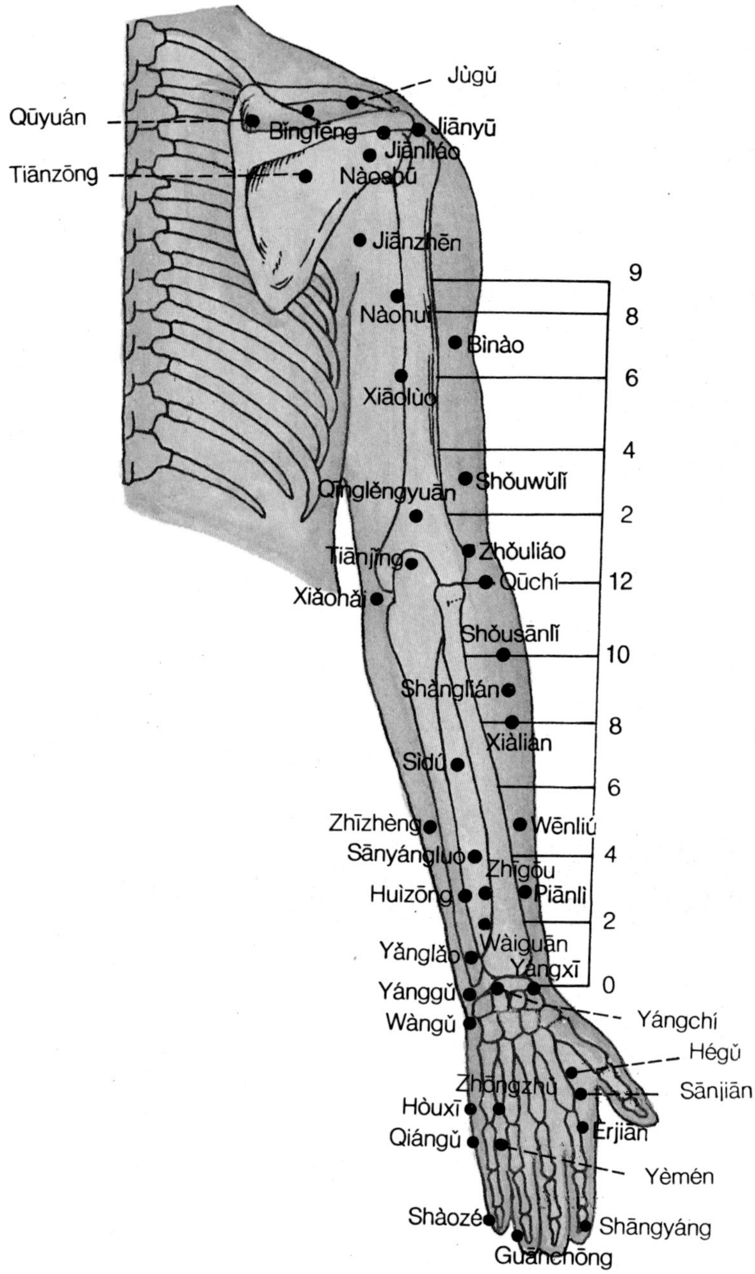

Fig. 14 Points of Three Yang Meridians of the Hand (Upper Limbs)

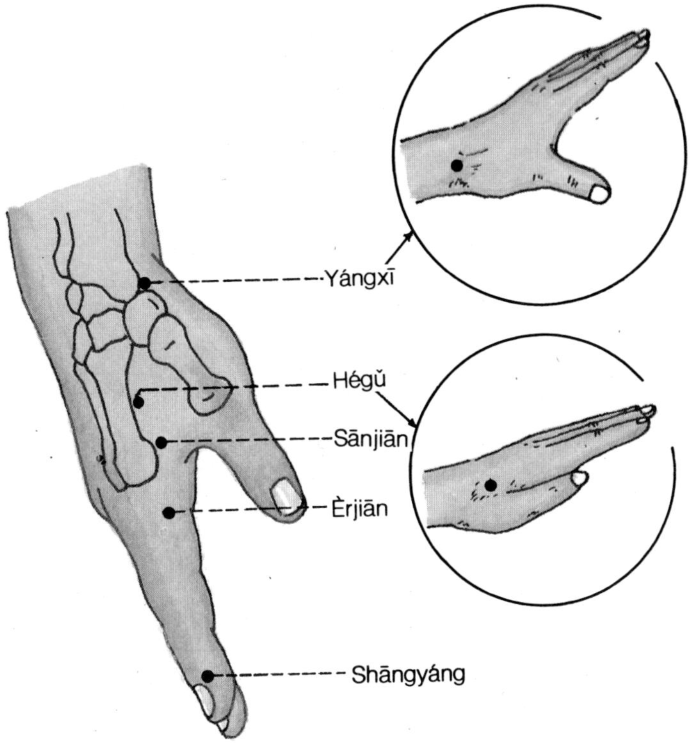

Fig. 15 Points of Large Intestine Meridian (Hand)

(LI 5) and Quchi (LI 11), 2 *cun* below the cubital crease (Figs. 14 & 16).

2. 2. 11 LI 11 Qūchí 曲池

With the elbow flexed, at the lateral end of the cubital crease, at the midpoint of the line connecting Chize (LU 5) and the external humeral epicondyle (Figs. 14 & 17).

2. 2. 12 LI 12 Zhǒuliáo 肘髎

With the elbow flexed, on the lateral side of the upper arm, 1 *cun* above Quchi (LI 11), on the border of the humerus (Figs. 14 & 17).

2. 2. 13 LI 13 Shǒuwǔlǐ 手五里

On the lateral side of the upper arm and on the line connecting Quchi (LI 11) and Jianyu (LI 15), 3 *cun* above Quchi (LI 11) (Figs. 14 & 17).

2. 2. 14 LI 14 Bìnào 臂臑

On the lateral side of the arm, at the insertion of the deltoid muscle and on the line connecting Quchi (LI 11) and Jianyu (LI 15), 7 *cun* above Quchi (LI 11) (Figs. 14 & 17).

2. 2. 15 LI 15 Jiānyú 肩髃

On the shoulder, superior to the deltoid muscle, in the depression anterior and inferior to the acromion when the arm is abducted or raised on the level of the shoulder (Figs. 14 & 17).

2. 2. 16 LI 16 Jùgǔ 巨骨

7 cun

5 cun

Qūchí
Shǒusānlǐ
Xiàlián
Shànglián
Wēnliú
Piānlì
Yángxī

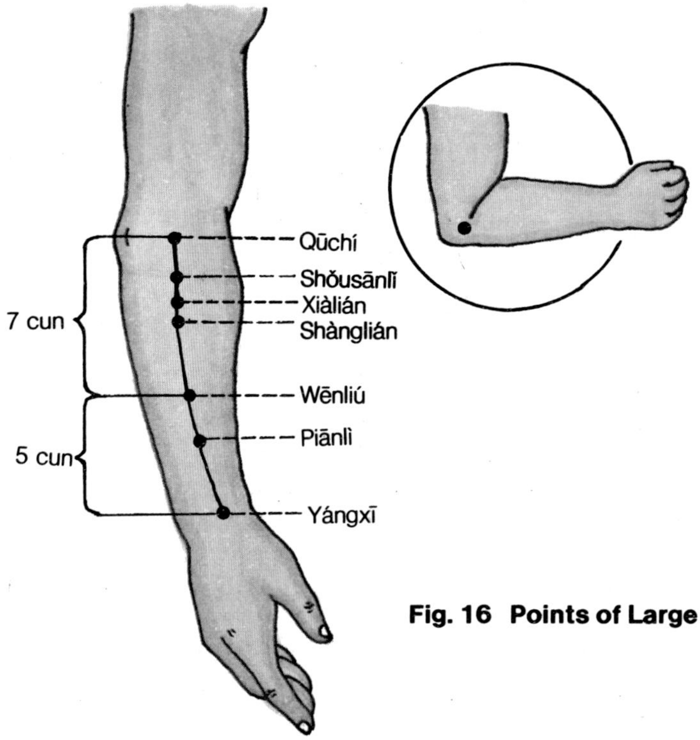

Fig. 16   Points of Large Intestine Meridian (Forearm)

Jiānyū
Bìnào
Shǒuwǔlǐ
Zhǒuliáo
Qūchí

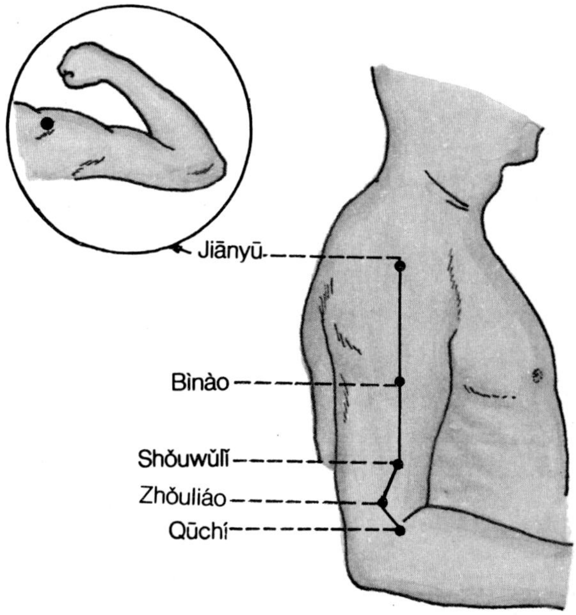

Fig. 17   Points of Large Intestine Meridian (Arm)

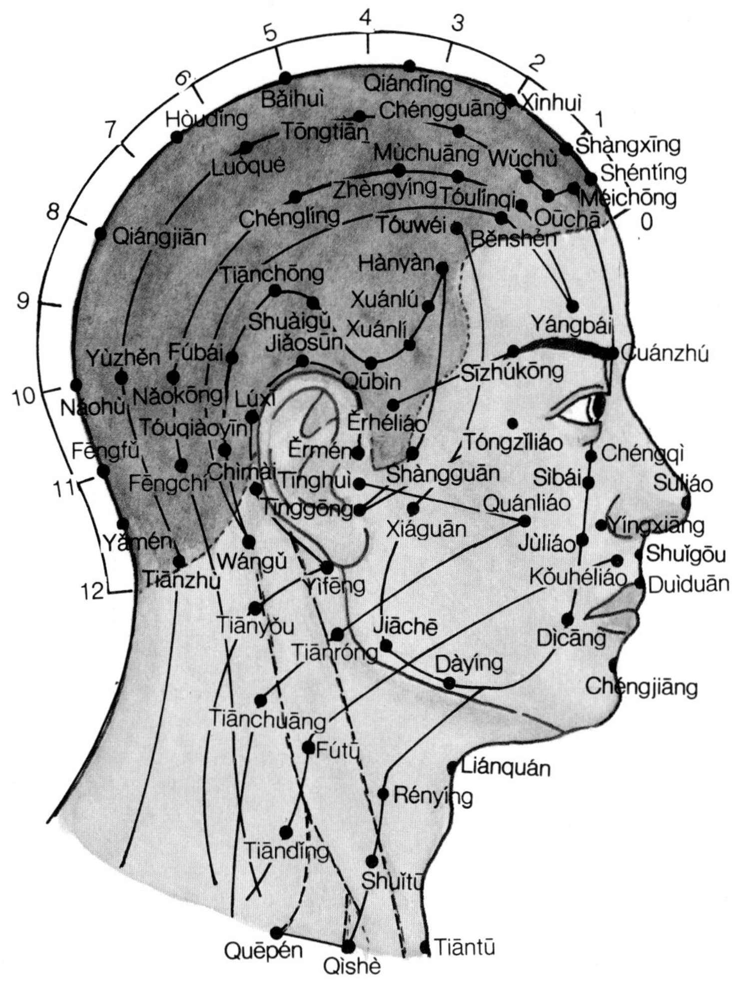

Fig. 7 Points on the Head (Side View)

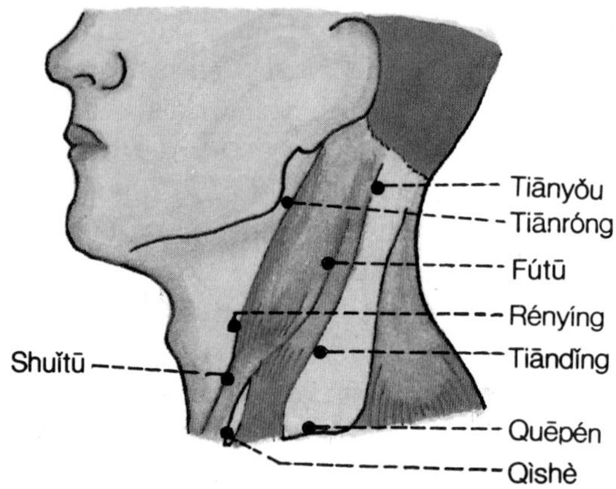

Fig. 18 Points of Large Intestine and Stomach Meridians (Neck)

On the shoulder, in the depression between the acromial extremity of the clavicle and scapular spine (Fig. 14).

2. 2. 17 LI 17 Tiāndǐng 天鼎

On the lateral side of the neck, at the posterior border of the sternocleidomastoid muscle beside the laryngeal protuberance, at the midpoint of the line connecting Futu (LI 18) and Quepen (ST 12) (Figs. 7 & 18).

2. 2. 18 LI 18 Fútū 扶突

On the lateral side of the neck, beside the laryngeal protuberance, between the anterior and posterior borders of the sternocleidomastoid muscle (Figs. 7 & 18).

2. 2. 19 LI 19 Kǒuhéliáo 口禾髎

On the upper lip, directly below the lateral border of the nostril, on the level of Shuigou (DU 26) (Figs. 7 & 18).

2. 2. 20 LI 20 Yíngxiāng 迎香

In the nasolabial groove, beside the midpoint of the lateral border of the nasal ala (Fig. 7 & 18).

2. 3 Points of the Stomach Meridian of Foot-Yangming, ST

足陽明胃經穴

Zúyángmíng Wèijīng Xué

2. 3. 1 ST 1 Chéngqì 承泣

On the face, directly below the pupil, between the eyeball and the infraorbital ridge (Figs. 7 & 19).

2. 3. 2 ST 2 Sìbái 四白

On the face, directly below the pupil, in the depression of the infraorbital foramen (Figs. 7 & 19).

2. 3. 3 ST 3 Jùliáo 巨髎

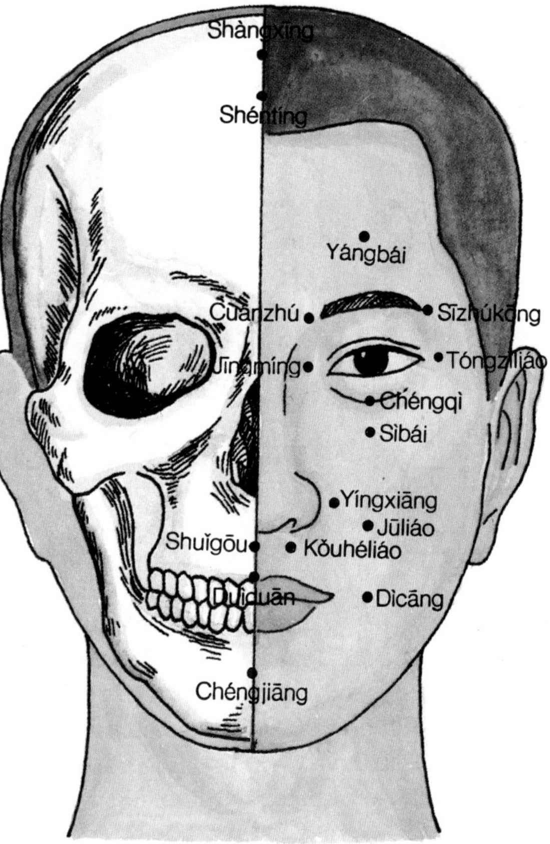

Fig. 19 Chéngqì, Sìbái, Jùliáo and Dìcāng Points

On the face, directly below the pupil, on the level of the lower border of the nasal ala, beside the nasolabial groove (Figs. 7 & 19).

2. 3. 4 ST 4 Dìcāng 地倉

On the face, directly below the pupil, beside the mouth angle (Figs. 7 & 19).

2. 3. 5 ST 5 Dàyíng 大迎

Anterior to the mandibular angle, on the anterior border of the masseter muscle, where the pulsation of the facial artery is palpable (Figs. 7 & 20).

2. 3. 6 ST 6 Jiáchē 頰車

On the cheek, one finger breadth (middle finger) anterior and superior to the mandibular angle, in the depression where the masseter muscle is prominent (Figs. 7 & 20).

2. 3. 7 ST 7 Xiàguān 下關

On the face, anterior to the ear, in the depression between the zygomatic arch and mandibular notch (Figs. 7 & 20).

2. 3. 8 ST 8 Tóuwéi 頭維

On the lateral side of the head, 0.5 *cun* above the anterior hairline at the corner of the forehead, and 4.5 *cun* lateral to the midline of the head (Figs. 7 & 20).

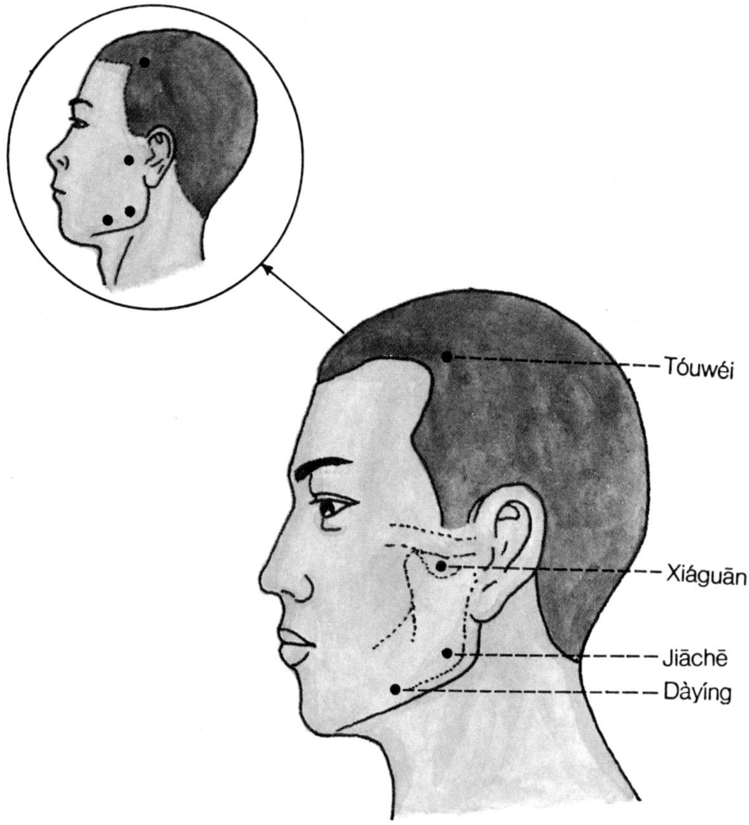

Fig. 20 Jiáchē, Xiàguān and Tóuwéi Points

2. 3. 9 ST 9 Rényíng 人迎

On the neck, beside the laryngeal protuberance, and on the anterior border of the sternocleidomastoid muscle where the pulsation of the common carotid artery is palpable (Figs. 7 & 18).

2. 3. 10 ST 10 Shuǐtū 水突

On the neck and on the anterior border of the sternocleidomastoid muscle, at the midpoint of the line connecting Renying (ST 9) and Qishe (ST 11) (Figs. 7 & 18).

2. 3. 11 ST 11 Qìshè 氣舍

On the neck and on the upper border of the medial end of the clavicle, between the sternal and clavicular heads of the sternocleidomastoid muscle (Figs. 7 & 18).

2. 3. 12 ST 12 Quēpén 缺盆

At the centre of the supraclavicular fossa, 4 *cun* lateral to the anterior midline (Figs. 7 & 18).

2. 3. 13 ST 13 Qìhù 氣户

On the chest, below the midpoint of the lower border of the clavicle, 4 *cun* lateral to the anterior midline (Fig. 8).

2. 3. 14 ST 14 Kùfáng 庫房

On the chest, in the 1st intercostal space, 4 *cun* lateral to the anterior midline (Fig. 8).

2. 3. 15 ST 15 Wūyì 屋翳

On the chest, in the 2nd intercostal space, 4 *cun* lateral to the anterior midline (Fig. 8).

2. 3. 16 ST 16 Yīngchuāng 膺窗

On the chest, in the 3rd intercostal space, 4 *cun* lateral to the anterior midline (Fig. 8).

2. 3. 17 ST 17 Rǔzhōng 乳中

On the chest, in the 4th intercostal space, at the centre of the nipple, 4 *cun* lateral to the anterior midline (Fig. 8).

2. 3. 18 ST 18 Rǔgēn 乳根

On the chest, directly below the nipple, on the lower border of the breast, in the 5th intercostal space, 4 *cun* lateral to the anterior midline (Figs. 8 & 21).

2. 3. 19 ST 19 Bùróng 不容

On the upper abdomen, 6 *cun* above the centre of the umbilicus and 2 *cun* lateral to the anterior midline (Figs. 8 & 21).

2. 3. 20 ST 20 Chéngmǎn 承滿

On the upper abdomen, 5 *cun* above the centre of the umbilicus and 2 *cun* lateral to the anterior midline (Figs. 8 & 21).

2. 3. 21 ST 21 Liángmén 梁門

On the upper abdomen, 4 *cun* above the centre of the umbilicus and 2 *cun* lateral to the anterior midline (Figs. 8 & 21).

2. 3. 22 ST 22 Guānmén 關門

On the upper abdomen, 3 *cun* above the centre of the umbilicus and 2 *cun* lateral to the anterior midline (Figs. 8 & 21).

2. 3. 23 ST 23 Tàiyǐ 太乙

On the upper abdomen, 2 *cun* above the centre of the umbilicus and 2 *cun* lateral to the anterior midline (Figs. 8 & 21).

2. 3. 24 ST 24 Huáròumén 滑肉門

On the upper abdomen, 1 *cun* above the centre of the umbilicus and 2 *cun* lateral to the anterior midline (Figs. 8 & 21).

2. 3. 25 ST 25 Tiānshū 天樞

On the middle abdomen, 2 *cun* lateral to the centre of the umbilicus (Figs. 8 & 21).

2. 3. 26 ST 26 Wàilíng 外陵

On the lower abdomen, 1 *cun* below the centre of the umbilicus and 2 *cun* lateral to the anterior midline (Figs. 8 & 21).

2. 3. 27 ST 27 Dàjù 大巨

On the lower abdomen, 2 *cun* below the centre of the umbilicus and 2 *cun* lateral to the anterior midline (Figs. 8 & 21).

2. 3. 28 ST 28 Shuǐdào 水道

On the lower abdomen, 3 *cun* below the centre of the umbilicus and 2 *cun* lateral to the anterior midline (Figs. 8 & 21).

2. 3. 29 ST 29 Guīlái 歸來

On the lower abdomen, 4 *cun* below the centre of the umbilicus and 2 *cun* lateral to the anterior midline (Figs. 8 & 21).

Rǔgēn
Bùróng
Chéngmǎn
Liángmén
Guānmén
Tàiyǐ
Huáròumén
Tiānshū
Wàilíng
Dàjù
Shuǐdào
Guīlái

8 cun

5 cun

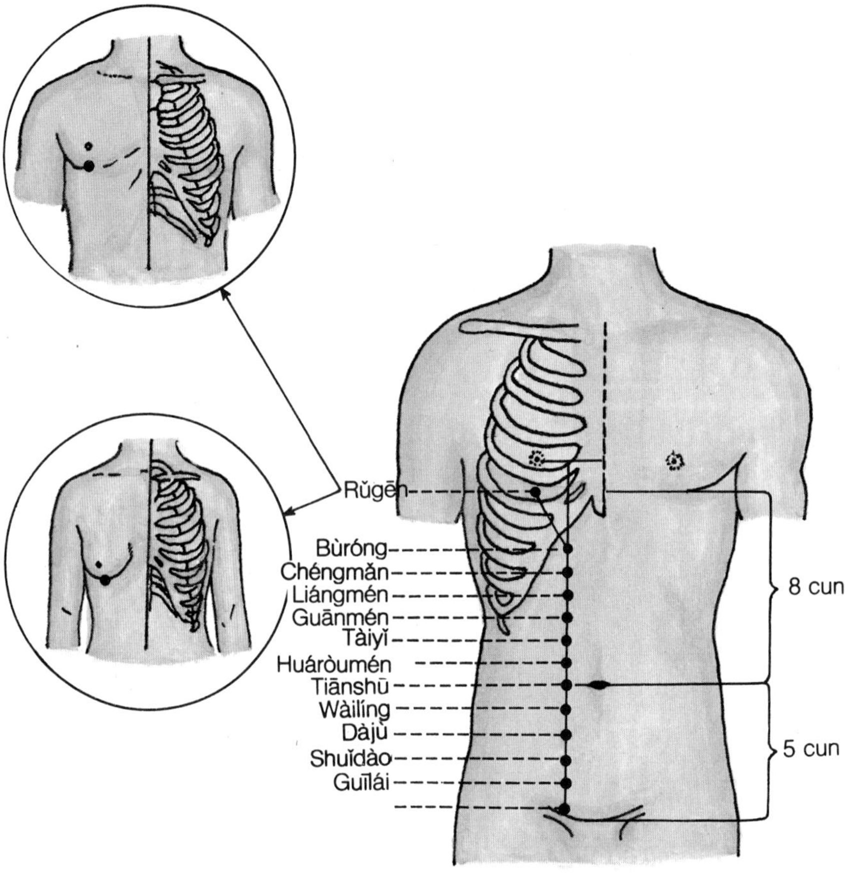

Fig. 21 Points of Stomach Meridian (Abdomen)

2. 3. 30 ST 30 Qìchōng 氣衝

Slightly above the inguinal groove, 5 *cun* below the centre of the umbilicus and 2 *cun* lateral to the anterior midline (Figs. 8 & 21).

2. 3. 31 ST 31 Bìguān 髀關

On the anterior side of the thigh and on the line connecting the anteriosuperior iliac spine and the superiolateral corner of the patella, on the level of the perineum when the thigh is flexed, in the depression lateral to the sartorius muscle (Figs. 22 & 23)

2. 3. 32 ST 32 Fútù 伏兔

On th anterior side of the thigh and on the line connecting the anteriosuperior iliac spine and the superiolateral corner of the patella, 6 *cun* above this corner (Figs. 22 & 23).

2. 3. 33 ST 33 Yīnshì 陰市

On the anterior side of the thigh and on the line connecting anteriosuperior iliac spine and the superiolateral corner of the patella, 3 *cun* above this corner (Figs. 22 & 23).

2. 3. 34 ST 34 Liángqīu 梁丘

With the knee flexed, on the anterior side of the thigh and on the line connecting the anteriosuperior iliac spine and the superiolateral corner of the patella, 2 *cun* above this corner (Figs. 22 & 23).

2. 3. 35 ST 35 Dúbí 犢鼻

With the knee flexed, on the knee, in the depression lateral to the patella and its ligament (Figs. 22 & 24).

2. 3. 36 ST 36 Zúsānlǐ 足三裏

On the anteriolateral side of the leg, 3 *cun* below Dubi (ST 35), one finger breadth (middle finger) from the anterior crest of the tibia (Figs. 22 & 24).

2. 3. 37 ST 37 Shàngjùxū 上巨虛

On the anteriolateral side of the leg, 6 *cun* below Dubi (ST 35), one finger breadth (middle finger) from the anterior crest of the tibia (Figs. 22 & 24).

2. 3. 38 ST 38 Tiáokǒu 條口

On the anteriolateral side of the leg, 8 *cun* below Dubi (ST 35), one finger breadth (middle finger) from the anterior crest of the tibia (Figs. 22 & 24).

2. 3. 39 ST 39 Xiàjùxū 下巨虛

On the anteriolateral side of the leg, 9 *cun* below Dubi (ST 35), one finger breadth (middle finger) from the anterior crest of the tibia (Figs. 22 & 24).

2. 3. 40 ST 40 Fēnglóng 豐隆

On the anteriolateral side of the leg, 8 *cun* above the tip of the external malleolus, lateral to Tiaokou (ST 38), and two finger breadths (middle finger) from the anterior crest of the tibia (Figs. 22 & 24).

2. 3. 41 ST 41 Jǐexī 解谿

In the central depression of the crease between the instep of the foot and leg, between the tendons of the long extensor muscle of the great toe and the long extensor muscle of the toes (Figs. 22 & 25).

2. 3. 42 ST 42 Chōngyáng 衝陽

On the dome of the instep of the foot, between the tendons of the long extensor muscle of the great toe and the long extensor muscle of the toes, where the pulsation of the dorsal artery of the foot is palpable (Figs. 22 & 25).

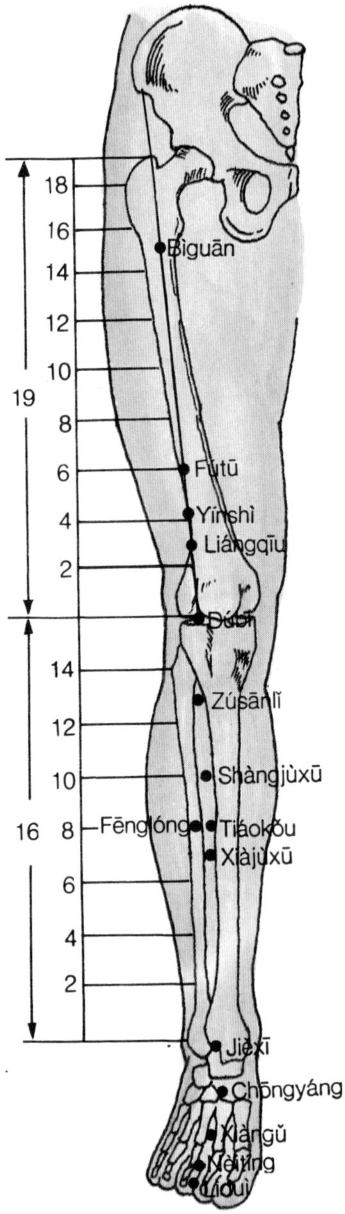

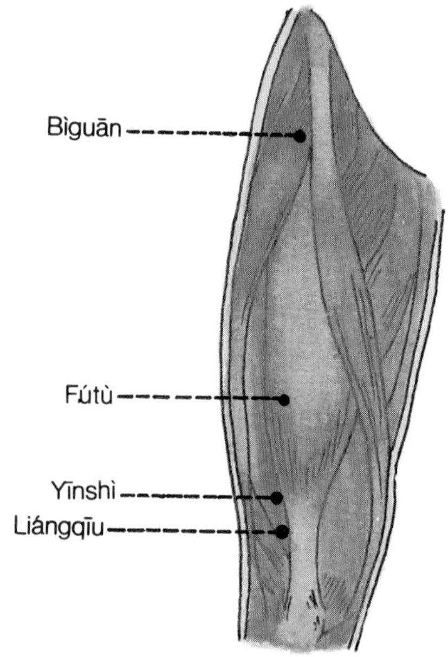

Fig. 23 Points of Stomach Meridian (Thigh)

Fig. 22 Points of Stomach Meridian (Lower Limbs)

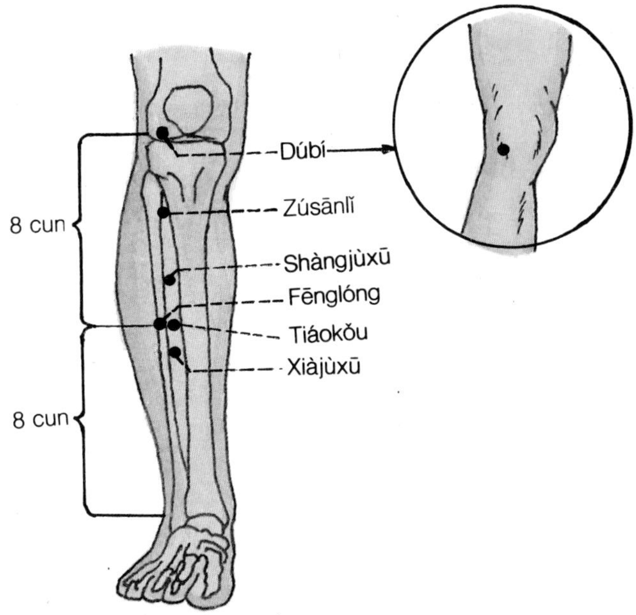

Fig. 24 Points of Stomach Meridian (Leg)

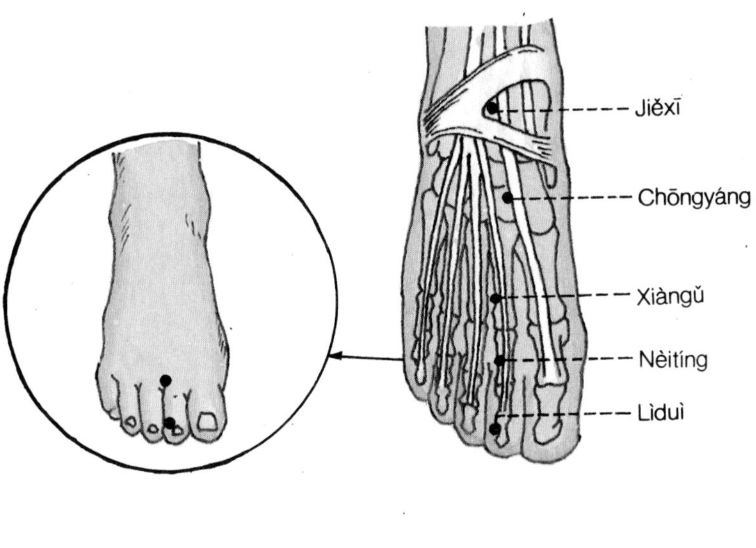

Fig. 25 Points of Stomach Meridian (Foot)

2. 3. 43 ST 43 Xiàngǔ 陷谷

On the instep of the foot, in the depression distal to the commissure of the 2nd and 3rd metatarsal bones (Figs. 22 & 25).

2. 3. 44 ST 44 Nèitíng 内庭

On the instep of the foot, at the junction of the red and white skin proximal to the margin of the web between the 2nd and 3rd toes (Figs. 22 & 25).

2. 3. 45 ST 45 Lìduì 厲兑

On the lateral side of the distal segment of the 2nd toe, 0.1 *cun* from the corner of the toenail (Figs. 22 & 25).

2. 4 Points of the Spleen Meridian of Foot-Taiyin, SP

足太陰脾經穴

Zútàiyīn Píjīng Xué

2. 4. 1 SP 1 Yǐnbái 隱白

On the medial side of the distal segment of the great toe, 0.1 *cun* from the corner of the toenail (Figs. 26 & 27).

2. 4. 2 SP 2 Dàdū 大都

On the medial border of the foot, in the depression of the junction of the red and white skin, anterior and inferior to the 1st metatarsophalangeal joint (Figs. 26 & 27).

2. 4. 3 SP 3 Tàibái 太白

On the medial border of the foot, in the depression of the junction of the red and white skin, posterior and inferior to the 1st metatarsophalangeal joint (Figs. 26 & 27).

2. 4. 4 SP 4 Gōngsūn 公孫

On the medial border of the foot, anterior and inferior to the proximal end of the 1st metatarsal bone (Figs 26 & 27).

2. 4. 5 SP 5 Shāngqiū 商丘

In the depression anterior and inferior to the medial malleolus, at the midpoint of the line connecting the tuberosity of the navicular bone and the tip of the medial malleolus (Figs. 26 & 27).

2. 4. 6 SP 6 Sānyīnjiāo 三陰交

On the medial side of the leg, 3 *cun* above the tip of the medial malleolus, posterior to the medial border of the tibia (Figs. 26 & 28).

2. 4. 7 SP 7 Lòugǔ 漏谷

On the medial side of the leg and on the line connecting the tip of the medial malleolus and Yinlingquan (SP 9), 6 *cun* from the tip of the medial malleolus, posterior to the medial border of the tibia (Figs. 26 & 28).

2. 4. 8 SP 8 Dìjī 地機

On the medial side of the leg and on the line connecting the tip of the medial malleolus and Yinlingquan (SP 9), 3 *cun* below Yinlingquan (SP 9) (Figs. 26 & 28).

2. 4. 9 SP 9 Yīnlíngqúan 陰陵泉

On the medial side of the leg, in the depression posterior and inferior to the medial condyle of the tibia (Figs, 26 & 28).

2. 4. 10 SP 10 Xuèhǎi 血海

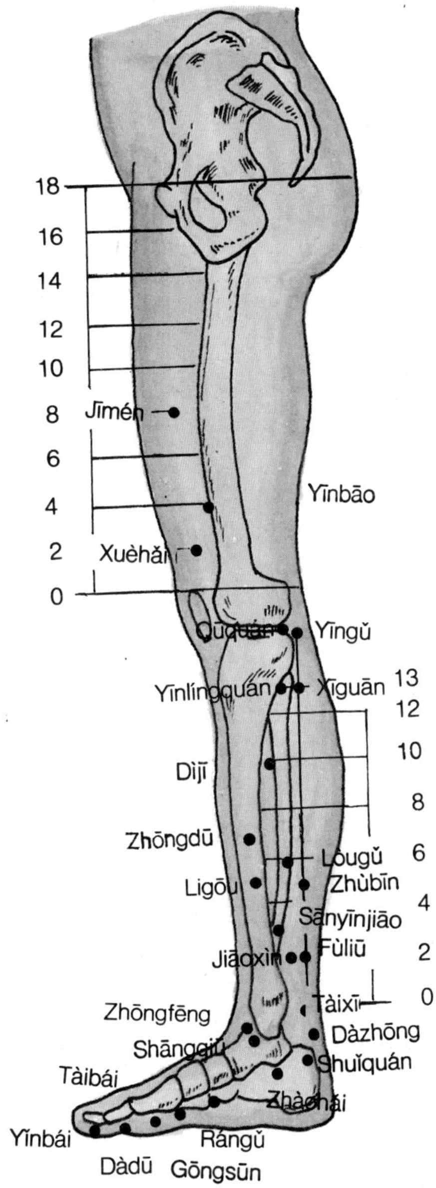

Fig. 26 Points of Three Yin Meridians of the Foot (Lower Limbs)

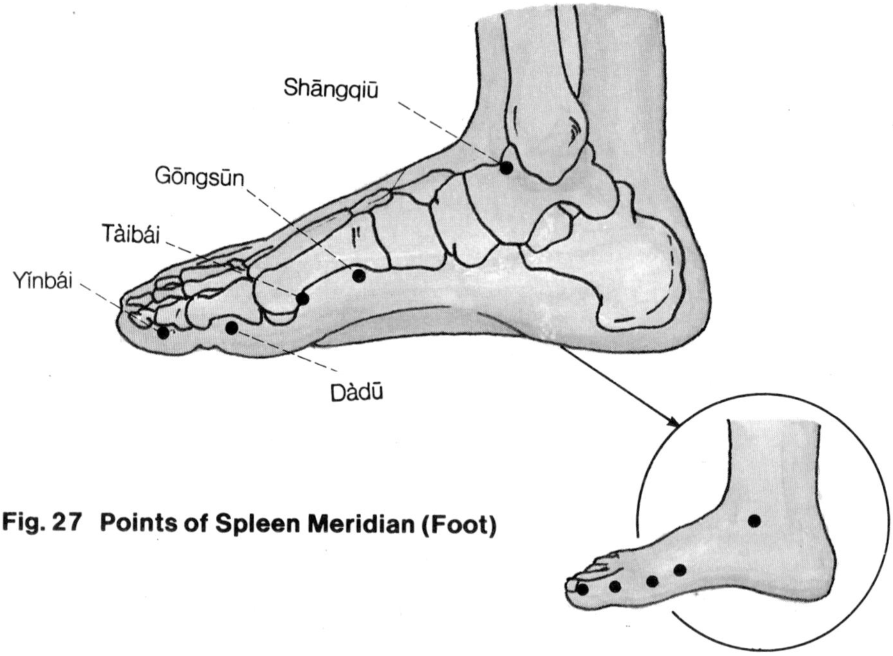

Fig. 27 Points of Spleen Meridian (Foot)

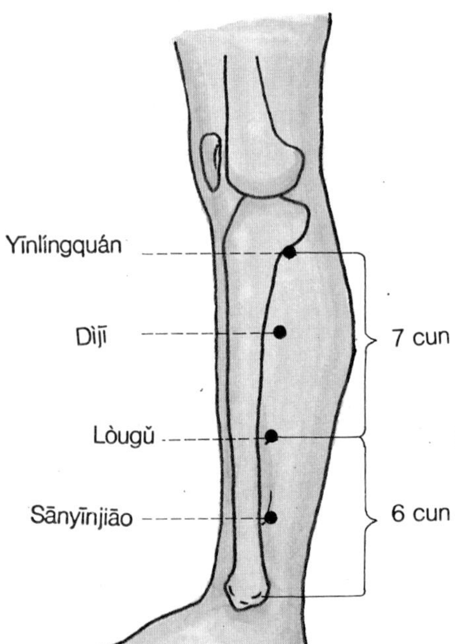

Fig. 28 Points of Spleen Meridian (Leg)

Xuèhǎi

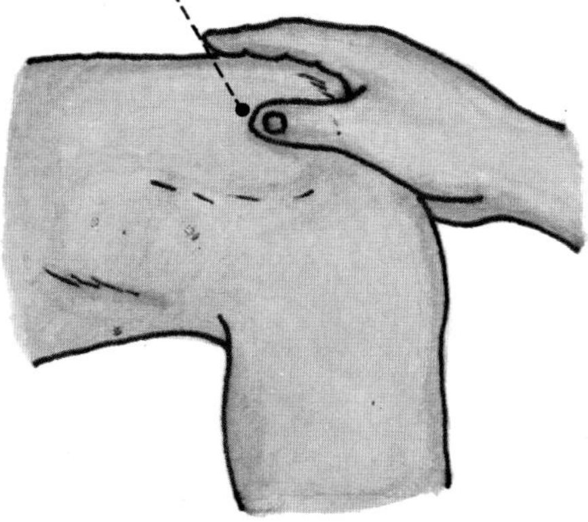

Fig. 29 Xùehǎi Point

Fù'āi

Dàhéng

Fùjié

Fúshè

Chōngmén

5 cun

3 cun

5 cun

Shénquè

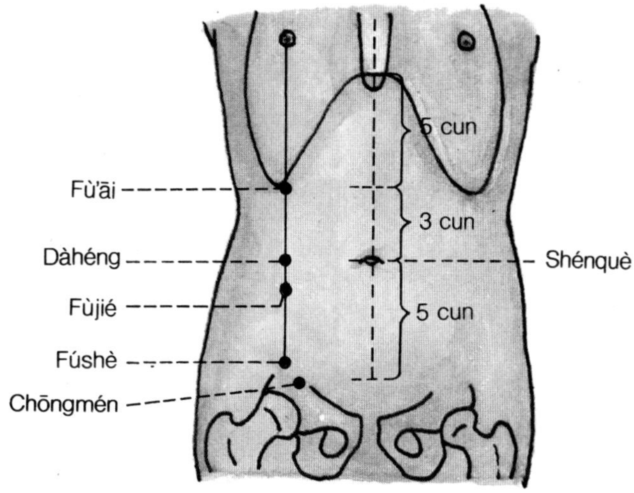

Fig. 30 Points of Spleen Meridian (Abdomen)

Zhōuróng

Xiōngxiāng

Tiānxī

Shídòu

Dàbāo

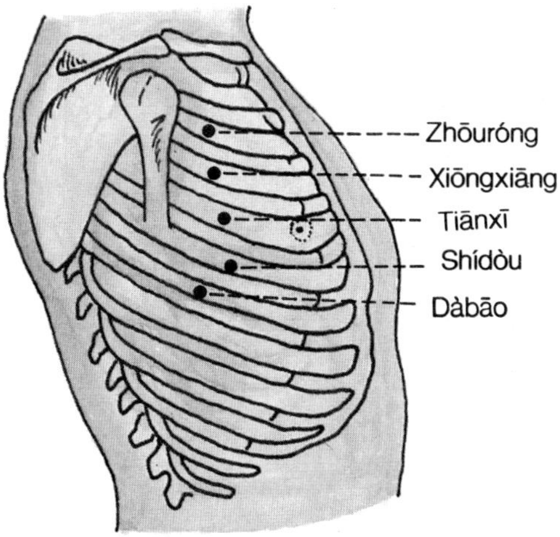

Fig. 31 Points of Spleen Meridian (Chest)

With the knee flexed, on the medial side of the thigh, 2 *cun* above the superior medial corner of the patella, on the prominence of the medial head of the quadriceps muscle of the thigh (Figs. 26 & 29).

2. 4. 11 SP 11 Jīmén 箕門

On the medial side of the thigh and on the line connecting Xuehai (SP 10) and Chongmen (SP 12), 6 *cun* above Xuehai (SP 10) (Fig. 26).

2. 4. 12 SP 12 Chōngmén 衝門

At the lateral end of the inguinal groove, 3.5 *cun* lateral to the midpoint of the upper border of the symphysis pubis, lateral to the pulsating external iliac artery (Figs. 8 & 30).

2. 4. 13 SP 13 Fùshè 府舍

On the lower abdomen, 4 *cun* below the centre of the umbilicus, 0.7 *cun* above Chongmen (SP 12), and 4 *cun* lateral to the anterior midline (Figs. 8 & 30).

2. 4. 14 SP 14 Fùjíe 腹結

On the lower abdomen, 1.3 *cun* below Daheng (SP 15), and 4 *cun* lateral to the anterior midline (Figs. 8 & 30).

2. 4. 15 SP 15 Dàhéng 大横

On the middle abdomen, 4 *cun* lateral to the centre of the umbilicus (Figs. 8 & 30).

2. 4. 16 SP 16 Fù'āi 腹哀

On the upper abdomen, 3 *cun* above the centre of the umbilicus, and 4 *cun* lateral to the anterior midline (Figs. 8 & 30).

2. 4. 17 SP 17 Shídòu 食竇

On the lateral side of the chest and in the 5th intercostal space, 6 *cun* lateral to the anterior midline (Figs. 8 & 31).

2. 4. 18 SP 18 Tiānxī 天谿

On the lateral side of the chest and in the 4th intercostal space, 6 *cun* lateral to the anterior midline (Figs. 8 & 31).

2. 4. 19 SP 19 Xiōngxiāng 胸鄉

On the lateral side of the chest and in the 3rd intercostal space, 6 *cun* lateral to the anterior midline (Figs. 8 & 31).

2. 4. 20 SP 20 Zhōuróng 周榮

On the lateral side of the chest and in the 2nd intercostal space, 6 *cun* lateral to the anterior midline (Figs. 8 & 31).

2. 4. 21 SP 21 Dàbāo 大包

On the lateral side of the chest and on the middle axillary line, in the 6th intercostal space (Figs. 10 & 31).

2. 5 Points of the Heart Meridian of Hand-Shaoyin, HT

手少陰心經穴

Shǒushàoyīn Xīnjīng Xué

2. 5. 1 HT 1 Jíquán 極泉

At the apex of the axillary fossa, where the pulsation of the axillary artery is palpable.

2. 5. 2 HT 2 Qīnglíng 青靈

On the medial side of the arm and on the line connecting Jiquan (HT 1) and Shaohai (HT 3), 3 *cun* above the cubital crease, in the groove medial to the biceps muscle of the arm (Fig. 11).

2. 5. 3 HT 3 Shàohǎi 少海

With the elbow flexed, at the midpoint of the line connecting the medial end of the cubital crease and the medial epicondyle of the humerus (Figs. 11 & 32).

2. 5. 4 HT 4 Língdào 靈道

On the palmar side of the forearm and on the radial side of the tendon of the ulnar flexor muscle of the wrist, 1.5 *cun* proximal to the crease of the wrist (Figs. 11 & 32).

2. 5. 5 HT 5 Tōnglǐ 通裏

On the palmar side of the forearm and on the radial side of the tendon of the ulnar flexor muscle of the wrist, 1 *cun* proximal to the crease of the wrist (Figs. 11 & 32).

2. 5. 6 HT 6 Yīnxì 陰郄

On the palmar side of the forearm and on the radial side of the tendon of the ulnar flexor muscle of the wrist, 0.5 *cun* proximal to the crease of the wrist (Figs. 11 & 32).

2. 5. 7 HT 7 Shénmén 神門

On the wrist, at the ulnar end of the crease of the wrist, in the depression of the radial side of the tendon of the ulnar flexor muscle of the wrist (Figs. 11 & 32).

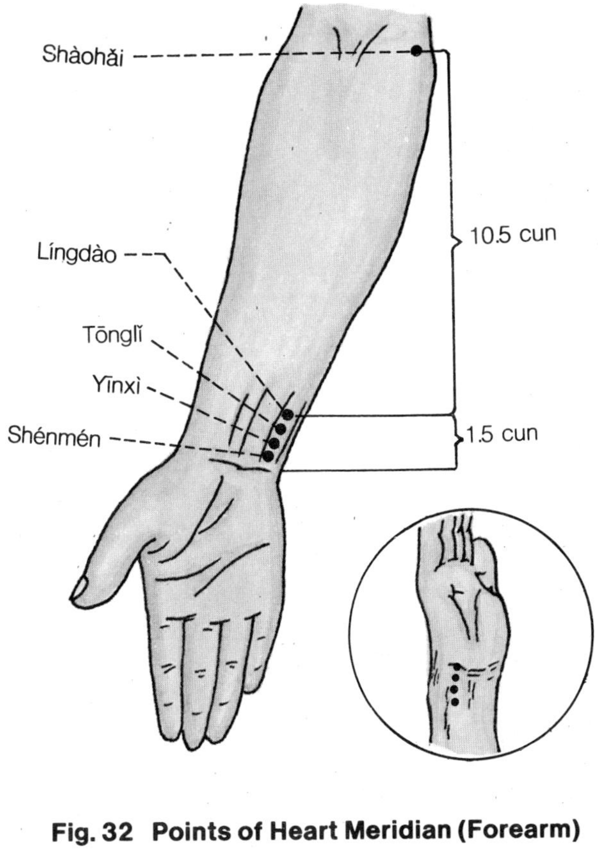

Fig. 32 Points of Heart Meridian (Forearm)

2. 5. 8 HT 8 **Shàofǔ** 少府

In the palm, between the 4th and 5th metacarpal bones, at the part of the palm touching the tip of the little finger when a fist is made (Figs. 11 & 33).

2. 5. 9 HT 9 Shàochōng 少衝

On the radial side of the distal segment of the little finger, 0.1 *cun* from the corner of the nail (Figs. 11 & 33).

2. 6 Points of the Small Intestine Meridian of Hand-Taiyang, SI
手太陽小腸經穴
Shǒutàiyáng Xiǎochángjīng Xúe

2. 6. 1 SI 1 Shàozé 少澤

On the ulnar side of the distal segment of the little finger, 0.1 *cun* from the corner of the nail (Figs. 14 & 34).

2. 6. 2 SI 2 Qiángǔ 前谷

At the junction of the red and white skin along the ulnar border of the hand, at the ulnar end of the crease of the 5th metacarpophalangeal joint when a loose fist is made (Figs. 14 & 34).

2. 6. 3 SI 3 Hòuxī 後谿

At the junction of the red and white skin along the ulnar border of the hand, at the ulnar end of the distal palmar crease, proximal to the 5th metacarpophalangeal joint when a hollow fist is made (Figs. 14 & 34).

2. 6. 4 SI 4 Wàngǔ 腕骨

On the ulnar border of the hand, in the depression between the proximal end of the 5th metacarpal bone and hamate bone, and at the junction of the red and white skin (Figs. 14 & 34).

2. 6. 5 SI 5 Yánggǔ 陽谷

On the ulnar border of the wrist, in the depression between the styloid process of the ulna and triangular bone (Figs. 14 & 34).

2. 6. 6 SI 6 Yǎnglǎo 養老

On the ulnar side of the posterior surface of the forearm, in the depression proximal to and on the radial side of the head of the ulna (Figs. 14 & 34).

2. 6. 7 SI 7 Zhīzhèng 支正

On the ulnar side of the posterior surface of the forearm and on the line connecting Yanggu (SI 5) and Xiaohai (SI 8), 5 *cun* proximal to the dorsal crease of the wrist (Fig. 14).

2. 6. 8 SI 8 Xiǎohǎi 小海

On the medial side of the elbow, in the depression between the olecranon of the ulna and the medial epicondyle of the humerus (Fig. 14).

2. 6. 9 SI 9 Jiānzhēn 肩貞

Posterior and inferior to the shoulder joint, 1 *cun* above the posterior end of the axillary fold with the arm adducted. (Figs. 9 & 35).

2. 6. 10 SI 10 Nàoshú 臑俞

On the shoulder, above the posterior end of the axillary fold, in the depression below the lower border of the scapular spine (Figs. 9 & 35).

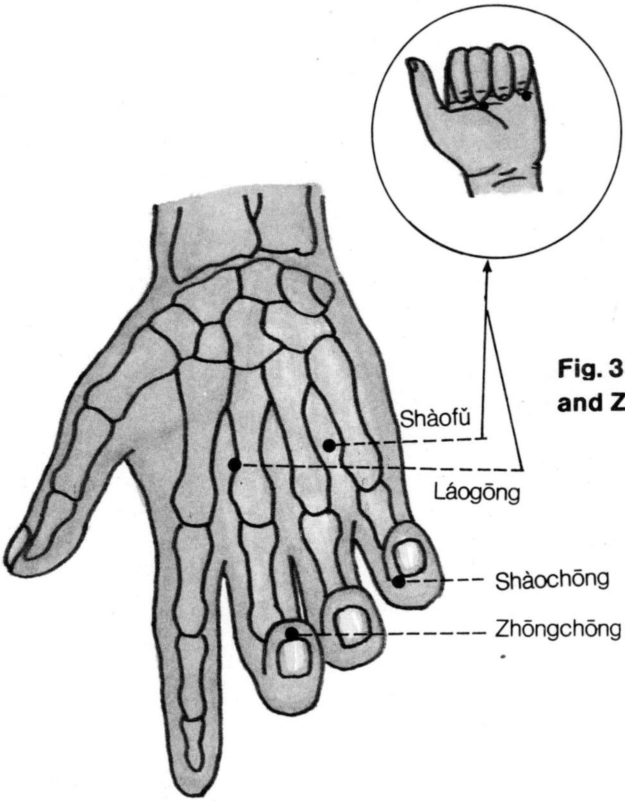

Fig. 33 Shàofǔ, Shàochōng, Laógōng and Zhōngchōng Points

Shàofǔ

Láogōng

Shàochōng

Zhōngchōng

Yǎnglǎo

Yánggǔ

Wàngǔ

Hòuxī

Qiángǔ

Shàozé

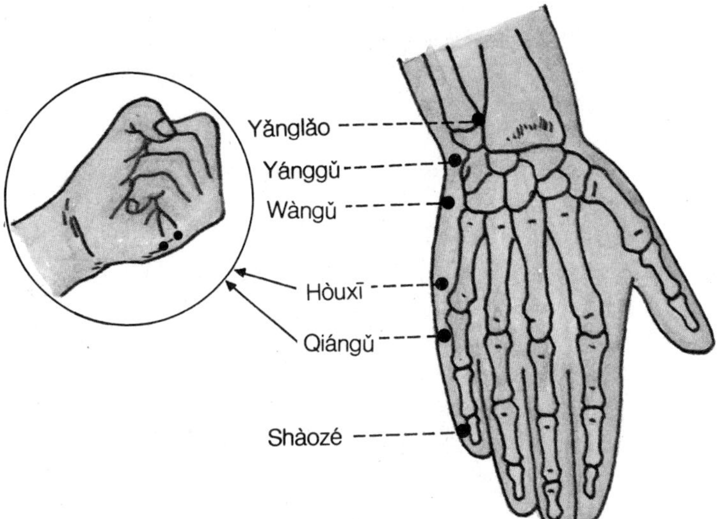

Fig. 34 Points of Small Intestine Meridian (Hand)

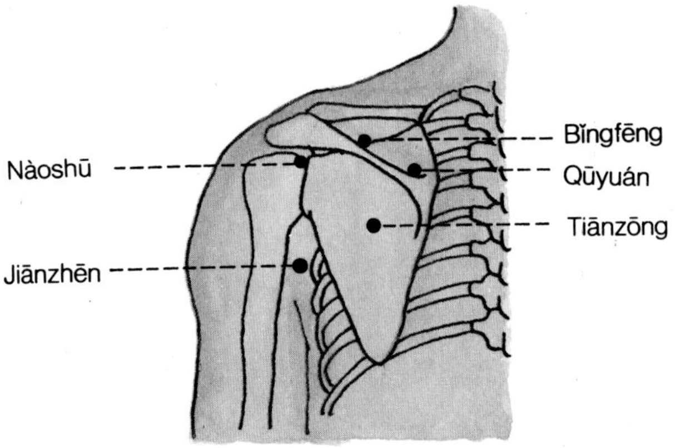

Fig. 35 Points of Small Intestine Meridian (Shoulder)

2. 6. 11 SI 11 Tiānzōng 天宗

On the scapula, in the depression of the centre of the subscapular fossa, and on the level of the 4th thoracic vertebra (Figs. 9 & 35).

2. 6. 12 SI 12 Bĭngfēng 秉風

On the scapula, at the centre of the suprascapular fossa, directly above Tianzong (SI 11), in the depression found when the arm is raised (Figs. 9 & 35).

2. 6. 13 SI 13 Qūyuán 曲垣

On the scapula, at the medial end of the suprascapular fossa, at the midpoint of the line connecting Naoshu (SI 10) and the spinous process of the 2nd thoracic vertebra (Figs. 9 & 35).

2. 6. 14 SI 14 Jiānwàishū 肩外俞

On the back, below the spinous process of the 1st thoracic vertebra, 3 ***cun*** lateral to the posterior midline (Fig. 9).

2. 6. 15 SI 15 Jiānzhōngshū 肩中俞

On the back, below the spinous process of the 7th cervical vertebra, 2 ***cun*** lateral to the posterior midline (Fig. 9).

2. 6. 16 SI 16 Tiānchuāng 天窗

On the lateral side of the neck, posterior to the sternocleidomastoid muscle and Futu (LI 18), on the level of the laryngeal protuberance.

2. 6. 17 SI 17 Tiānróng 天容

On the lateral side of the neck, posterior to the mandibular angle, in the depression of the anterior border of the sternocleidomastoid muscle (Figs. 7 & 18).

2. 6. 18 SI 18 Quánliáo 顴髎

On the face, directly below the outer canthus, in the depression below the zygomatic bone (Fig. 7).

2. 6. 19 SI 19 Tīnggōng 聽宫

On the face, anterior to the tragus and posterior to the mandibular condyloid process, in the depression found when the mouth is open (Fig. 7).

2. 7 Points of the Bladder Meridian of Foot-Taiyang, BL

足太陽膀胱經穴

Zútàiyáng Pángguāngjīng Xué

2. 7. 1 BL 1 Jīngmíng 睛明

On the face, in the depression slightly above the inner canthus (Figs. 7 & 19).

2. 7. 2 BL 2 Cuánzhú 攢竹

On the face, in the depression of the medial end of the eyebrow, at the supraorbital notch (Figs. 7 & 19).

2. 7. 3 BL 3 Méichōng 眉衝

On the head, directly above Cuanzhu (BL 2), 0.5 *cun* above the anterior hairline, on the line connecting Shenting (DU 24) and Qucha (BL 4) (Fig. 7).

2. 7. 4 BL 4 Qūchā 曲差

On the head, 0.5 *cun* directly above the midpoint of the anterior hairline and 1.5 *cun* lateral to the midline, at the junction of the midial third and middle third of the line connecting Shenting (DU 24) and Touwei (ST 8) (Fig. 7).

2. 7. 5 BL 5 Wǔchù 五處

On the head, 1 *cun* directly above the midpoint of the anterior hairline and 1.5 *cun* lateral to the midline (Fig. 7).

2. 7. 6 BL 6 Chéngguāng 承光

On the head, 2.5 *cun* directly above the midpoint of the anterior hairline and 1.5 *cun* lateral to the midline (Fig. 7).

2. 7. 7 BL 7 Tōngtiān 通天

On the head, 4 *cun* directly above the midpoint of the anterior hairline and 1.5 *cun* lateral to the midline (Fig. 7).

2. 7. 8 BL 8 Luòquè 絡卻

On the head, 5.5 *cun* directly above the midpoint of the anterior hairline and 1.5 *cun* lateral to the midline (Figs. 7 & 36).

2. 7. 9 BL 9 Yùzhěn 玉枕

On the occiput, 2.5 *cun* directly above the midpoint of the posterior hairline and 1.3 *cun* lateral to the midline, in the depression on the level of the upper border of the external occipital protuberance (Figs. 7 & 36).

2. 7. 10 BL 10 Tiānzhù 天柱

On the nape, in the depression of the lateral border of the trapezius muscle and 1.3 *cun* lateral to the midpoint of the posterior hairline (Figs. 7 & 36).

2. 7. 11 BL 11 Dàzhù 大杼

On the back, below the spinous process of the 1st thoracic vertebra, 1.5 *cun* lateral to the posterior midline (Fig. 9).

2. 7. 12 BL 12 Fēngmén 風門

On the back, below the spinous process of the 2nd thoracic vertebra, 1.5 *cun* lateral to the posterior midline (Fig. 9).

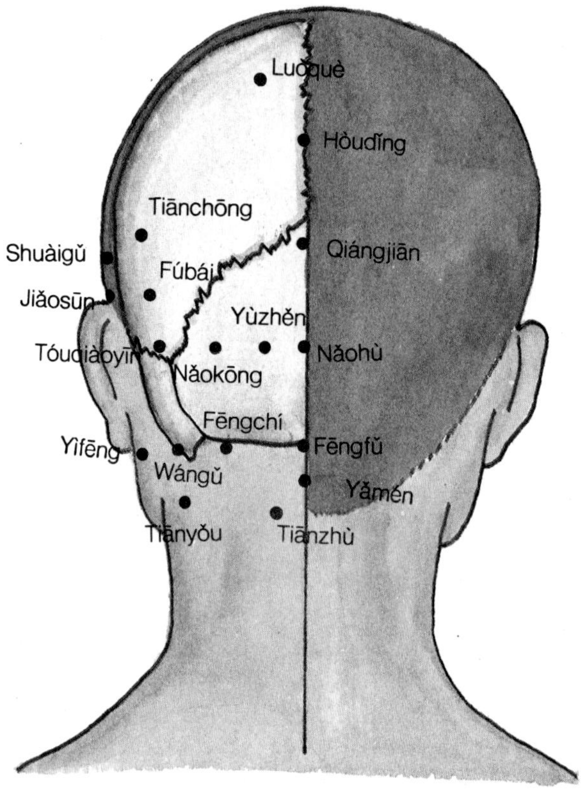

Fig. 36 Points of the Occiput

2. 7. 13 BL 13 Fèishū 肺俞

On the back, below the spinous process of the 3rd thoracic vertebra, 1.5 *cun* lateral to the posterior midline (Fig. 9).

2. 7. 14 BL 14 Júeyīnshū 厥陰俞

On the back, below the spinous process of the 4th thoracic vertebra, 1.5 *cun* lateral to the posterior midline (Fig. 9).

2. 7. 15 BL 15 Xīnshū 心俞

On the back, below the spinous process of the 5th thoracic vertebra, 1.5 *cun* lateral to the posterior midline (Fig. 9).

2. 7. 16 BL 16 Dūshū 督俞

On the back, below the spinous process of the 6th thoracic vertebra, 1.5 *cun* lateral to the posterior midline (Fig. 9).

2. 7. 17 BL 17 Géshū 隔俞

On the back, below the spinous process of the 7th thoracic vertebra, 1.5 *cun* lateral to the posterior midline (Fig. 9).

2. 7. 18 BL 18 Gānshū 肝俞

On the back, below the spinous process of the 9th thoracic vertebra, 1.5 *cun* lateral to the

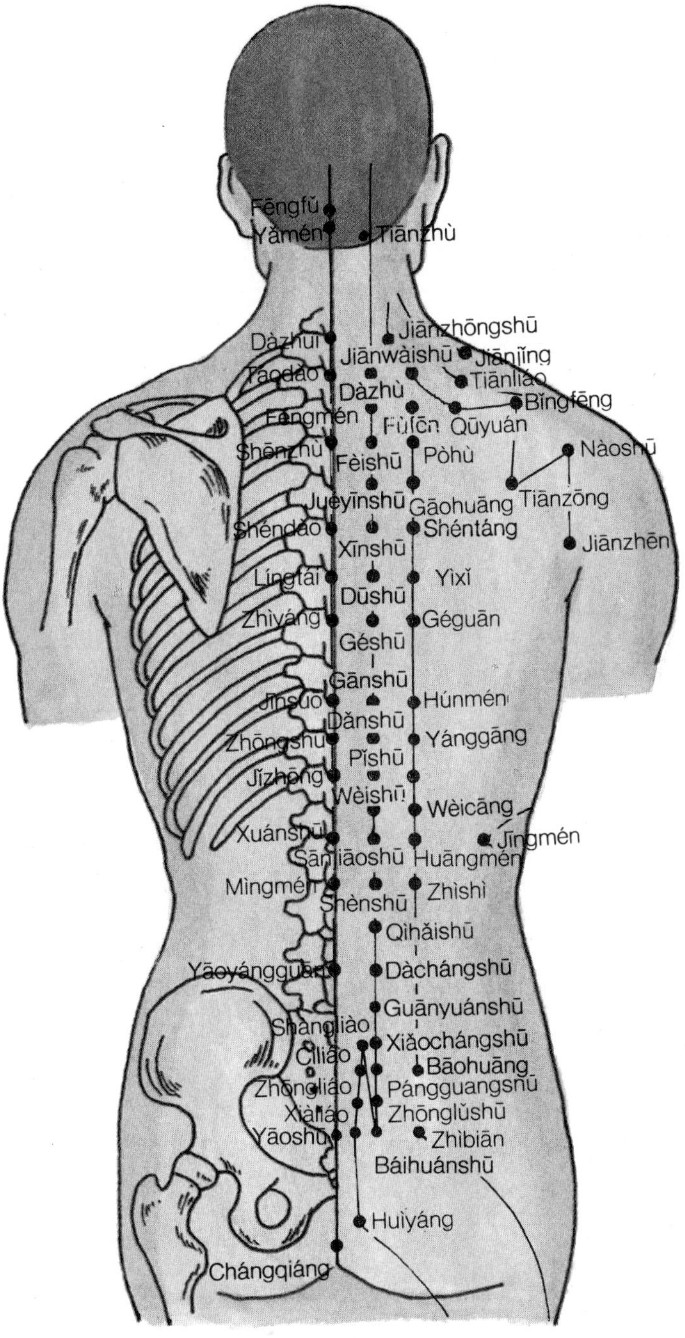

Fig. 9 Points on the Back

posterior midline (Fig. 9).

2. 7. 19 BL 19 Dǎnshū 膽俞

On the back, below the spinous process of the 10th thoracic vertebra, 1.5 *cun* lateral to the posterior midline (Fig. 9).

2. 7. 20 BL 20 Píshū 脾俞

On the back, below the spinous process of the 11th thoracic vertebra, 1.5 *cun* lateral to the posterior midline (Fig. 9).

2. 7. 21 BL 21 Wèishū 胃俞

On the back, below the spinous process of the 12th thoracic vertebra, 1.5 *cun* lateral to the posterior midline (Fig. 9).

2. 7. 22 BL 22 Sānjiāoshū 三焦俞

On the low back, below the spinous process of the 1st lumbar vertebra, 1.5 *cun* lateral to the posterior midline (Fig. 9).

2. 7. 23 BL 23 Shènshū 腎俞

On the low back, below the spinous process of the 2nd lumbar vertebra, 1.5 *cun* lateral to the posterior midline (Fig. 9).

2. 7. 24 BL 24 Qìhǎishū 氣海俞

On the low back, below the spinous process of the 3rd lumbar vertebra, 1.5 *cun* lateral to the posterior midline (Fig. 9).

2. 7. 25 BL 25 Dàchángshū 大腸俞

On the low back, below the spinous process of the 4th lumbar vertebra, 1.5 *cun* lateral to the posterior midline (Fig. 9).

2. 7. 26 BL 26 Guānyuánshū 關元俞

On the low back, below the spinous process of the 5th lumbar vertebra, 1.5 *cun* lateral to the posterior midline (Fig. 9).

2. 7. 27 BL 27 Xiǎochángshū 小腸俞

On the sacrum and on the level of the 1st posterior sacral foramen, 1.5 *cun* lateral to the median sacral crest (Fig. 9).

2. 7. 28 BL 28 Pángguāngshū 膀胱俞

On the sacrum and on the level of the 2nd posterior sacral foramen, 1.5 *cun* lateral to the median sacral crest (Fig. 9).

2. 7. 29 BL 29 Zhōnglǚshū 中膂俞

On the sacrum and on the level of the 3rd posterior sacral foramen, 1.5 *cun* lateral to the median sacral crest (Fig. 9).

2. 7. 30 BL 30 Báihuánshū 白環俞

On the sacrum and on the level of the 4th posterior sacral foramen, 1.5 *cun* lateral to the median sacral crest (Fig. 9).

2. 7. 31 BL 31 Shàngliáo 上髎

On the sacrum, at the midpoint between the posteriosuperior iliac spine and the posterior midline, just at the 1st posterior sacral foramen (Fig. 9).

2. 7. 32 BL 32 Cìliáo 次髎

On the sacrum, medial and inferior to the posteriosuperior iliac spine, just at the 2nd posterior sacral foramen (Fig. 9).

2. 7. 33 BL 33 Zhōngliáo 中髎

On the sacrum, medial and inferior to Ciliao (BL 32), just at the 3rd posterior sacral foramen (Fig. 9).

2. 7. 34 BL 34 Xiàliaó 下髎

On the sacrum, medial and inferior to Zhongliao (BL 33), just at the 4th posterior sacral foramen (Fig. 9).

2. 7. 35 BL 35 Huìyáng 會陽

On the sacrum, 0.5 *cun* lateral to the tip of the coccyx (Fig. 9).

2. 7. 36 BL 36 Chéngfú 承扶

On the posterior side of the thigh, at the midpoint of the inferior gluteal crease (Fig. 37).

2. 7. 37 BL 37 Yīnmén 殷門

On the posterior side of the thigh and on the line connecting Chengfu (BL 36) and Weizhong (BL 40), 6 *cun* below Chengfu (BL 36) (Fig. 37).

2. 7. 38 BL 38 Fúxì 浮郄

At the lateral end of the popliteal crease, 1 *cun* above Weiyang (BL 39), medial to the tendon of the biceps muscle of the thigh (Fig. 37).

2. 7. 39 BL 39 Wěiyáng 委陽

At the lateral end of the popliteal crease, medial to the tendon of the biceps muscle of the thigh (Figs. 37 & 38).

2. 7. 40 BL 40 Wěizhōng 委中

At the midpoint of the popliteal crease, between the tendons of the biceps muscle of the thigh and the semitendinous muscle (Figs. 37 & 38).

2. 7. 41 BL 41 Fùfēn 附分

On the back, below the spinous process of the 2nd thoracic vertebra, 3 *cun* lateral to the posterior midline (Fig. 9).

2. 7. 42 BL 42 Pòhù 魄户

On the back, below the spinous process of the 3rd thoracic vertebra, 3 *cun* lateral to the posterior midline (Fig. 9).

2. 7. 43 BL 43 Gāohuāng 膏肓

On the back, below the spinous process of the 4th thoracic vertebra, 3 *cun* lateral to the posterior midline (Fig. 9).

2. 7. 44 BL 44 Shéntáng 神堂

On the back, below the spinous process of the 5th thoracic vertebra, 3 *cun* lateral to the posterior midline (Fig. 9).

2. 7. 45 BL 45 Yìxǐ 譩譆

On the back, below the spinous process of the 6th thoracic vertebra, 3 *cun* lateral to the posterior midline (Fig. 9).

2. 7. 46 BL 46 Géguān 膈關

On the back, below the spinous process of the 7th thoracic vertebra, 3 *cun* lateral to the posterior midline (Fig. 9).

2. 7. 47 BL 47 Húnmén 魂門

On the back, below the spinous process of the 9th thoracic vertebra, 3 *cun* lateral to the posterior midline (Fig. 9).

2. 7. 48 BL 48 Yánggāng 陽綱

On the back, below the spinous process of the 10th thoracic vertebra, 3 *cun* lateral to the

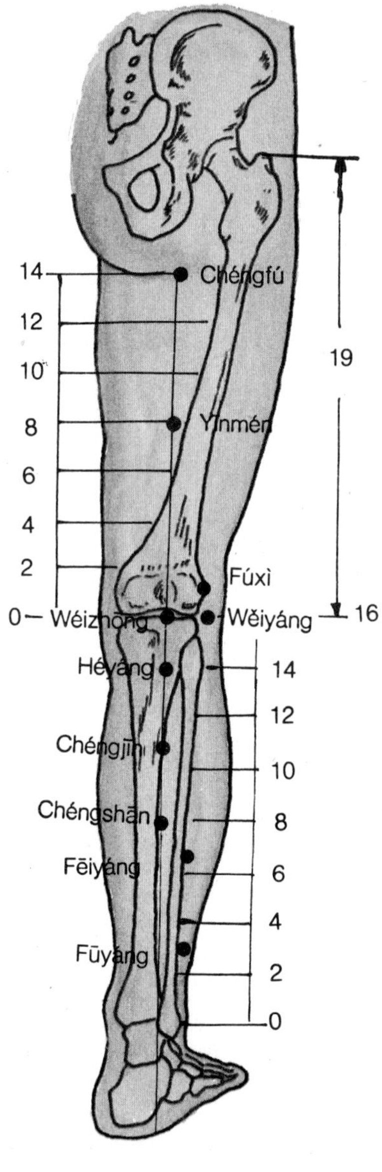

Fig. 37 Points of Bladder Meridian (Lower Limbs)

posterior midline (Fig. 9).

2. 7. 49 BL 49 Yìshè 意舍

On the back, below the spinous process of the 11th thoracic vertebra, 3 *cun* lateral to the posterior midline (Fig. 9).

2. 7. 50 BL 50 Wèicāng 胃倉

On the back, below the spinous process of the 12th thoracic vertebra, 3 *cun* lateral to the posterior midline (Fig. 9).

2. 7. 51 BL 51 Huāngmén 肓門

On the low back, below the spinous process of the 1st lumbar vertebra, 3 *cun* lateral to the posterior midline (Fig. 9).

2. 7. 52 BL 52 Zhìshì 志室

On the low back, below the spinous process of the 2nd lumbar vertebra, 3 *cun* lateral to the posterior midline (Fig. 9).

2. 7. 53 BL 53 Bāohuāng 胞肓

On the buttock and on the level of the 2nd posterior sacral foramen, 3 *cun* lateral to the median sacral crest (Fig. 9).

2. 7. 54 BL 54 Zhìbiān 秩邊

On the buttock and on the level of the 4th posterior sacral foramen, 3 *cun* lateral to the median sacral crest (Fig. 9).

2. 7. 55 BL 55 Héyáng 合陽

On the posterior side of the leg and on the line connecting Weizhong (BL 40) and Chengshan (BL 57), 2 *cun* below Weizhong (BL 40) (Figs. 37 & 38).

2. 7. 56 BL 56 Chéngjīn 承筋

On the posterior side of the leg and on the line connecting Weizhong (BL 40) and Chengshan (BL 57), at the centre of the gastrocnemius muscle belly, 5 *cun* below Weizhong (BL 40) (Figs. 37 & 38).

2. 7. 57 BL 57 Chéngshān 承山

On the posterior midline of the leg, between Weizhong (BL 40) and Kunlun (BL 60), in a pointed depression formed below the gastrocnemius muscle belly when the leg is stretched or the heel is lifted (Figs. 37 & 38).

2. 7. 58 BL 58 Fēiyáng 飛揚

On the posterior side of the leg, 7 *cun* directly above Kunlun (BL 60) and 1 *cun* lateral and inferior to Chengshan (BL 57) (Figs. 37 & 38).

2. 7. 59 BL 59 Fūyáng 跗陽

On the posterior side of the leg, posterior to the lateral malleolus, 3 *cun* directly above Kunlun (BL 60) (Fig. 37).

2. 7. 60 BL 60 Kūnlún 昆侖

Posterior to the lateral malleolus, in the depression between the tip of the external malleolus and Achilles tendon (Fig. 39).

2. 7. 61 BL 61 Púcān 僕參

On the lateral side of the foot, posterior and inferior to the external malleolus, directly below Kunlun (BL 60), lateral to the calcaneum, at the junction of the red and white skin (Fig. 39).

2. 7. 62 BL 62 Shēnmài 申脈

Wéizhōng

Wěiyáng

Héyáng

Chéngjīn(

Chéngshān

Fēiyáng

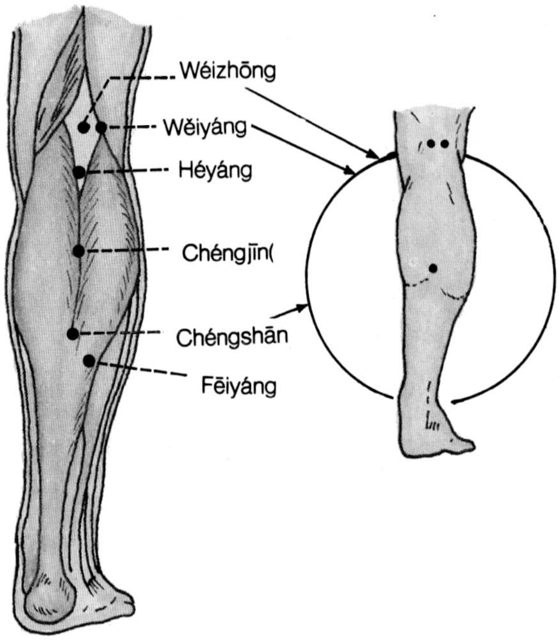

Fig. 38 Points of Bladder Meridian (Leg)

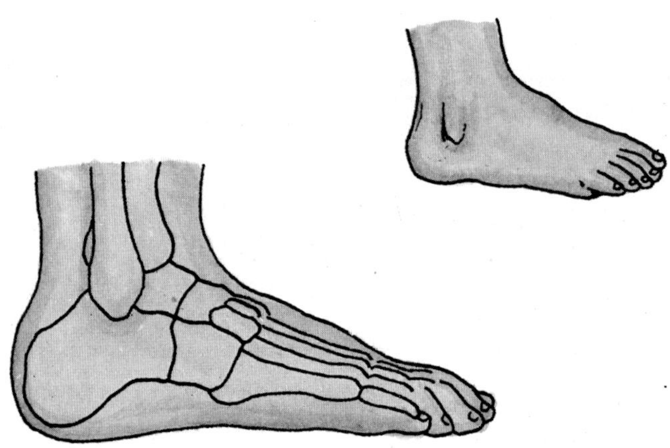

Fig. 39 Points of Bladder Meridian (Foot)

On the lateral side of the foot, in the depression directly below the external malleolus (Fig. 39).

2. 7. 63 BL 63 Jīnmén 金門

On the lateral side of the foot, directly below the anterior border of the external malleolus, on the lower border of the cuboid bone (Fig. 39).

2. 7. 64 BL 64 Jīnggǔ 京骨

On the lateral side of the foot, below the tuberosity of the 5th metatarsal bone, at the junction of the red and white skin (Fig. 39).

2. 7. 65 BL 65 Shùgǔ 束骨

On the lateral side of the foot, posterior to the 5th metatarsophalangeal joint, at the junction of the red and white skin (Fig. 39).

2. 7. 66 BL Zútōnggǔ 足通谷

On the lateral side of the foot, anterior to the 5th metatarsophalangeal joint, at the junction of the red and white skin (Fig. 39).

2. 7. 67 BL 67 Zhìyīn 至陰

On the lateral side of the distal segment of the little toe, 0.1 *cun* from the corner of the toenail (Fig. 39).

2. 8 Points of the Kidney Meridian of Foot-Shaoyin, KI

足少陰腎經穴

Zúshàoyīn Shènjīng Xúe

2. 8. 1 KI 1 Yǒngquán 涌泉

On the sole, in the depression appearing on the anterior part of the sole when the foot is in the plantar flexion, approximately at the junction of the anterior third and posterior two-thirds of the line connecting the base of the 2nd and 3rd toes and the heel (Fig. 40).

2. 8. 2 KI 2 Rángǔ 然谷

On the medial border of the foot, below the tuberosity of the navicular bone, and at the junction of the red and white skin (Figs. 26 & 41).

2. 8. 3 KI 3 Tàixī 太谿

On the medial side of the foot, posterior to the medial malleolus, in the depression between the tip of the medial malleolus and Achilles tendon (Figs. 26 & 41).

2. 8. 4 KI 4 Dàzhōng 大鐘

On the medial side of the foot, posterior and inferior to the medial malleolus, in the depression of the medial side of and anterior to the attachment of the Achilles tendon (Figs. 26 & 41).

2. 8. 5 KI 5 Shuǐquán 水泉

On the medial side of the foot, posterior and inferior to the medial malleolus, 1 *cun* directly below Taixi (KI 3), in the depression of the medial side of the tuberosity of the calcaneum (Figs. 26 & 41).

2. 8. 6 KI 6 Zhàohǎi 照海

On the medial side of the foot, in the depression below the tip of the medial malleolus

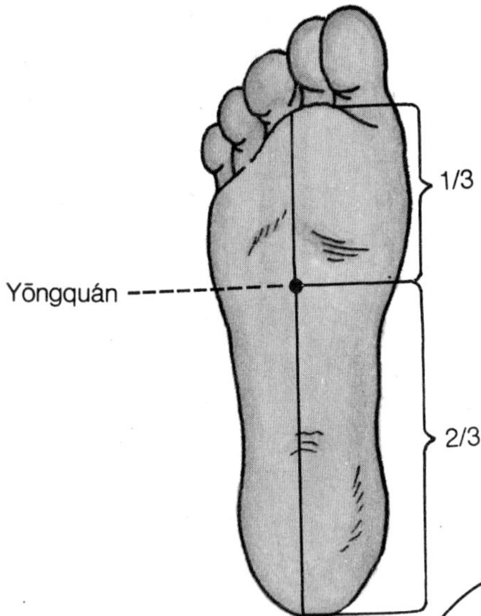

Fig. 40 Yǒngquán Point

Fig. 41 Points of Kidney Meridian (Foot)

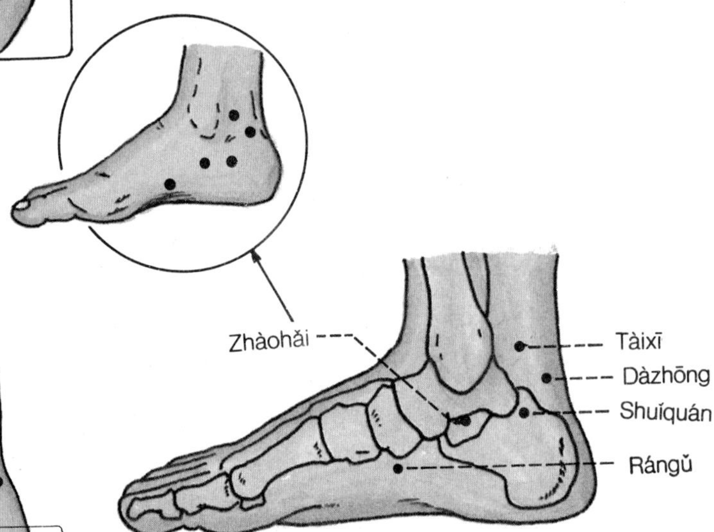

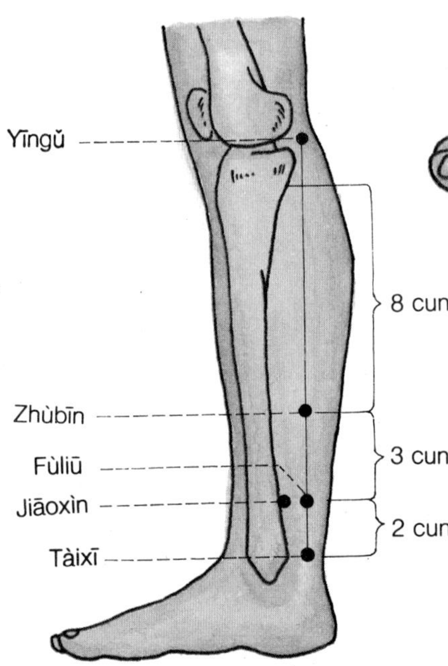

Fig. 42 Points of Kidney Meridian (Leg)

(Figs. 26 & 41).

2. 8. 7 KI 7 Fùliū 複溜

On the medial side of the leg, 2 *cun* directly above Taixi (KI 3), anterior to the Achilles tendon (Figs. 26 & 42).

2. 8. 8 KI 8 Jiāoxìn 交信

On the medial side of the leg, 2 *cun* above Taixi (KI 3) and 0.5 *cun* anterior to Fuliu (KI 7), posterior to the medial border of the tibia (Figs. 26 & 42).

2. 8. 9 KI 9 Zhùbīn 築賓

On the medial side of the leg and on the line connecting Taixi (KI 3) and Yingu (KI 10), 5 *cun* above Taixi (KI 3), medial and inferior to the gastrocnemius muscle belly (Figs. 26 & 42).

2. 8. 10 KI 10 Yīngǔ 陰谷

On the medial side of the popliteal fossa, between the tendons of the semitendinous and semimembranous muscles when the knee is flexed (Figs. 26 & 42).

2. 8. 11 KI 11 Hénggǔ 横骨

On the lower abdomen, 5 *cun* below the centre of the umbilicus and 0.5 *cun* lateral to the anterior midline (Fig. 8).

2. 8. 12 KI 12 Dàhè 大赫

On the lower abdomen, 4 *cun* below the centre of the umbilicus and 0.5 *cun* lateral to the anterior midline (Fig. 8).

2. 8. 13 KI 13 Qìxúe 氣穴

On the lower abdomen, 3 *cun* below the centre of the umbilicus and 0.5 *cun* lateral to the anterior midline (Fig. 8).

2. 8. 14 KI 14 Sìmǎn 四滿

On the lower abdomen, 2 *cun* below the centre of the umbilicus and 0.5 *cun* lateral to the anterior midline (Fig. 8).

2. 8. 15 KI 15 Zhōngzhù 中注

On the lower abdomen, 1 *cun* below the centre of the umbilicus and 0.5 *cun* lateral to the anterior midline (Fig. 8).

2. 8. 16 KI 16 Huāngshū 肓俞

On the middle abdomen, 0.5 *cun* lateral to the centre of the umbilicus (Fig. 8).

2. 8. 17 KI 17 Shāngqū 商曲

On the upper abdomen, 2 *cun* above the centre of the umbilicus, and 0.5 *cun* lateral to the anterior midline (Fig. 8).

2. 8. 18 KI 18 Shíguān 石關

On the upper abdomen, 3 *cun* above the centre of the umbilicus and 0.5 *cun* lateral to the anterior midline (Fig. 8).

2. 8. 19 KI 19 Yīndū 陰都

On the upper abdomen, 4 *cun* above the centre of the umbilicus and 0.5 *cun* lateral to the anterior midline (Fig. 8).

2. 8. 20 KI 20 Fùtōnggǔ 腹通谷

On the upper abdomen, 5 *cun* above the centre of the umbilicus and 0.5 *cun* lateral to the anterior midline (Fig. 8).

2. 8. 21 KI 21 Yōumén 幽門

On the upper abdomen, 6 *cun* above the centre of the umbilicus and 0.5 *cun* lateral to the anterior midline (Fig. 8).

2. 8. 22 KI 22 Bùláng 步廊

On the chest, in the 5th intercostal space, 2 *cun* lateral to the anterior midline (Fig. 8).

2. 8. 23 KI 23 Shénfēng 神封

On the chest, in the 4th intercostal space, 2 *cun* lateral to the anterior midline (Fig. 8).

2. 8. 24 KI 24 Língxū 靈墟

On the chest, in the 3rd intercostal space, 2 *cun* lateral to the anterior midline (Fig. 8).

2. 8. 25 KI 25 Shéncáng 神藏

On the chest, in the 2nd intercostal space, 2 *cun* lateral to the anterior midline (Fig. 8).

2. 8. 26 KI 26 Yùzhōng 彧中

On the chest, in the 1st intercostal space, 2 *cun* lateral to the anterior midline (Fig. 8).

2. 8. 27 KI 27 Shūfǔ 俞府

On the chest, below the lower border of the clavicle, 2 *cun* lateral to the midline (Fig. 8).

2. 9 Points of the Pericardium Meridian of Hand-Jueyin, PC
手厥陰心包經穴
Shǒujúeyīn Xīnbāojīng Xué

2. 9. 1 PC 1 Tiānchí 天池

On the chest, in the 4th intercostal space, 1 *cun* lateral to the nipple and 5 *cun* lateral to the anterior midline (Fig. 8).

2. 9. 2 PC 2 Tiānquán 天泉

On the medial side of the arm, 2 *cun* below the anterior end of the axillary fold, between the long and short heads of the biceps muscle of the arm (Fig. 11).

2. 9. 3 PC 3 Qūzé 曲澤

At the midpoint of the cubital crease, on the ulnar side of the tendon of the biceps muscle of the arm (Figs 11 & 43).

2. 9. 4 PC 4 Xīmén 郄門

On the palmar side of the forearm and on the line connecting Quze (PC 3) and Daling (PC 7), 5 *cun* above the crease of the wrist (Figs 11 & 43).

2. 9. 5 PC 5 Jiānshǐ 間使

On the palmar side of the forearm and on the line connecting Quze (PC 3) and Daling (PC 7), 3 *cun* above the crease of the wrist, between the tendons of the long palmar muscle and radial flexor muscle of the wrist (Figs. 11 & 43).

2. 9. 6 PC 6 Nèiguān 內關

On the palmar side of the forearm and on the line connecting Quze (PC 3) and Daling (PC 7), 2 *cun* above the crease of the wrist, between the tendons of the long palmar muscle and radial flexor muscle of the wrist (Figs. 11 & 43)

2. 9. 7 PC 7 Dàlíng 大陵

At the midpoint of the crease of the wrist, between the tendons of the long palmar muscle and radial flexor muscle of the wrist (Figs. 11 & 43).

2. 9. 8 PC 8 Láogōng 勞宮

At the centre of the palm, between the 2nd and 3rd metacarpal bones, but close to the

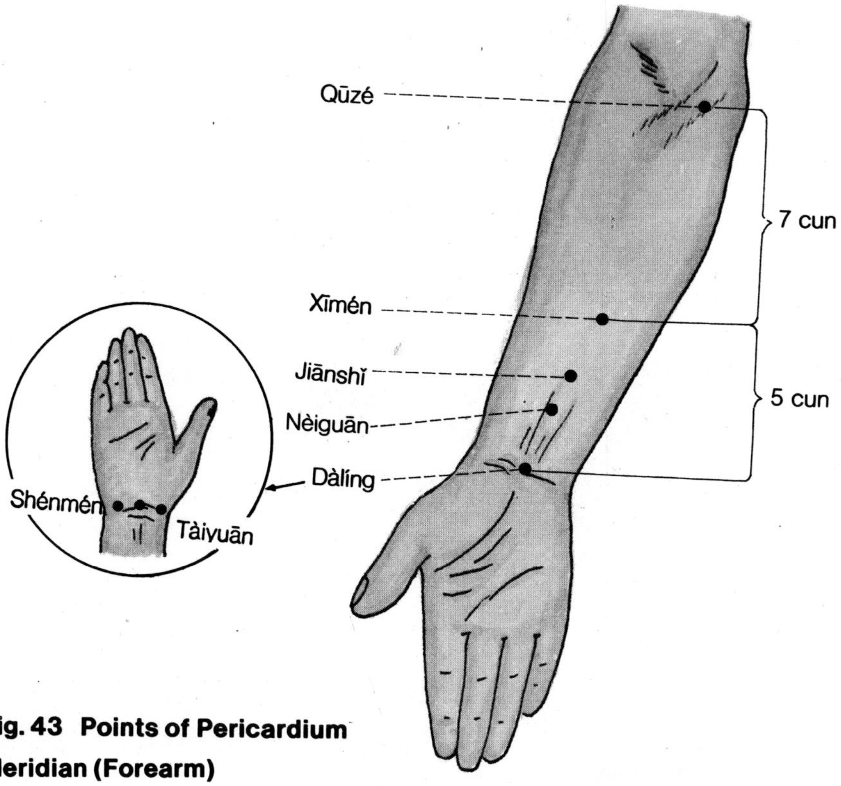

Fig. 43 Points of Pericardium Meridian (Forearm)

latter, and in the part touching the tip of the middle finger when a fist is made (Figs. 11 & 33).

2. 9. 9 PC 9 Zhōngchōng 中衝

At the centre of the tip of the middle finger (Figs. 11 & 33).

2. 10 Points of the Sanjiao (Triple Energizer) Meridian of Hand-Shaoyang, SJ (TE)

手少陽三焦經穴

Shǒushàoyáng Sānjiāojīng Xué

2. 10. 1 SJ 1 Guānchōng 關衝

On the ulnar side of the distal segment of the 4th finger, 0.1 *cun* from the corner of the nail (Figs. 14 & 44).

2. 10. 2 SJ 2 Yèmén 液門

On the dorsum of the hand, between the 4th and 5th fingers, at the junction of the red and white skin, proximal to the margin of the web (Figs. 14 & 44).

2. 10. 3 SJ 3 Zhōngzhǔ 中渚

On the dorsum of the hand, proximal to the 4th metacarpophalangeal joint, in the depression between the 4th and 5th metacarpal bones (Figs. 14 & 44).

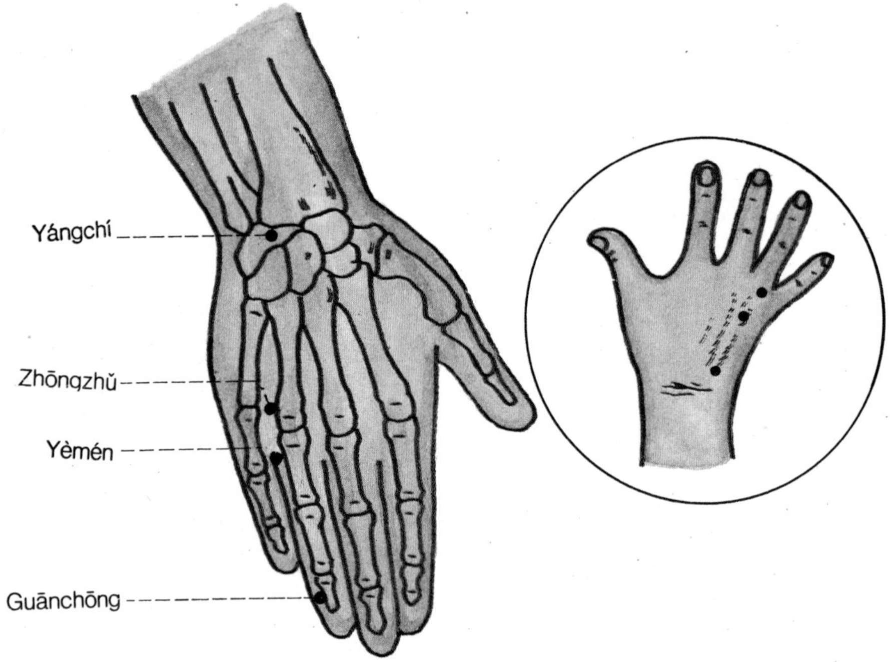

Fig. 44 Points of Sānjiāo Meridian (Hand)

2. 10. 4 SJ 4 Yángchí 陽池

At the midpoint of the dorsal crease of the wrist, in the depression on the ulnar side of the tendon of the extensor muscle of the fingers (Figs. 14 & 44).

2. 10. 5 SJ 5 Wàiguān 外關

On the dorsal side of the forearm and on the line connecting Yangchi (SJ 4) and the tip of the olecranon, 2 *cun* proximal to the dorsal crease of the wrist, between the radius and ulna (Figs 14 & 45).

2. 10. 6 SJ 6 Zhīgōu 支溝

On the dorsal side of the forearm and on the line connecting Yangchi (SJ 4) and the tip of the olecranon, 3 *cun* proximal to the dorsal crease of the wrist, between the radius and ulna (Figs. 14 & 45).

2. 10. 7 SJ 7 Huìzōng 會宗

On the dorsal side of the forearm, 3 *cun* proximal to the dorsal crease of the wrist, on the ulnar side of Zhigou (SJ 6) and on the radial border of the ulna (Figs. 14 & 45).

2. 10. 8 SJ 8 Sānyángluò 三陽絡

On the dorsal side of the forearm, 4 *cun* proximal to the dorsal crease of the wrist, between the radius and ulna (Figs. 14 & 45).

2. 10. 9 SJ 9 Sìdú 四瀆

On the dorsal side of the forearm and on the line connecting Yangchi (SJ 4) and the tip of the olecranon, 5 *cun* distal to the tip of the olecranon, between the radius and ulna (Figs. 14 & 45).

2. 10. 10 SJ 10 Tiānjǐng 天井

On the lateral side of the upper arm, in the depression 1 *cun* proximal to the tip of the olecranon when the elbow is flexed (Figs. 14 & 46).

2. 10. 11 SJ 11 Qīnglěngyūan 清冷淵

With the elbow flexed, on the lateral side of the upper arm, 2 *cun* above the tip of the olecranon and 1 *cun* above Tianjing (SJ 10) (Figs. 14 & 46).

2. 10. 12 SJ 12 Xiāoluò 消濼

On the lateral side of the upper arm, at the midpoint of the line connecting Qinglengyuan (SJ 11) and Naohui (SJ 13) (Figs. 14 & 46).

2. 10. 13 SJ 13 Nàohuì 臑會

On the lateral side of the upper arm and on the line connecting the tip of the olecranon and Jianliao (SJ 14), 3 *cun* below Jianliao (SJ 14), and on the posterioinferior border of the deltoid muscle (Figs. 14 & 46).

2. 10. 14 SJ 14 Jiānliáo 肩髎

On the shoulder, posterior to Jianyu (LI 15), in the depression inferior and posterior to the acromion when the arm is abducted (Figs. 14 & 46).

2. 10. 15 SJ 15 Tiānliáo 天髎

On the scapula, at the midpoint between Jianjing (GB 21) and Quyuan (SI 13), at the superior angle of the scapula (Figs. 9 & 47).

2. 10. 16 SJ 16 Tiānyǒu 天牖

On the lateral side of the neck, directly below the posterior border of the mastoid process, on the level of the mandibular angle, and on the posterior border of the sternocleidomastoid muscle (Figs. 7 & 18).

2. 10. 17 SJ 17 Yìfēng 翳風

Posterior to the ear lobe, in the depression between the mastoid process and mandibular angle (Figs. 7 & 48).

2. 10. 18 SJ 18 Chìmài 瘈脈

On the head, at the centre of the mastoid process, and at the junction of the middle third and lower third of the line connecting Jiaosun (SJ 20) and Yifeng (SJ 17) along the curve of the ear helix (Fig. 7).

2. 10. 19 SJ 19 Lúxī 顱息

On the head, at the junction of the upper third and middle third of the line connecting Jiaosun (SJ 20) and Yifeng (SJ 17) along the curve of the ear helix (Fig. 7).

2. 10. 20 SJ 20 Jiǎosūn 角孫

On the head, above the ear apex within the hairline (Figs. 7 & 48).

2. 10. 21 SJ 21 Ěrmén 耳門

On the face, anterior to the supratragic notch, in the depression behind the posterior border of the condyloid process of the mandible (Fig. 7).

2. 10. 22 SJ 22 Ěrhéliáo 耳和髎

On the lateral side of the head, on the posterior margin of the temples, anterior to the anterior border of the root of the ear auricle and posterior to the superficial temporal artery (Fig. 7).

2. 10. 23 SJ 23 Sīzhúkōng 絲竹空

On the face, in the depression of the lateral end of the eyebrow (Figs. 7 & 48).

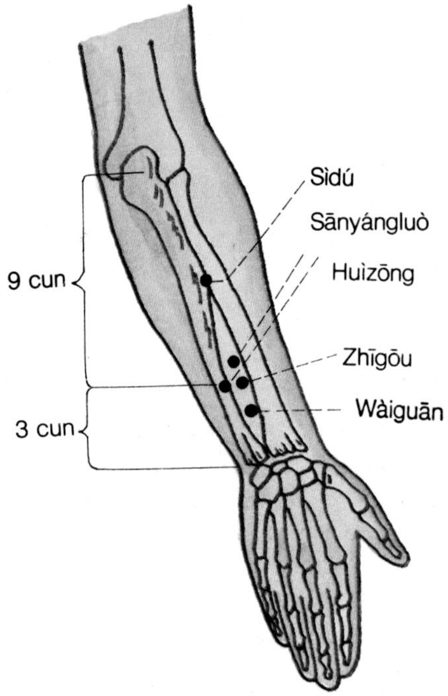

Fig. 45 Points of Sānjiāo Meridian (Forearm)

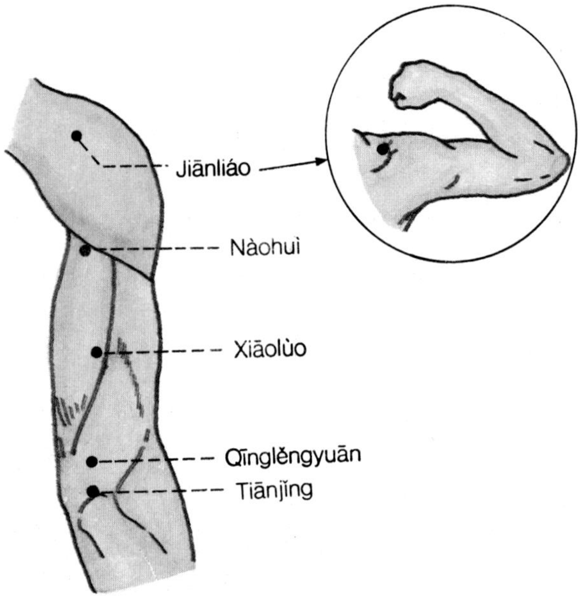

Fig. 46 Points of Sānjiāo Meridian (Arm)

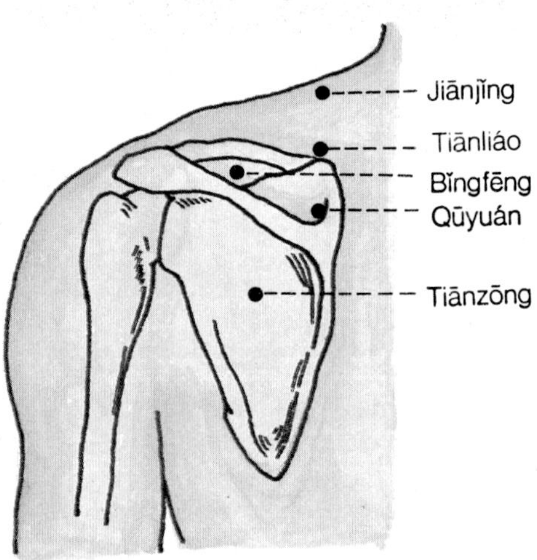

Fig. 47 Points of Sānjiāo Meridian (Shoulder)

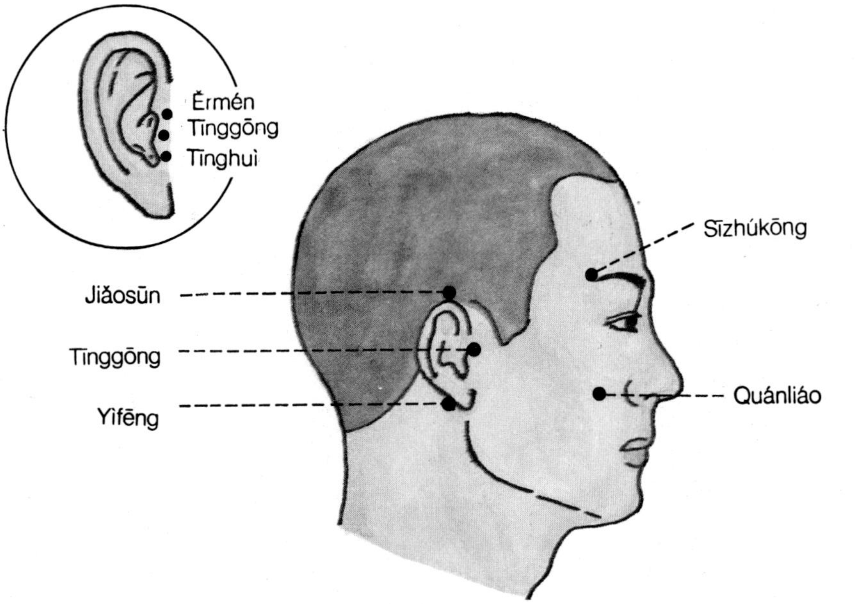

Fig. 48 Points of Sānjiāo and Small Intestine Meridian (Head and Face)

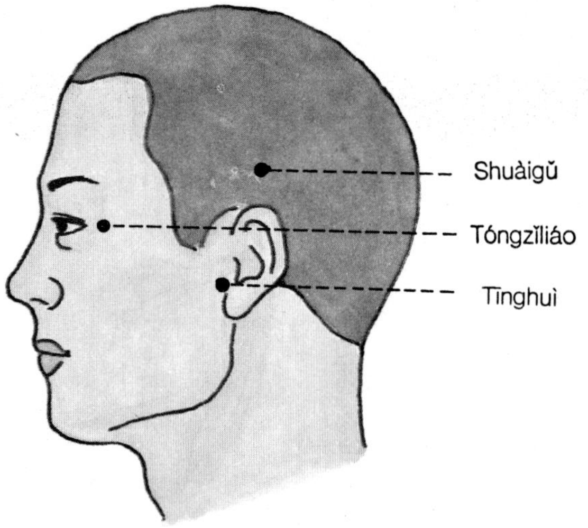

Fig. 49 Tóngzǐlíao, Tīnghuì and Shuàigǔ Points

2. 11 Points of the Gallbladder Meridian of Foot-Shaoyang, GB

足少陽膽經穴

Zúshàoyáng Dǎnjīng Xué

2. 11. 1 GB 1 Tóngzǐliáo 瞳子髎

On the face, lateral to the outer canthus, on the lateral border of the orbit (Figs. 7 & 49).

2. 11. 2 GB 2 Tīnghuì 聽會

On the face, anterior to the intertragic notch, in the depression posterior to the condyloid process of the mandible when the mouth is open (Figs. 7 & 49).

2. 11. 3 GB 3 Shàngguān 上關

Anterior to the ear, directly above Xiaguan (ST 7), in the depression above the upper border of the zygomatic arch (Fig. 7).

2. 11. 4 GB 4 Hǎnyàn 頷厭

On the head, in the hair above the temples, at the junction of the upper fourth and lower three fourths of the curved line connecting Touwei (ST 8) and Qubin (GB 7) (Fig. 7).

2. 11. 5 GB 5 Xuánlú 懸顱

On the head, in the hair above the temples, at the midpoint of the curved line connecting Touwei (ST 8) and Qubin (GB 7) (Fig. 7).

2. 11. 6 GB 6 Xuánlí 懸釐

On the head, in the hair above the temples, at the junction of the upper three fourths and lower fourth of the curved line connecting Touwei (ST 8) and Qubin (GB 7) (Fig. 7).

2. 11. 7 GB 7 Qūbìn 曲鬢

On the head, at a crossing point of the vertical posterior border of the temples and horizontal line through the ear apex. (Fig. 7).

2. 11. 8 GB 8 Shuàigǔ 率谷

On the head, directly above the ear apex, 1.5 *cun* above the hairline, directly above Jiaosun (SJ 20) (Figs. 7 & 49).

2. 11. 9 GB 9 Tiānchōng 天衝

On the head, directly above the posterior border of the ear root, 2 *cun* above the hairline and 0.5 *cun* posterior to Shuaigu (GB 8) (Figs. 7 & 36).

2. 11. 10 GB 10 Fúbái 浮白

On the head, posterior and superior to the mastoid process, at the junction of the middle third and upper third of the curved line connecting Tianchong (GB 9) and Wangu (GB 12) (Figs. 7 & 36).

2. 11. 11 GB 11 Tóuqiàoyīn 頭竅陰

On the head, posterior and superior to the mastoid process, at the junction of the middle third and lower third of the curved line connecting Tianchong (GB 9) and Wangu (GB 12) (Figs. 7 & 36).

2. 11. 12 GB 12 Wángǔ 完骨

On the head, in the depression posterior and inferior to the mastoid process (Figs. 7 & 36).

2. 11. 13 GB 13 Běnshén 本神

On the head, 0.5 *cun* above the anterior hairline, 3 *cun* lateral to Shenting (DU 24), at the junction of the medial two thirds and lateral third of the line connecting Shenting (DU 24) and

Touwei (ST 8) (Fig. 7).

2. 11. 14 GB 14 Yángbái 陽白

On the forehead, directly above the pupil, 1 *cun* above the eyebrow (Figs. 7 & 19).

2. 11. 15 GB 15 Tóulínqì 頭臨泣

On the head, directly above the pupil and 0.5 *cun* above the anterior hairline, at the midpoint of the line connecting Shenting (DU 24) and Touwei (ST 8) (Fig. 7).

2. 11. 16 GB 16 Mùchuāng 目窗

On the head, 1.5 *cun* above the anterior hairline and 2.25 *cun* lateral to the midline of the head (Fig. 7).

2. 11. 17 GB 17 Zhèngyíng 正營

On the head, 2.5 *cun* above the anterior hairline and 2.25 *cun* lateral to the midline of the head (Fig. 7).

2. 11. 18 GB 18 Chénglíng 承靈

On the head, 4 *cun* above the anterior hairline and 2.25 *cun* lateral to the midline of the head (Fig. 7).

2. 11. 19 GB 19 Nǎokōng 腦空

On the head and on the level of the upper border of the external occipital protuberance or Naohu (DU 17), 2.25 *cun* lateral to the midline of the head (Figs. 7 & 36).

2. 11. 20 GB 20 Fēngchí 風池

On the nape, below the occipital bone, on the level of Fengfu (DU 16), in the depression between the upper ends of the sternocleidomastoid and trapezius muscles (Figs. 7 & 36).

2. 11. 21 GB 21 Jiānjǐng 肩井

On the shoulder, directly above the nipple, at the midpoint of the line connecting Dazhui (DU 14) and the acromion (Figs. 9 & 47).

2. 11. 22 GB 22 Yuānyè 淵腋

On the lateral side of the chest, on the midaxillary line when the arm is raised, 3 *cun* below the axilla, in the 4th intercostal space (Figs. 10 & 50).

2. 11. 23 GB 23 Zhéjīn 輒筋

On the lateral side of the chest, 1 *cun* anterior to Yuanye (GB 22), on the level of the nipple, and in the 4th intercostal space (Figs. 10 & 50).

2. 11. 24 GB 24 Rìyuè 日月

On the upper abdomen, directly below the nipple, in the 7th intercostal space, 4 *cun* lateral to the anterior midline (Figs. 8 & 10).

2. 11. 25 GB 25 Jīngmén 京門

On the lateral side of the waist, 1.8 *cun* posterior to Zhangmen (LR 13), below the free end of the 12th rib (Figs. 10 & 50).

2. 11. 26 GB 26 Dàimài 帶脈

On the lateral side of the abdomen, 1.8 *cun* below Zhangmen (LR 13), at the crossing point of a vertical line through the free end of the 11th rib and a horizontal line through the umbilicus (Figs. 10 & 50).

2. 11. 27 GB 27 Wǔshū 五樞

On the lateral side of the abdomen, anterior to the anteriosuperior iliac spine, 3 *cun* below the level of the umbilicus (Figs. 8 & 51).

2. 11. 28 GB 28 Wéidào 維道

Jíquán
Yúnmén
Zhōngfǔ
Zhōuróng
Yuānyè
Xiōngxiāng
Zhéjīn
Tiānxī
Shídòu
Dàbāo
Rìyuè
Jīngmén
Fù'āi
Zhāngmén
Dàimài
Dàhéng
Fùjié
Wèishū
Wéidào
Fúshè
Jùliáo
Huántiào

**Fig. 10 Points on the Lateral Side
of the Chest and Abdomen**

Yuānyè
Zhéjīn
Dàbāo
Zhāngmén
Jīngmén
Dàimài

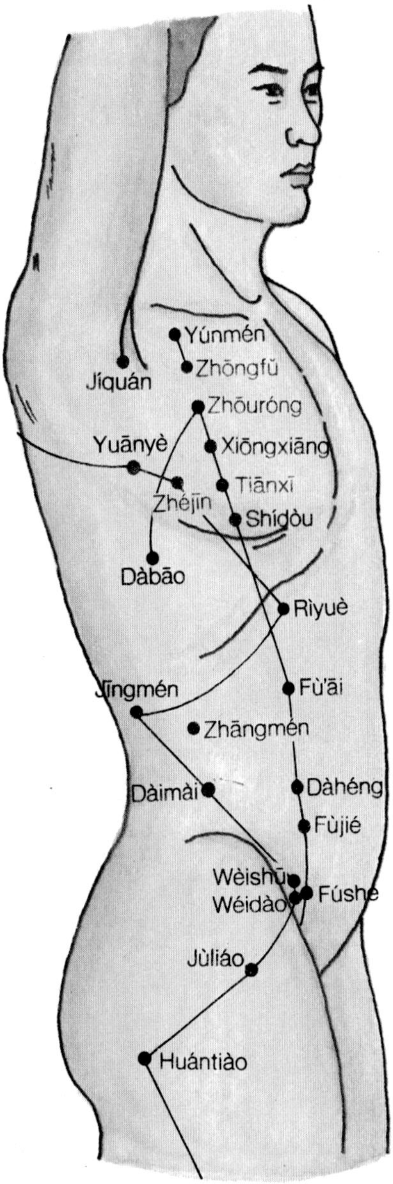

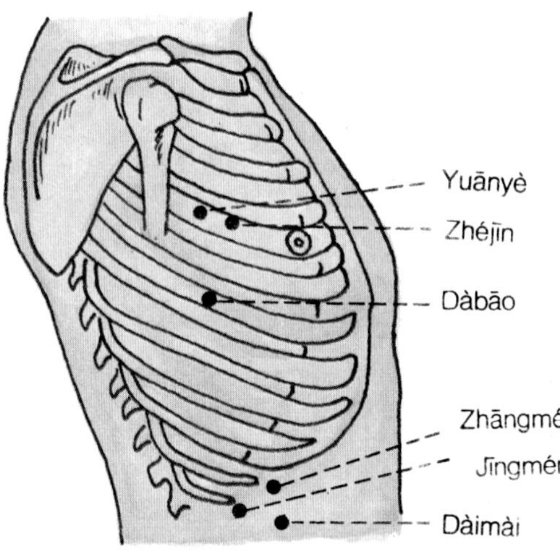

**Fig. 50 Yúanyè, Zhéjīn, Jīngmén
and Dàimài Points**

On the lateral side of the abdomen, anterior and inferior to the anteriosuperior iliac spine, 0.5 *cun* anterior and inferior to Wushu (GB 27) (Figs. 8 & 51).

2. 11. 29 GB 29 Jūliáo 居髎

On the hip, at the midpoint of the line connecting the anteriosuperior iliac spine and the prominence of the great trochanter (Figs. 10 & 51).

2. 11. 30 GB 30 Huántiào 環跳

On the lateral side of the thigh, at the junction of the middle third and lateral third of the line connecting the prominence of the great trochanter and the sacral hiatus when the patient is in a lateral recumbent position with the thigh flexed (Figs. 10 & 52).

2. 11. 31 GB 31 Fēngshì 風市

On the lateral midline of the thigh, 7 *cun* above the popliteal crease, or at the place touching the tip of the middle finger when the patient stands erect with the arms hanging down freely (Figs. 53 & 54).

2. 11. 32 GB 32 Zhōngdú 中瀆

On the lateral side of the thigh, 2 *cun* below Fengshi (GB 31), or 5 *cun* above the popliteal crease, between the lateral vastus muscle and biceps muscle of the thigh (Figs. 53 & 54).

2. 11. 33 GB 33 Xīyángguān 膝陽關

On the lateral side of the knee, 3 *cun* above Yanglingquan (GB 34), in the depression above the external epicondyle of the femur (Figs. 53 & 54).

2. 11. 34 GB 34 Yánglíngquán 陽陵泉

On the lateral side of the leg, in the depression anterior and inferior to the head of the fibula (Figs. 53 & 55).

2. 11. 35 GB 35 Yángjiāo 陽交

On the lateral side of the leg, 7 *cun* above the tip of the external malleolus, on the posterior border of the fibula (Figs. 53 & 55).

2. 11. 36 GB 36 Wàiqiū 外丘

On the lateral side of the leg, 7 *cun* above the tip of the external malleolus, on the anterior border of the fibula and on the level of Yangjiao (BG 35) (Figs. 53 & 55).

2. 11. 37 GB 37 Guāngmíng 光明

On the lateral side of the leg, 5 *cun* above the tip of the external malleolus, on the anterior border of the fibula (Figs. 53 & 55).

2. 11. 38 GB 38 Yángfǔ 陽輔

On the lateral side of the leg, 4 *cun* above the tip of the external malleolus, slightly anterior to the anterior border of the fibula (Figs. 53 & 55).

2. 11. 39 GB 39 Xuánzhōng 懸鍾

On the lateral side of the leg, 3 *cun* above the tip of the external malleolus, on the anterior border of the fibula (Figs. 53 & 55).

2. 11. 40 GB 40 Qiūxū 丘墟

Anterior and inferior to the external malleolus, in the depression lateral to the tendon of the long extensor muscle of the toes (Figs. 53 & 56).

2. 11. 41 GB 41 Zúlínqì 足臨泣

On the lateral side of the instep of the foot, posterior to the 4th metatarsophalangeal joint, in the depression lateral to the tendon of the extensor muscle of the little toe (Figs. 53 & 56).

2. 11. 42 GB 42 Dìwǔhuì 地五會

Wǔshū

Wéidào

Jūliáo

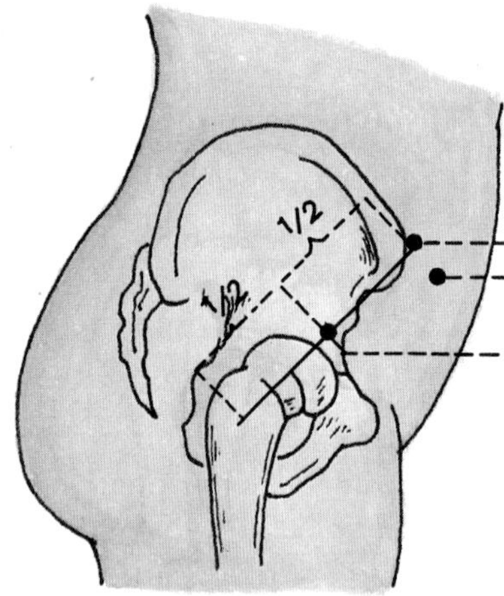

Fig. 51 Wǔshū, Wéidào and Jūliáo Points

Huántiào

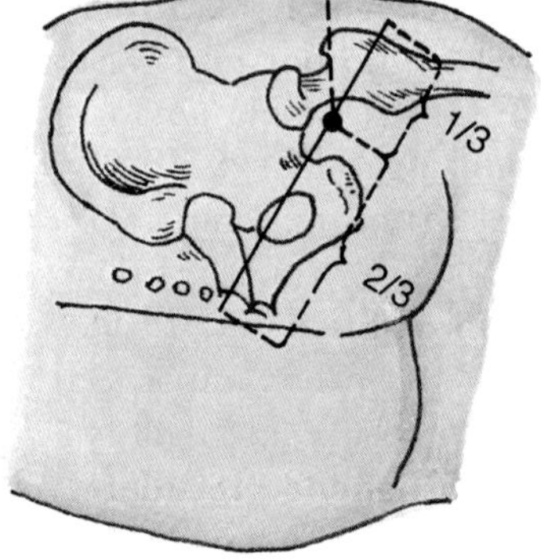

Fig. 52 Huántiào Point

Fēngshì

Zhōngdú

Xīyángguān

Yánglíngquán

Yángjiāo

Wàiqiū

Guāngmíng

Yángfǔ

Xuánzhōng

Qiūxū

Zúlínqì Xiáxī

Dìwǔhuì Zúqiàobyīn

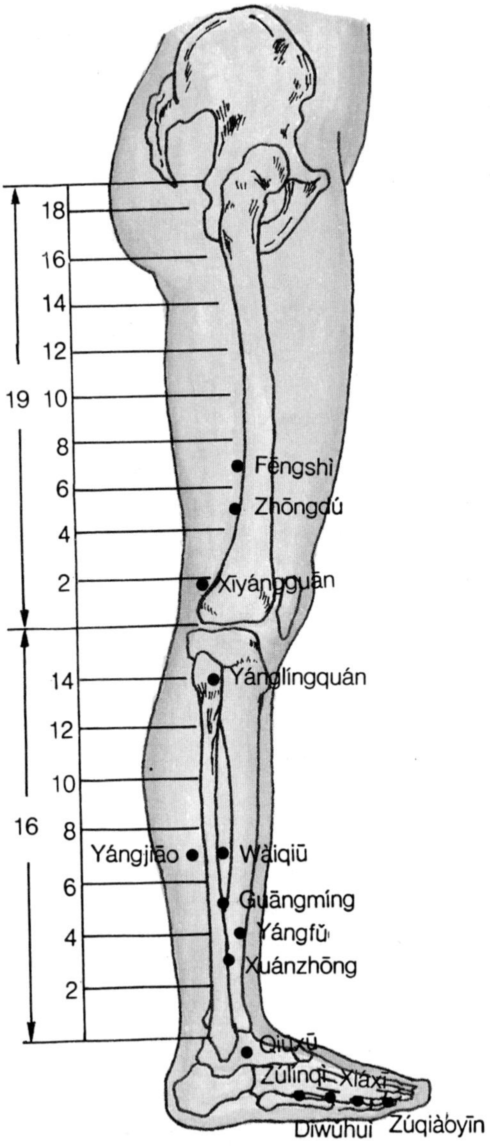

Fig. 53 Points of Gallbladder

Meridian (Lower Limbs)

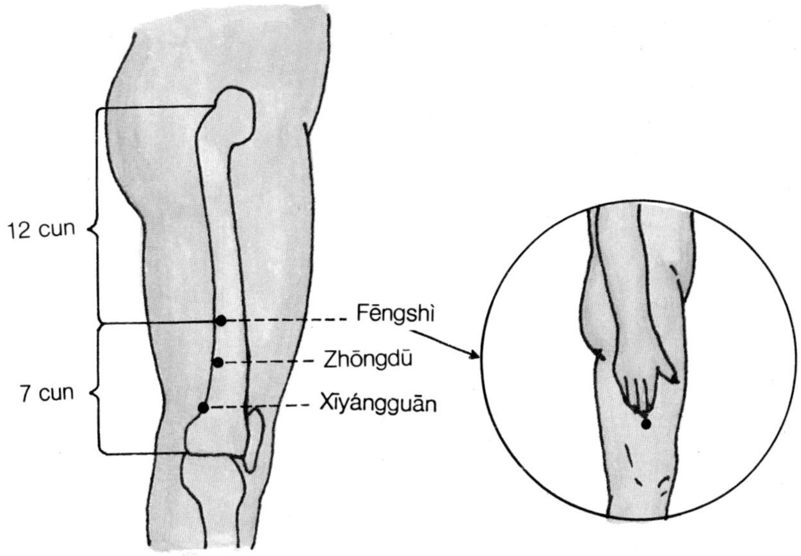

Fig. 54 Points of Gallbladder Meridian (Thigh)

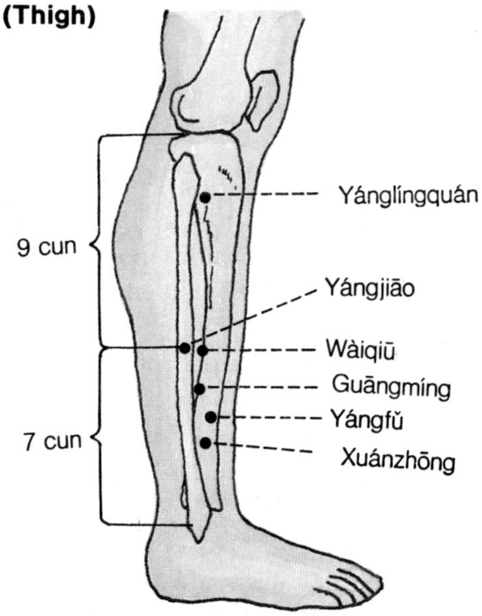

Fig. 55 Points of Gallbladder Meridian (Leg)

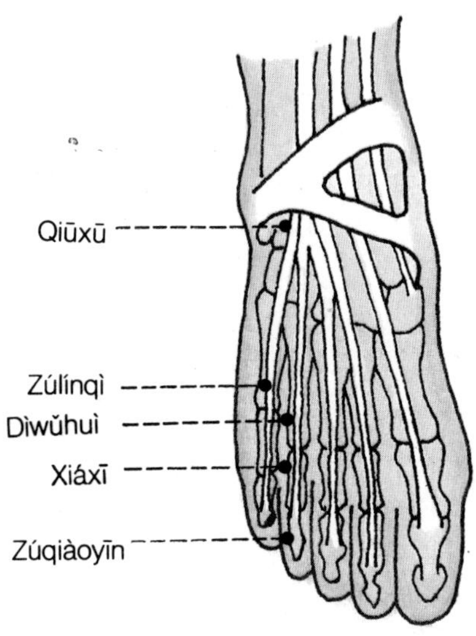

Fig. 56 Points of Gallbladder Meridian (Foot)

On the lateral side of the instep of the foot, posterior to the 4th metatarsophalangeal joint, between the 4th and 5th metatarsal bones, medial to the tendon of the extensor muscle of the little toe (Figs. 53 & 56).

2. 11. 43 GB 43 Xiáxī 俠谿

On the lateral side of the instep of the foot, between the 4th and 5th toes, at the junction of the red and white skin, proximal to the margin of the web (Figs. 53 & 56).

2. 11. 44 GB 44 Zúqiàoyīn 足竅陰

On the lateral side of the distal segment of the 4th toe, 0.1 *cun* from the corner of the toenail (Figs. 53 & 56).

2. 12 Points of the Liver Meridian of Foot-Jueyin, LR

足厥陰肝經穴

Zújuéyīn Gānjīng Xué

2. 12. 1 LR 1 Dàdūn 大敦

On the lateral side of the distal segment of the great toe, 0.1 *cun* from the corner of the toenail (Fig. 57).

2. 12. 2 LR 2 Xíngjiān 行間

On the instep of the foot, between the 1st and 2nd toes, at the junction of the red and white skin proximal to the margin of the web (Fig. 57).

2. 12. 3 LR 3 Tàichōng 太衝

On the instep of the foot, in the depression of the posterior end of the 1st interosseous metatarsal space (Fig. 57).

2. 12. 4 LR 4 Zhōngfēng 中封

On the instep of the foot, anterior to the medial malleolus, on the line connecting Shangqiu (SP 5) and Jiexi (ST 41), in the depression medial to the tendon of the anterior tibial muscle (Figs. 26 & 57).

2. 12. 5 LR 5 Lígōu 蠡溝

On the medial side of the leg, 5 *cun* above the tip of the medial malleolus, on the midline of the medial surface of the tibia (Figs. 26 & 58).

2. 12. 6 LR 6 Zhōngdū 中都

On the medial side of the leg, 7 *cun* above the tip of the medial malleolus, on the midline of the medial surface of the tibia (Figs. 26 & 58).

2. 12. 7 LR 7 Xīguān 膝關

On the medial side of the leg, posterior and inferior to the medial epicondyle of the tibia, 1 *cun* posterior to Yinlingquan (SP 9), at the upper end of the medial head of the gastrocnemius muscle (Figs. 26 & 58).

2. 12. 8 LR 8 Qūquán 曲泉

On the medial side of the knee, at the medial end of the popliteal crease when the knee is flexed, posterior to the medial epicondyle of the tibia, in the depression of the anterior border of the insertions of the semimembranous and semitendinous muscles (Figs. 26 & 59).

2. 12. 9 LR 9 Yīnbāo 陰包

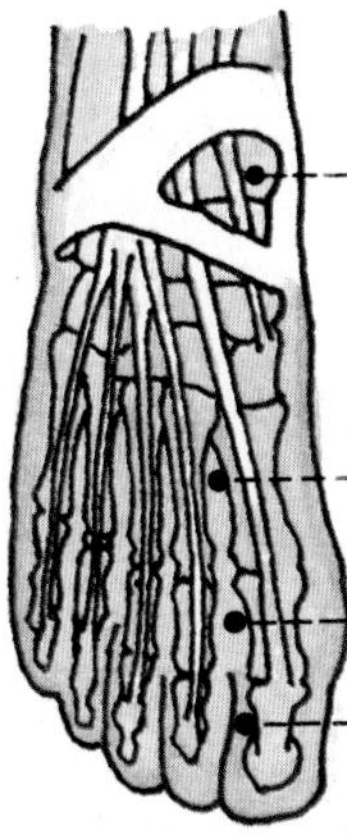

Fig. 57 Points of Liver Meridian (Foot)

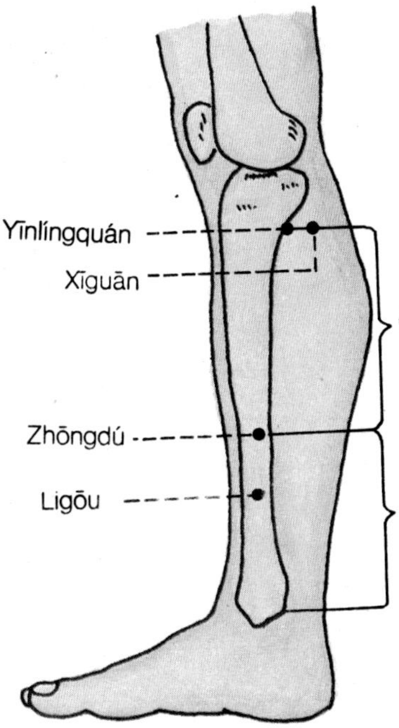

Fig. 58 Points of Liver Meridian (Leg)

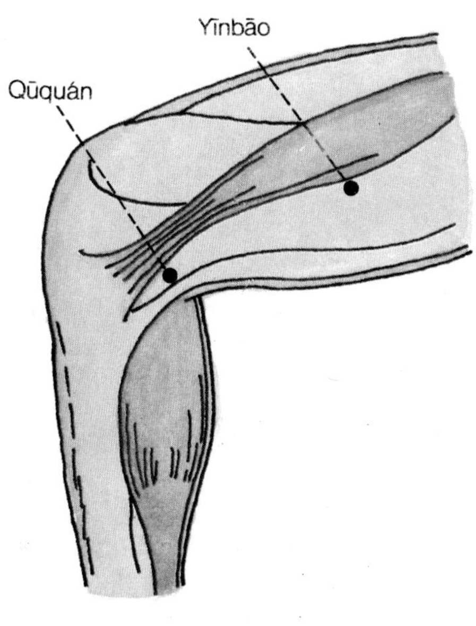

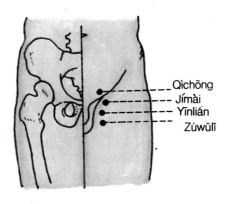

Fig. 59 Qūquán and Yīnbāo Points

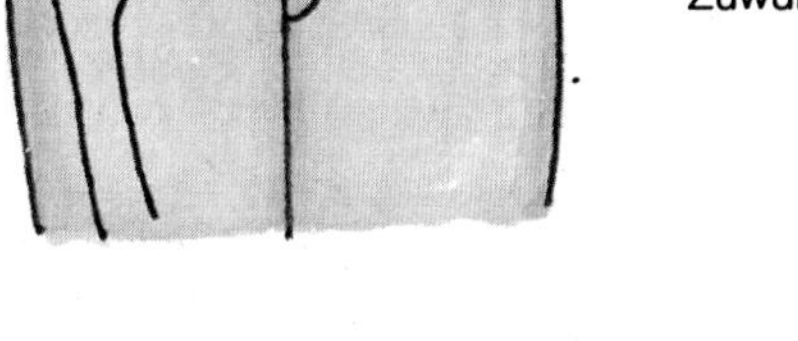

Fig. 60 Zúsānlǐ, Yīnlian and Jímài Points

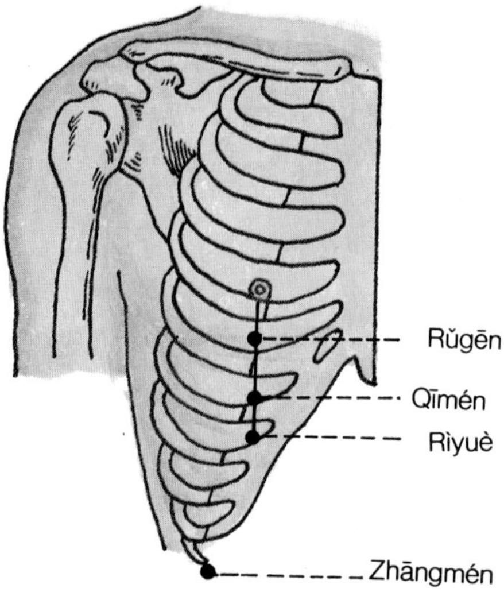

Fig. 61 Zhāngmén and Qīmén Points

On the medial side of the thigh, 4 *cun* above the medial epicondyle of the femur, between the medial vastus muscle and sartorius muscle (Figs. 26 & 59).

2. 12. 10 LR 10 Zúwǔlǐ 足五裏

On the medial side of the thigh, 3 *cun* directly below Qichong (ST 30), at the proximal end of the thigh, below the pubic tubercle and on the lateral border of the long abductor muscle of the thigh (Fig. 60).

2. 12. 11 LR 11 Yīnlían 陰廉

On the medial side of the thigh, 2 *cun* directly below Qichong (ST 30), at the proximal end of the thigh, below the pubic tubercle and on the lateral border of the long abductor muscle of the thigh (Fig. 60).

2. 12. 12 LR 12 Jímài 急脈

Lateral to the pubic tubercle, lateral and inferior to Qichong (ST 30), in the inguinal groove where the pulsation of the femoral artery is palpable, 2.5 *cun* lateral to the anterior midline (Figs. 8 & 60).

2. 12. 13 LR 13 Zhāngmén 章門

On the lateral side of the abdomen, below the free end of the 11th rib (Figs. 8 & 61).

2. 12. 14 LR 14 Qīmén 期門

On the chest, directly below the nipple, in the 6th intercostal space, 4 *cun* lateral to the anterior midline (Figs. 8 & 61).

2. 13 Points of the Du Meridian (Governor Vessel), Du (GV)

督脈穴

Dūmài Xué

2. 13. 1 DU 1 Chángqiáng 長强

Below the tip of the coccyx, at the midpoint of the line connecting the tip of the coccyx and anus (Figs. 62 & 64).

2. 13. 2 DU 2 Yāoshū 腰俞

On the sacrum and on the posterior midline, just at the sacral hiatus (Figs. 63 & 64).

2. 13. 3 DU 3 Yāoyángguān 腰陽關

On the low back and on the posterior midline, in the depression below the spinous process of the 4th lumbar vertebra (Figs. 63 & 64).

2. 13. 4 DU 4 Mìngmén 命門

On the low back and on the posterior midline, in the depression below the spinous process of the 2nd lumbar vertebra (Figs. 63 & 64).

2. 13. 5 DU 5 Xuánshū 懸樞

On the low back and on the posterior midline, in the depression below the spinous process of the 1st lumbar vertebra (Figs. 63 & 64).

2. 13. 6 DU 6 Jĭzhōng 脊中

On the back and on the posterior midline, in the depression below the spinous process of the 11th thoracic vertebra (Figs. 63 & 64).

2. 13. 7 DU 7 Zhōngshū 中樞

On the back and on the posterior midline, in the depression below the spinous process of the 10th thoracic vertebra (Figs. 63 & 64).

2. 13. 8 DU 8 Jīnsuō 筋縮

On the back and on the posterior midline, in the depression below the spinous process of the 9th thoracic vertebra (Figs. 63 & 64).

2. 13. 9 DU 9 Zhìyáng 至陽

On the back and on the posterior midline, in the depression below the spinous process of the 7th thoracic vertebra (Figs. 63 & 64).

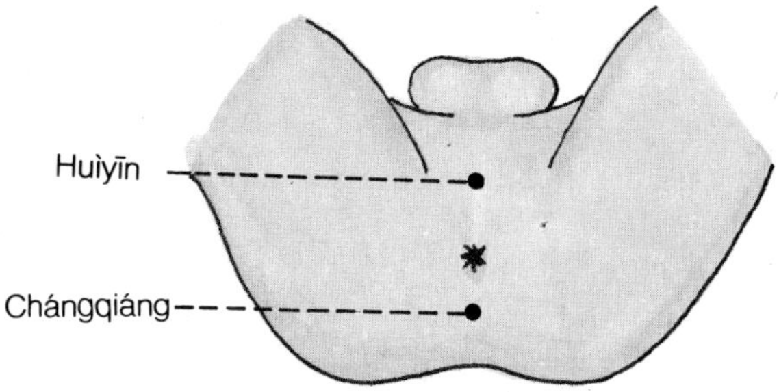

Fig. 62 Chángqiáng and Hùiyīn Points

- Dàzhūi
- Táodào
- Shēnzhù
- Shéndào
- Língtái
- Zhìyáng
- Jīnsuō
- Zhōngshū
- Jǐzhōng
- Xuánshū
- Mìngmén
- Yāoyángguān
- Yāoshū
- Chángqiáng

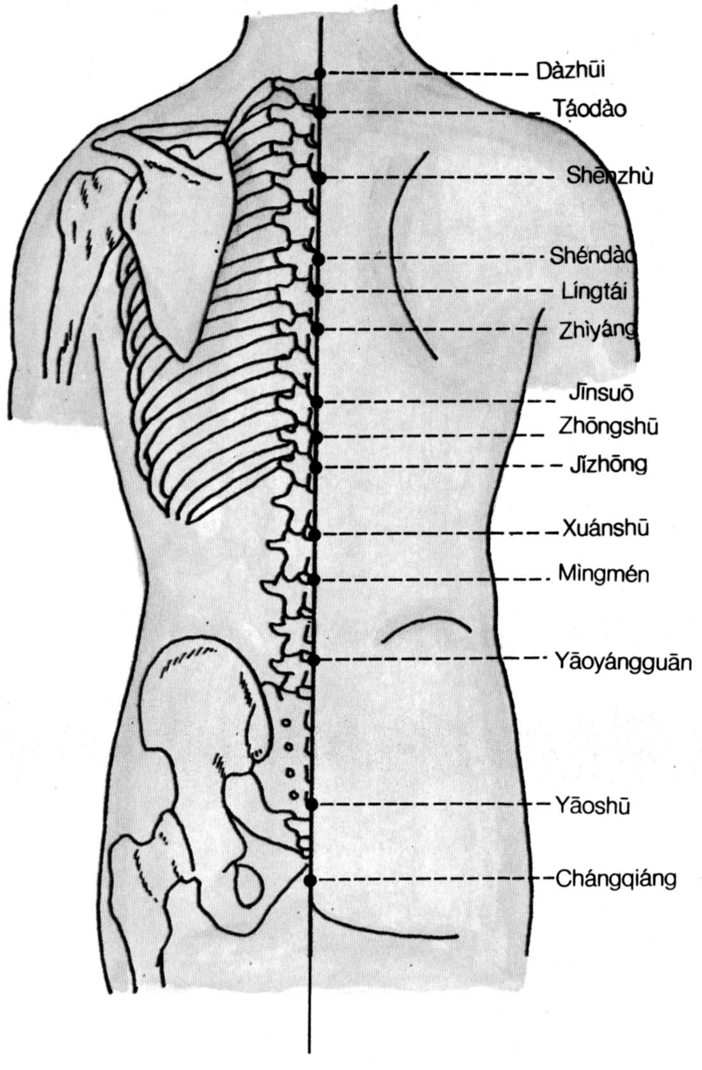

Fig. 63 Points of Du Meridian (Back View)

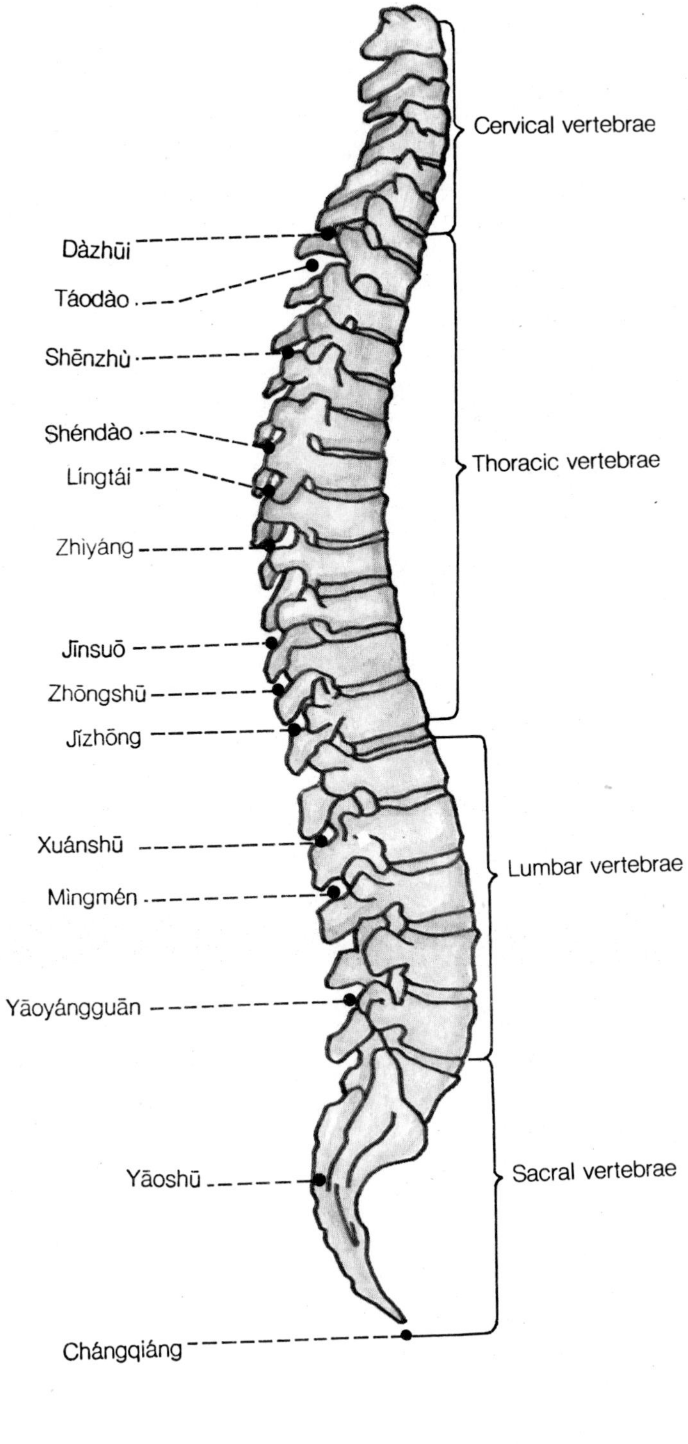

Fig. 64 Points of Du Meridian

2. 13. 10 DU 10 **Língtái** 靈台

On the back and on the posterior midline, in the depression below the spinous process of the 6th thoracic vertebra (Figs. 63 & 64).

2. 13. 11 DU 11 **Shéndào** 神道

On the back and on the posterior midline, in the depression below the spinous process of the 5th thoracic vertebra (Figs. 63 & 64).

2. 13. 12 DU 12 **Shēnzhù** 身柱

On the back and on the posterior midline, in the depression below the spinous process of the 3rd thoracic vertebra (Figs. 63 & 64).

2. 13. 13 DU 13 **Táodào** 陶道

On the back and on the posterior midline, in the depression below the spinous process of the 1st thoracic vertebra (Figs. 63 & 64).

2. 13. 14 DU 14 **Dàzhuī** 大椎

On the posterior midline, in the depression below the 7th cervical vertebra (Figs. 63 & 64).

2. 13. 15 DU 15 **Yǎmén** 啞門

On the nape, 0.5 *cun* directly above the midpoint of the posterior hairline, below the 1st cervical vertebra (Figs. 7 & 9).

2. 13. 16 DU 16 **Fēngfǔ** 風府

On the nape, 1 *cun* directly above the midpoint of the posterior hairline, directly below the external occipital protuberance, in the depression between the trapezius muscle of both sides (Figs. 7 & 9).

2. 13. 17 DU 17 **Nǎohù** 腦户

On the head, 2.5 *cun* directly above the midpoint of the posterior hairline, 1.5 *cun* above Fengfu (DU 16), in the depression on the upper border of the external occipital protuberance (Figs. 7 & 36).

2. 13. 18 DU 18 **Qiángjiān** 强間

On the head, 4 *cun* directly above the midpoint of the posterior hairline and 1.5 *cun* above Naohu (Du 17) (Figs. 7 & 36).

2. 13. 19 DU 19 **Hòudǐng** 後頂

On the head, 5.5 *cun* directly above the midpoint of the posterior hairline and 3 *cun* above Naohu (Du 17) (Figs. 7 & 36).

2. 13. 20 DU 20 **Bǎihuì** 百會

On the head, 5 *cun* directly above the midpoint of the anterior hairline, at the midpoint of the line connecting the apexes of both ears (Fig. 7).

2. 13. 21 DU 21 **Qiándǐng** 前頂

On the head, 3.5 *cun* directly above the midpoint of the anterior hairline and 1.5 *cun* anterior to Baihui (DU 20) (Fig. 7).

2. 13. 22 DU 22 **Xìnhuì** 顖會

On the head, 2 *cun* directly above the midpoint of the anterior hairline and 3 *cun* anterior to Baihui (DU 20) (Fig. 7).

2. 13. 23 DU 23 **Shàngxīng** 上星

On the head, 1 *cun* directly above the midpoint of the anterior hairline (Figs. 7 & 19).

2. 13. 24 DU 24 **Shéntíng** 神庭

On the head, 0.5 *cun* directly above the midpoint of the anterior hairline (Figs. 7 & 19).

2. 13. 25 DU 25 Sùliáo 素髎

On the face, at the centre of the nose apex (Figs. 7 & 8).

2. 13. 26 DU 26 Shuǐgōu 水溝

On the face, at the junction of the upper third and middle third of the philtrum (Figs. 7 & 8).

2. 13. 27 DU 27 Duìduān 兑端

On the face, on the labial tubercle of the upper lip, on the vermilion border between the philtrum and upper lip (Figs. 7 & 19).

2. 13. 28 DU 28 Yínjiāo 齦交

Inside of the upper lip, at the junction of the labial frenum and upper gum (Fig. 65).

2. 14 Points of the Ren Meridian (Conception Vessel), RN (CV)

任脈穴

Rènmài Xué

2. 14. 1 RN 1 Huìyīn 會陰

On the perineum, at the midpoint between the posterior border of the scrotum and anus in male, and between the posterior commissure of the large labia and anus in female (Fig. 62).

2. 14. 2 RN 2 Qūgǔ 曲骨

On the lower abdomen and on the anterior midline, at the midpoint of the upper border of the pubic symphysis (Fig. 8).

2. 14. 3 RN 3 Zhōngjí 中極

On the lower abdomen and on the anterior midline, 4 *cun* below the centre of the umbilicus (Fig. 8).

2. 14. 4 RN 4 Guānyuán 關元

On the lower abdomen and on the anterior midline, 3 *cun* below the centre of the umbilicus (Fig. 8).

2. 14. 5 RN 5 Shímén 石門

On the lower abdomen and on the anterior midline, 2 *cun* below the centre of the umbilicus (Fig. 8).

2. 14. 6 RN 6 Qìhǎi 氣海

On the lower abdomen and on the anterior midline, 1.5 *cun* below the centre of the umbilicus (Fig. 8).

2. 14. 7 RN 7 Yīnjiāo 陰交

On the lower abdomen and on the anterior midline, 1 *cun* below the centre of the umbilicus (Fig. 8).

2. 14. 8 RN 8 Shénquè 神闕

On the middle abdomen and at the centre of the umbilicus (Figs. 8 & 66).

2. 14. 9 RN 9 Shuǐfēn 水分

On the upper abdomen and on the anterior midline, 1 *cun* above the centre of the umbilicus (Figs 8 & 66).

2. 14. 10 RN 10 Xiàwǎn 下脘

On the upper abdomen and on the anterior midline, 2 *cun* above the centre of the umbilicus

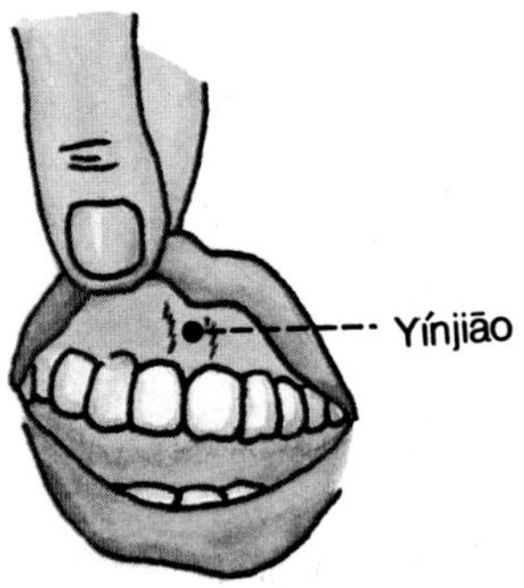

Fig. 65 Yínjiāo Point

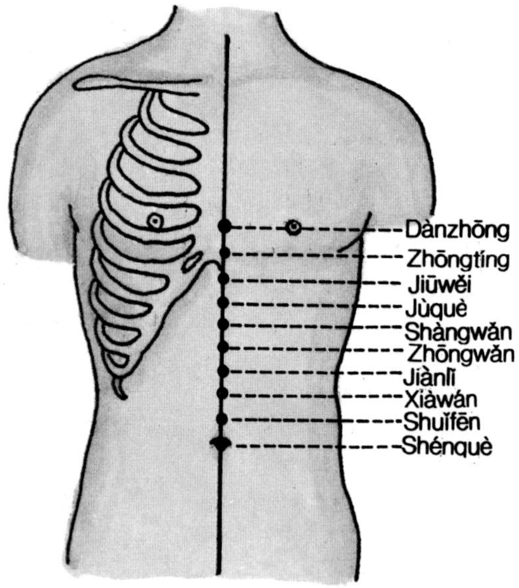

Fig. 66 Point of Ren Meridian (Abdomen)

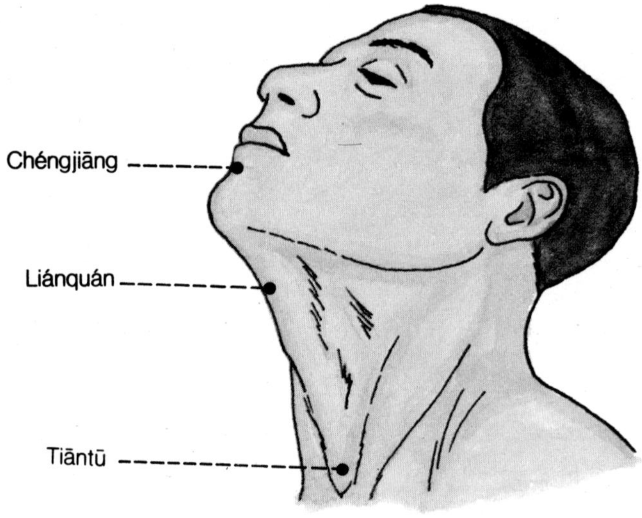

Fig. 67 Tiāntū, Liánquán and Chéngjiāng Points

(Figs 8 & 66).

2. 14. 11 RN 11 Jiànlǐ 建裏

On the upper abdomen and on the anterior midline, 3 *cun* above the centre of the umbilicus (Figs 8 & 66).

2. 14. 12 RN 12 Zhōngwǎn 中脘

On the upper abdomen and on the anterior midline, 4 *cun* above the centre of the umbilicus (Figs 8 & 66).

2. 14. 13 RN 13 Shàngwǎn 上脘

On the upper abdomen and on the anterior midline, 5 *cun* above the centre of the umbilicus (Figs 8 & 66).

2. 14. 14 RN 14 Jùquè 巨闕

On the upper abdomen and on the anterior midline, 6 *cun* above the centre of the umbilicus (Figs 8 & 66).

2. 14. 15 RN 15 Jiūwěi 鳩尾

On the upper abdomen and on the anterior midline, 1 *cun* below the xiphisternal synchondrosis (Figs. 8 & 66).

2. 14. 16 RN 16 Zhōngtíng 中庭

On the chest and on the anterior midline, on the level of the 5th intercostal space, on the xiphosternal synchondrosis (Figs. 8 & 66).

2. 14. 17 RN 17 Dànzhōng 膻中

On the chest and on the anterior midline, on the level of the 4th intercostal space, at the midpoint of the line connecting both nipples (Figs. 8 & 66).

2. 14. 18 RN 18 Yùtáng 玉堂

On the chest and on the anterior midline, on the level of the 3rd intercostal space (Fig. 8).

2. 14. 19 RN 19 Zǐgōng 紫宫

On the chest and on the anterior midline, on the level of the 2nd intercostal space (Fig. 8).

2. 14. 20 RN 20 Huágài 華蓋

On the chest and on the anterior midline, on the level of the 1st intercostal space (Fig. 8).

2. 14. 21 RN 21 Xuànjī 璇璣

On the chest and on the anterior midline, 1 *cun* below Tiantu (RN 22) (Fig. 8).

2. 14. 22 RN 22 Tiāntū 天突

On the neck and on the anterior midline, at the centre of the suprasternal fossa (Figs. 8 & 67).

2. 14. 23 RN 23 Liánquán 廉泉

On the neck and on the anterior midline, above the laryngeal protuberance, in the depression above the upper border of the hyoid bone (Figs. 8 & 67).

2. 14. 24 RN 24 Chéngjiāng 承漿

On the face, in the depression at the midpoint of the mentolabial sulcus (Figs. 8 & 67).

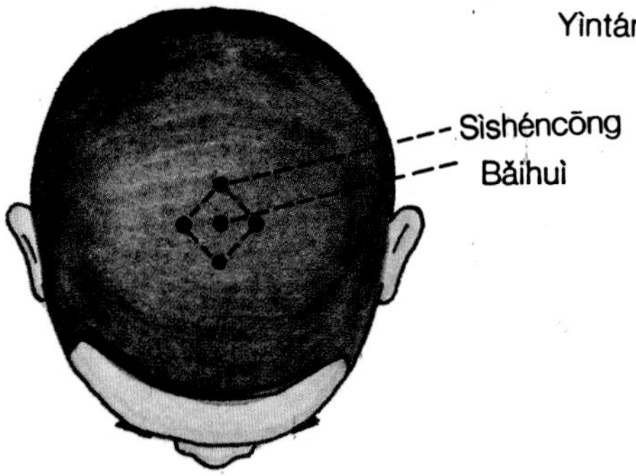

Fig. 68 Sìshéncōng Point

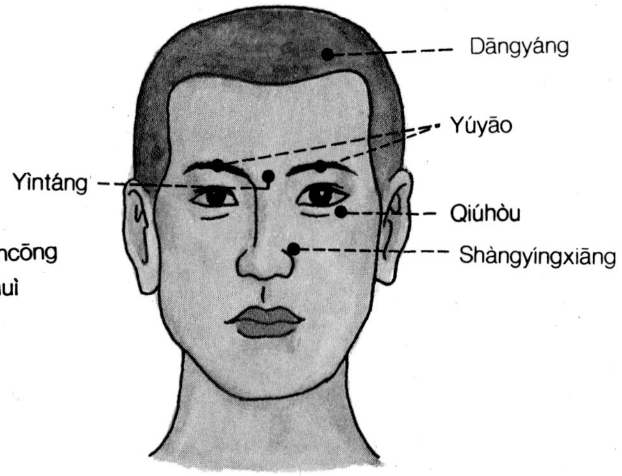

Fig. 69 Extra Points (Head and Face)

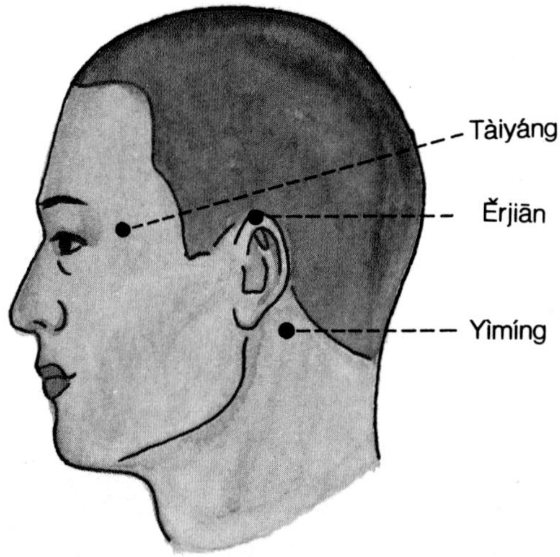

Fig. 70 Tàiyáng, Ěrjiān and Yìmíng Points

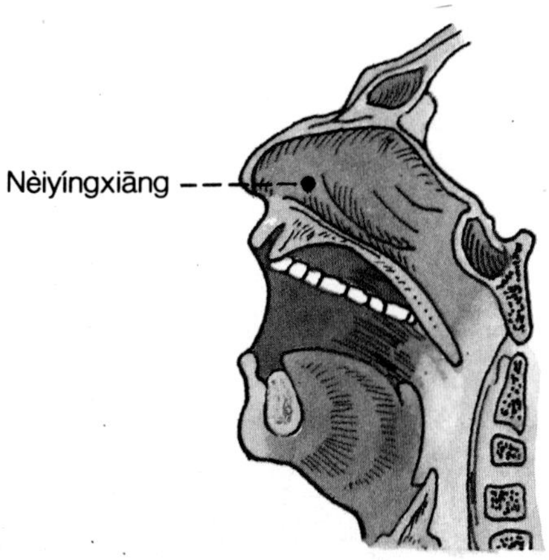

Fig. 71 Nèiyíngxiāng Point

3. Standard Locations of the Extra Points, EX

經外穴

Jīngwài Xué

3. 1 Points of the Head and Neck, EX-HN

頭頸部穴

Tóujǐngbù Xué

3. 1. 1 EX-HN 1 Sìshéncōng 四神聰

Four points on the vertex of the head, 1 *cun* anterior, posterior and lateral to Baihui (DU 20) (Fig. 68).

3. 1. 2 EX-HN 2 Dāngyáng 當陽

At the frontal part of the head, directly above the pupil, 1 *cun* above the anterior hairline (Fig. 69).

3. 1. 3 EX-HN 3 Yìntáng 印堂

On the forehead, at the midpoint between the eyebrows (Fig. 69).

3. 1. 4 EX-HN 4 Yúyāo 魚腰

On the forehead, directly above the pupil, in the eyebrow (Fig. 69).

3. 1. 5 EX-HN 5 Tàiyáng 太陽

At the temporal part of the head, between the lateral end of the eyebrow and the outer canthus, in the depression one finger breadth behind them (Fig. 70).

3. 1. 6 EX-HN 6 Ěrjiān 耳尖

Above the apex of the ear auricle, at the tip of the auricle when the ear is folded forward (Fig. 70).

3. 1. 7 EX-HN 7 Qíuhòu 球後

On the face, at the junction of the lateral fourth and medial three fourths of the infraorbital margin (Fig. 69).

3. 1. 8 EX-HN 8 Shàngyíngxiāng 上迎香

On the face, at the junction of the alar cartilage of the nose and the nasal concha, near the upper end of the nasolabial groove (Fig. 69).

3. 1. 9 EX-HN 9 Nèiyíngxiāng 内迎香

In the nostril, at the junction between the mucosa of the alar cartilage of the nose and the nasal concha (Fig. 71).

3. 1. 10 EX-HN 10 Jùquán 聚泉

In the mouth, at the midpoint of the dorsal midline of the tongue (Fig. 72).

3. 1. 11 EX-HN 11 Hǎiquán 海泉

In the mouth, at the midpoint of the frenulum of the tongue (Fig. 73).

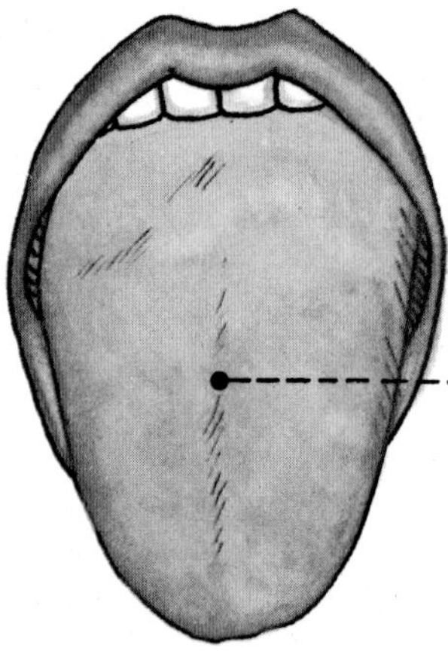

Fig. 72 Jùquán Point

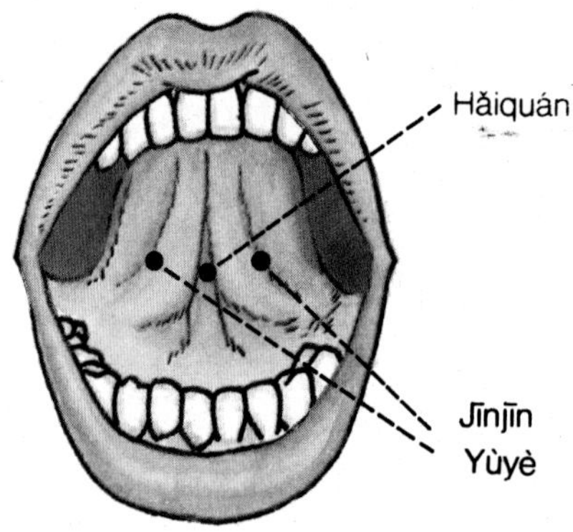

Fig. 73 Hǎiquán, Jīnjīn and Yùyè Points

3. 1. 12 EX-HN 12 Jīnjīn 金津
In the mouth, on the vein in the left side of the frenulum of the tongue (Fig. 73).
3. 1. 13 EX-HN 13 Yùyè 玉液
In the mouth, on the vein in the right side of the frenulum of the tongue (Fig. 73).
3. 1. 14 EX-HN 14 Yìmíng 翳明
On the nape, 1 *cun* posterior to Yifen (SJ 17) (Fig. 70).
3. 1. 15 EX-HN 15 Jǐngbǎiláo 頸百勞
On the nape, 2 *cun* directly above Dazhui (Du 14) and 1 *cun* lateral to the posterior midline (Fig. 74).

3. 2 Points of the Chest and Abdomen, EX-CA
胸腹部穴
Xiōngfùbù Xué

3. 2. 1 EX-CA 1 Zǐgōng 子宫
On the lower abdomen, 4 *cun* below the centre of the umbilicus and 3 *cun* lateral to Zhongji (RN 3) (Fig. 75).

3. 3 Points of the Back, EX-B
背部穴
Bèibù Xué

3. 3. 1 EX-B 1 Dìngchuǎn 定喘
On the back, below the spinous process of the 7th cervical vertebra, 0.5 *cun* lateral to the posterior midline (Fig. 76).

Fig. 74 Extra Points (Back View)

Jǐngbǎiláo

Wèiwǎnxiàshū

Pǐgēn

Xiàjíshū

Yāoyǎn

Shíqīzhuī

Yāoqí

Yāoyí

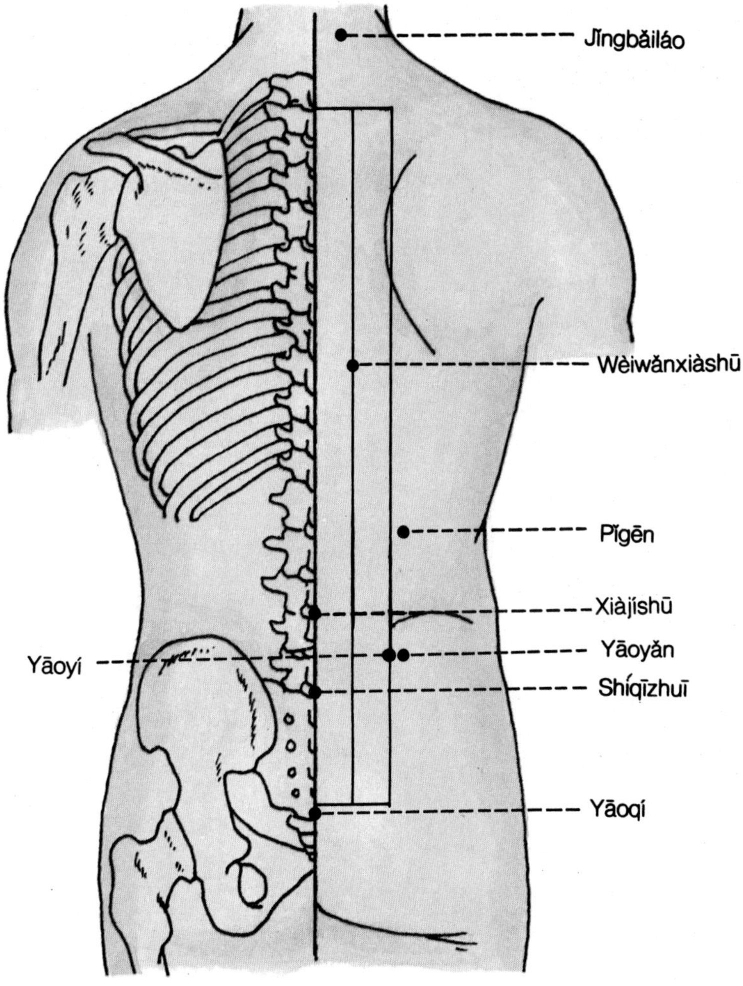

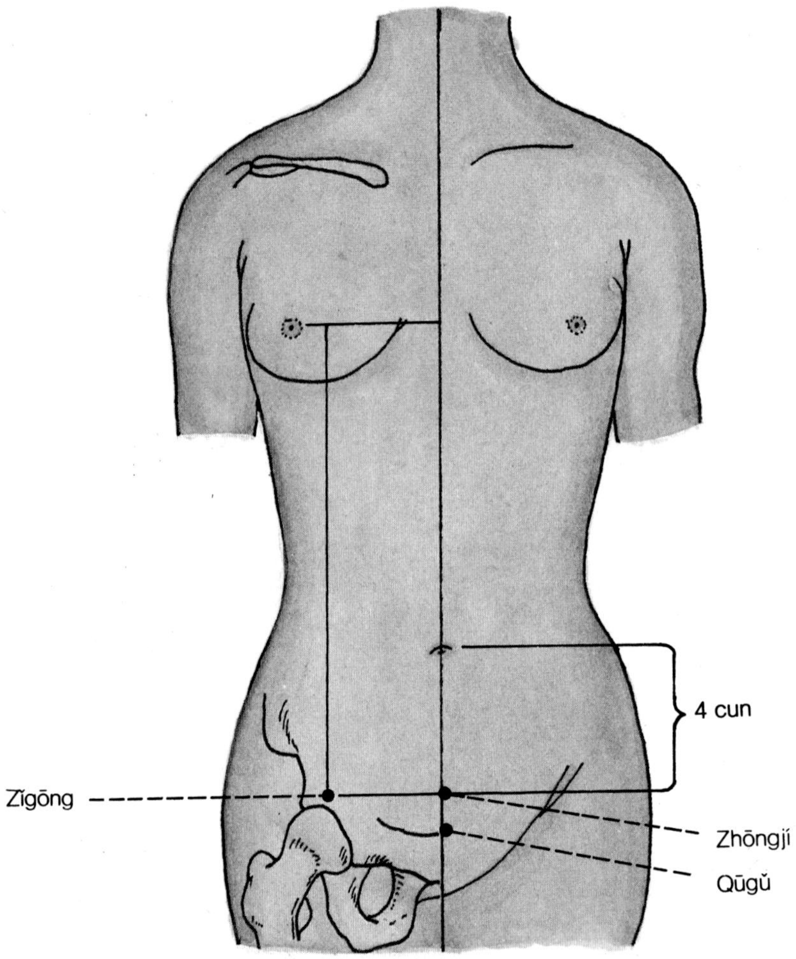

Fig. 75 Zǐgōng Point

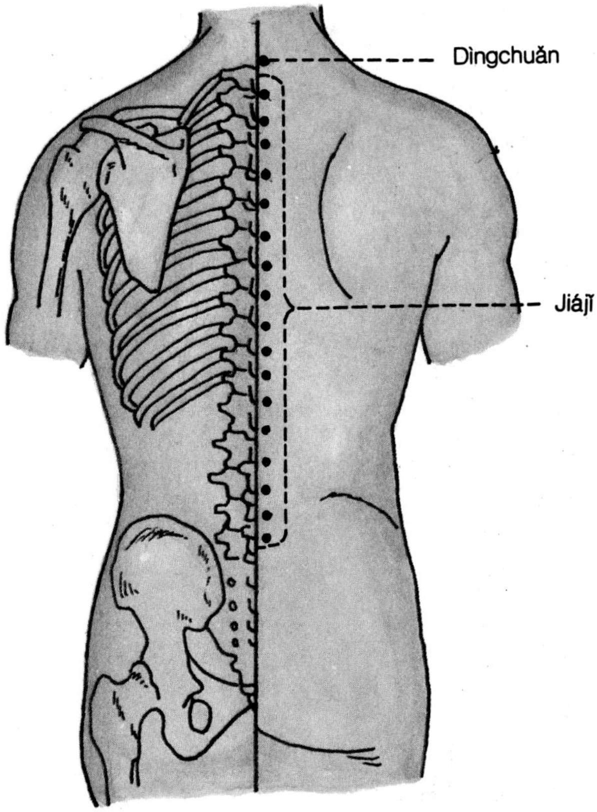

Fig. 76 Dìngchuǎn and Jiájǐ Points

3. 3. 2 EX-B 2 Jiájǐ 夾脊

On the back and low back, 17 points on each side, below the spinous processes from the 1st thoracic to the 5th lumbar vertebrae, 0.5 *cun* lateral to the posterior midline (Fig. 76).

3. 3. 3 EX-B 3 Wèiwǎnxiàshū 胃脘下俞

On the back, below the spinous process of the 8th thoracic vertebra, 1.5 *cun* lateral to the posterior midline (Fig. 74).

3. 3. 4 EX-B 4 Pǐgēn 痞根

On the low back, below the spinous process of the 1st lumbar vertebra, 3.5 *cun* lateral to the posterior midline (Fig. 74).

3. 3. 5 EX-B 5 Xiàjíshū 下極俞

On the midline of the low back, below the spinous process of the third lumbar vertebra.

3. 3. 6 EX-B 6 Yāoyí 腰宜

On the low back, below the spinous process of the 4th lumbar vertebra, 3 *cun* lateral to the posterior midline (Fig. 74).

3. 3. 7 EX-B 7 Yāoyǎn 腰眼

On the low back, below the spinous process of the 4th lumbar vertebra, in the depression 3.5 *cun* lateral to the posterior midline (Fig. 74).

3. 3. 8 EX-B 8 Shíqīzhuī 十七椎

On the low back and on the posterior midline, below the spinous process of the 5th lumbar vertebra (Fig. 74).

3. 3. 9 EX-B 9 Yāoqí 腰奇

On the low back, 2 *cun* directly above the tip of the coccyx, in the depression between the sacral horns (Fig. 74).

3. 4 Points of the Upper Extremities, EX-UE

上肢穴

Shàngzhī Xué

3. 4. 1 EX-UE 1 Zhǒujiān 肘尖

On the posterior side of the elbow, at the tip of the olecranon when the elbow is flexed (Fig. 77).

3. 4. 2 EX-UE 2 Èrbái 二白

Two points on the palmar side of each forearm, 4 *cun* proximal to the crease of the wrist, on each side of the tendon of the radial flexor muscle of the wrist (Fig. 78).

3. 4. 3 EX-UE 3 Zhōngquán 中泉

On the dorsal crease of the wrist, in the depression on the radial side of the tendon of the common extensor muscle of the fingers (Fig. 79).

3. 4. 4 EX-UE 4 Zhōngkuí 中魁

On the dorsal side of the middle finger, at the centre of the proximal interphalangeal joint (Fig. 79).

3. 4. 5 EX-UE 5 Dàgǔkōng 大骨空

On the dorsal side of the thumb, at the centre of the interphalangeal joint (Fig. 79).

3. 4. 6 EX-UE 6 Xiǎogǔkōng 小骨空

Zhǒujiān

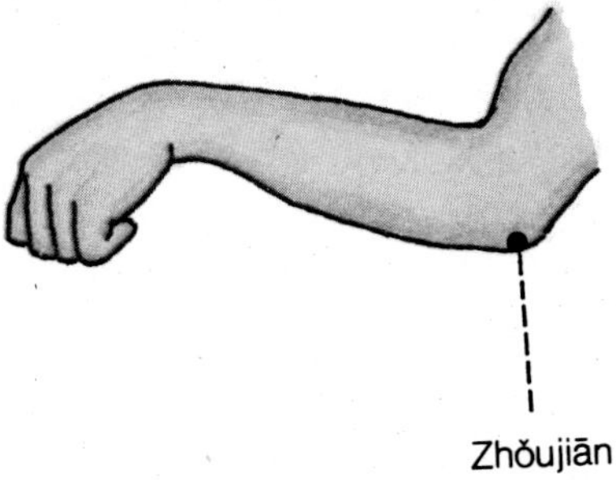

Fig. 77 Zhǒujiān Point

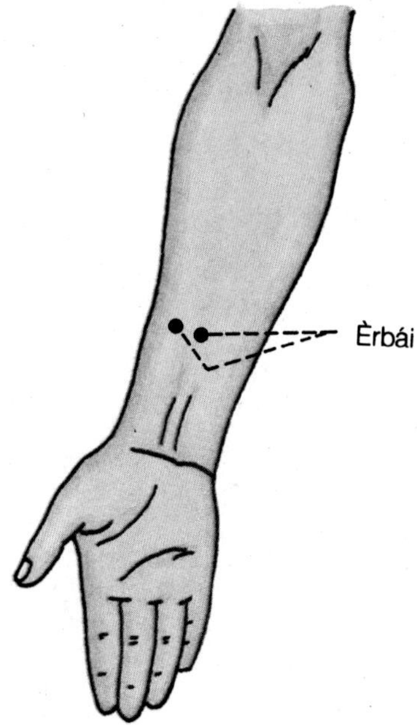

Èrbái

Fig. 78 Erbái Point

Zhōngkuí

Xiǎogǔkōng

Bāxié

Dàgǔkōng

Zhōngquán

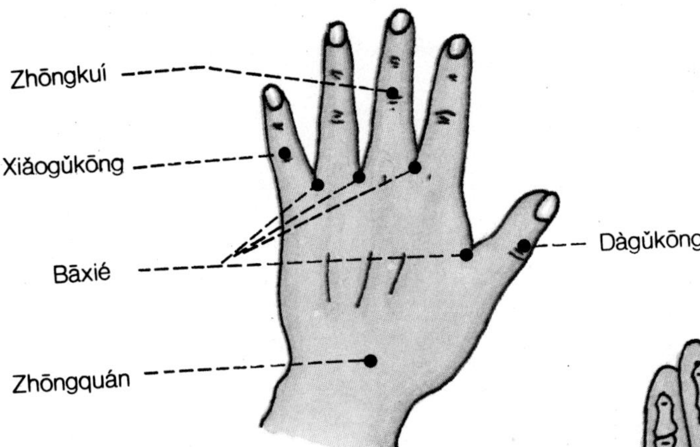

Fig. 79 Extra Points (Dorsum of the Hand)

Wàiláogōng

Yāotòngdiǎn

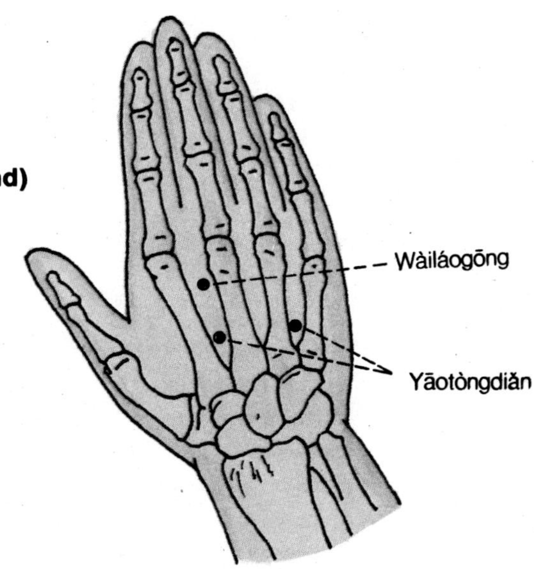

Fig. 80 Yāotòngdiǎn and Wàiláogōng Points

On the dorsal side of the little finger, at the centre of the proximal interphalangeal joint (Fig. 79).

3. 4. 7 EX-UE 7 Yāotòngdiǎn 腰痛點

Two points on the dorsum of each hand, between the 1st and 2nd and between the 3rd and 4th metacarpal bones, and at the midpoint between the dorsal crease of the wrist and the metacarpophalangeal joint (Fig. 80).

3. 4. 8 EX-UE 8 Wàiláogōng 外勞宮

On the dorsum of the hand, between the 2nd and 3rd metacarpal bones, and 0.5 *cun* proximal to the metacarpophalangeal joint (Fig. 80).

3. 4. 9 EX-UE 9 Bāxié 八邪

Four points on the dorsum of each hand, at the junction of the red and white skin proximal to the margin of the webs between each two of the five fingers of a hand (Fig. 79).

3. 4. 10 EX-UE 10 Sìfèng 四縫

Four points on each hand, on the palmar side of the 2nd to 5th fingers and at the centre of the proximal interphalangeal joints (Fig. 81).

3. 4. 11 EX-UE 11 Shíxuān 十宣

Ten points on both hands, at the tips of the 10 fingers, 0.1 *cun* from the free margin of the nails (Fig. 81).

3. 5 Points of the Lower Extremities, EX-LE

下肢穴

Xiàzhī Xué

3. 5. 1 EX-LE 1 Kuāngǔ 髖骨

Two points on each thigh, in the lower part of the anterior surface of the thigh, 1.5 *cun* lateral and medial to Liangqiu (ST 34) (Fig. 82).

3. 5. 2 EX-LE 2 Hèdǐng 鹤頂

Above the knee, in the depression of the midpoint of the upper border of the patella (Fig. 82).

3. 5. 3 EX-LE 3 Bǎichóngwō 百蟲窩

3 *cun* above the medial superior corner of the petella of the thigh with the knee flexed, i.e. 1 *cun* above Xuehai (SP 10).

3. 5. 4 EX-LE 4 Nèixīyǎn 内膝眼

In the depression medial to the patellar ligament when the knee is flexed (Figs. 82 & 83).

3. 5. 5 EX-LE 5 Xīyǎn 膝眼

In the depression on both sides of the patellar ligament when the knee is flexed. The medial and lateral points are named "Neixiyan" and "Waixiyan" respectively (Fig. 82).

3. 5. 6 EX-LE 6 Dǎnnáng 膽囊

At the upper part of the lateral surface of the leg, 2 *cun* directly below the depression anterior and inferior to the head of the fibula [Yanglingquan (GB 34)] (Fig. 84).

3. 5. 7 EX-LE 7 Lánwěi 闌尾

At the upper part of the anterior surface of the leg, 5 *cun* below Dubi (ST 35), one finger breadth lateral to the anterior crest of the tibia (Fig. 82).

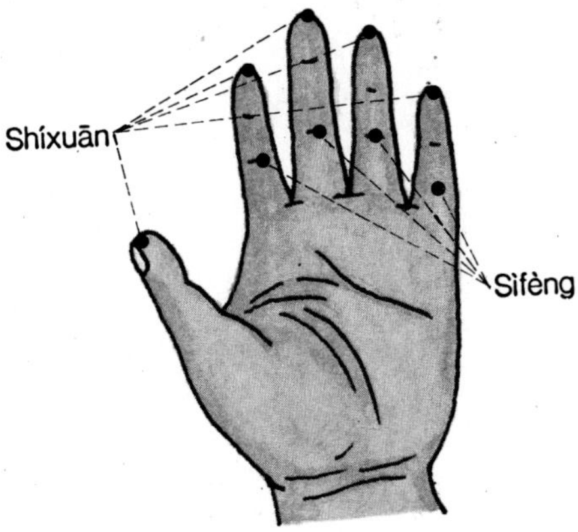

Fig. 81 Sìfèng and Shíxuān Points

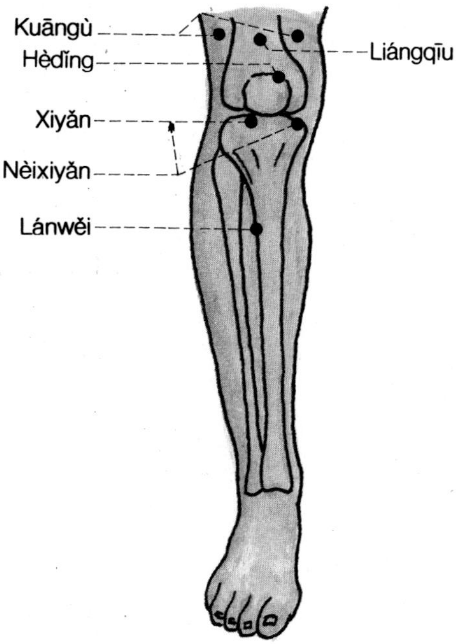

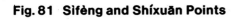

Fig. 82 Kuāngǔ, Hèdǐng, Xīyǎn and Lánwěi Points

3. 5. 8 EX-LE 8 Nèihuáijiān 内踝尖

On the medial side of the foot, at the tip of the medial malleolus (Fig. 83).

3. 5. 9 EX-LE 9 Wàihuáijiān 外踝尖

On the lateral side of the foot, at the tip of the lateral malleolus (Fig. 84).

3. 5. 10 EX-LE 10 Bāfēng 八風

Eight points on the instep of both feet, at the junction of the red and white skin proximal to the margin of the webs between each two neighbouring toes (Fig. 85).

3. 5. 11 EX-LE 11 Dúyīn 獨陰

On the plantar side of the 2nd toe, at the centre of the distal interphalangeal joint (Fig. 86).

3. 5. 12 EX-LE 12 Qìduān 氣端

Ten points at the tips of the 10 toes of both feet, 0.1 *cun* from the free margin of each toenail (Fig. 85).

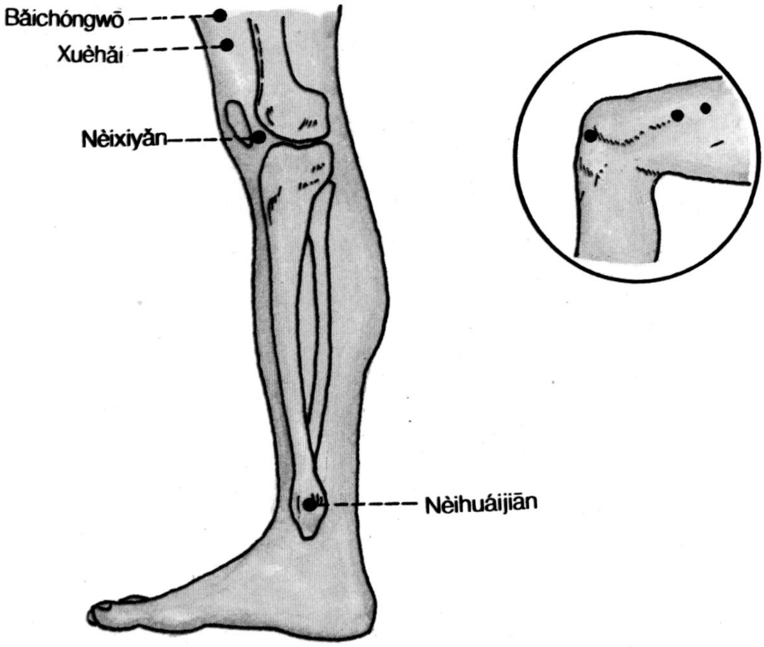

Fig. 83 Xīnèi, Nèixīyǎn and Nèihuáijiān Points

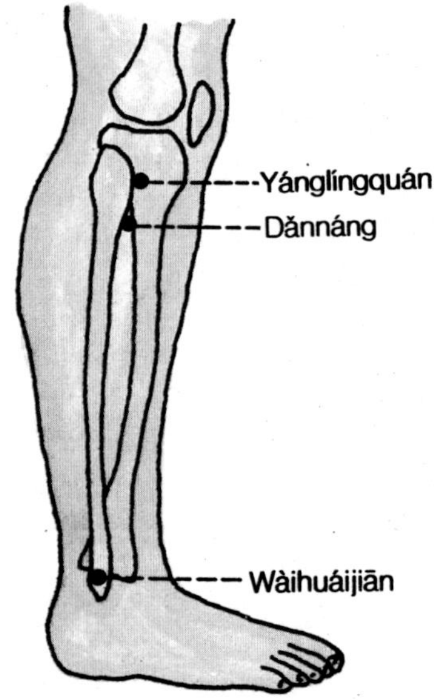

Fig. 84 Dǎnnáng and Wàihuáijiān Points

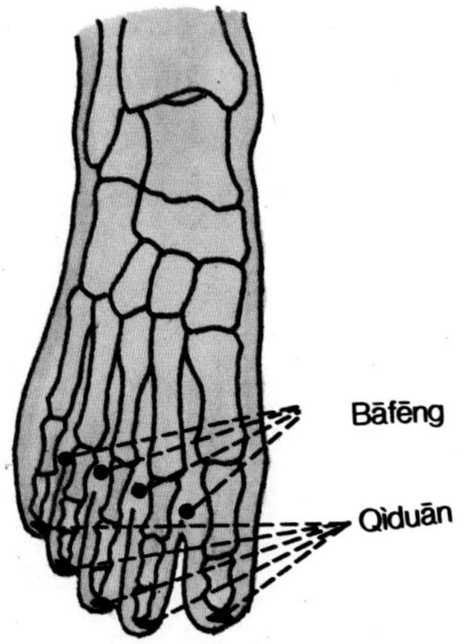

Fig. 85 Bāfēng and Qìduān Points

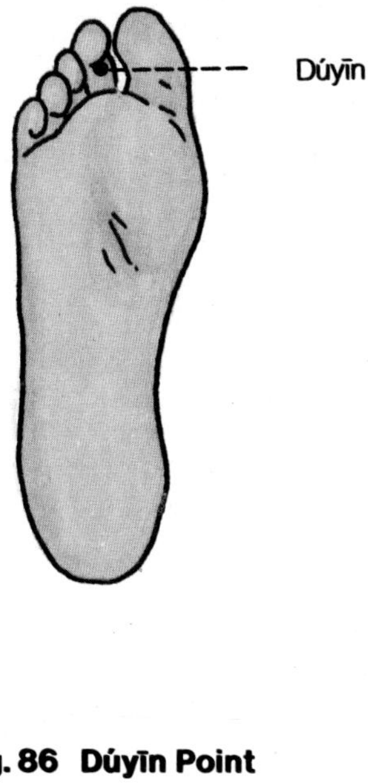

Fig. 86 Dúyīn Point

PART TWO

1. Introduction

As the basis for the location of the points, the following medical books have been consulted. They are *Miraculous Pivot* (*Ling Shu*), *Plain Questions* (*Su Wen*, annotated by Wang Bing), *The Classic of Questions* (*Nan Jing*), *The Classic of Sphygmology* (*Mai Jing*), *A-B Classic of Acupuncture and Moxibustion* (*Zhen Jiu Jia Yi Jing*), *A Handbook of Prescriptions for Emergencies* (*Zhou Hou Bei Ji Fang*), *Essential Treasured Prescriptions for Emergencies* (*Qian Jin Yao Fang*), *Supplement to Essential Treasured Prescriptions* (*Yi Fang*), *Clandestine Essentials from the Imperial Library* (*Wai Tai Mi Yao*), *Imperial Benevolent Prescriptions* (*Tai Ping Sheng Hui Fang*), *Illustrated Manual of Points for Acupuncture and Moxibustion on a Bronze Statue with Acupoints* (*Tong Ren Shu Xue Zhen Jiu Tu Jing*), *Acupuncture-Moxibustion Classic for Saving Life* (*Zhen Jiu Zi Sheng Jing*), *Bianque's Jade Dragon Classics of Acupuncture and Moxibustion* (*Zhen Jiu Yu Long Jing*), *An Elaboration of the Fourteen Meridians* (*Shi Si Jing Fa Hui*), *Classic of God Merit* (*Sheng Ying Jing*), *Essentials of Acupuncture and Moxibustion* (*Zhen Jiu Ju Ying*), *A Great Compendium of Acupuncture and Moxibustion* (*Zhen Jiu Da Cheng*), *Six Collections of Acupuncture Prescriptions* (*Zhen Fang Liu Ji*), *Studies on Acupoints Along Meridians* (*Xun Jing Kao Xue Bian*), *Gold Mirror of Orthodox Medical Lineage* (*Yi Zong Jin Jian*), *The Origin of Acupuncture and Moxibustion* (*Zhen Jiu Feng Yuan*), etc. In some books the locations of points are described in detail, but in other books simply, and changes have been made in later ages. Therefore, it is necessary to make a comprehensive analysis and to locate points in accordance with clinical experience. The present book, in which quotations from those renowned medical literature are listed with the analysis of different views and collations, attempts to provide a correct basis for point location.

2. Records on Methods of the Location of Points

Anatomical Landmarks

"When the muscles, depressions of joints and other clefts are pressed by hand, patients feel better." (*Qian Jin*,* Chapter 29)

Note: *Jia Yi* often describes points lying in the "depressions" or the "clefts" formed between muscles, bones and joints. For example, Hegu (LI 4) is in the depression between the 1st and 2nd metacarpal bones and Neiguan (PC 6) between the "two tendons."

Bone-Proportional Measurement

1. Longitudinal Measurement of the Head

1) "It is 12 *cun* from the anterior hairline to the posterior hairline." (*Ling Shu*)

2) "The distance from the midpoint between the eyebrows to the anterior hairline is 3 *cun*; the distance between Dazhui (DU 14) and the posterior hairline is also 3 *cun*." (*Sheng Hui*)

Note: This is the evidence for the distance of 12 *cun* from the anterior hairline to the posterior hairline shown in the medical classics. If the anterior hairline is not present, 3 *cun* is added from the midpoint between the eyebrows. In case the posterior hairline is not present, 3 *cun* is added from the spinous process of the 7th cervical vertebra (Dazhui DU 14). This is the way to locate points on the head and nape.

2. Transverse Measurement of the Head

1) "The distance between the two mastoid processes is 9 *cun*." (*Ling Shu*)

2) "Shenting (DU 24) is on the anterior hairline, directly above the nose; Qucha (BL 4) is 1.5 *cun* lateral to Shenting (DU 24); Benshen (GB 13) is on the hairline of the forehead, 1.5 *cun* lateral to Qucha (BL 4). Touwei (ST 8) is on the anterior hairline and at the corner of the forehead, 1.5 *cun* lateral to Benshen (GB 13)." (*Jia Yi*)

Note: The distance between the two mastoid processes is 9 *cun*, corresponding to the distance between bilateral Touwei (ST 8); the distance between Shenting (DU 24), Qucha (BL 4), Benshen (GB 13) and Touwei (ST 8) is 1.5 *cun* respectively, making 4.5 *cun* in all, or 9 *cun* bilaterally. This is the way for the transverse measurement of the points on the head.

3. Longitudinal Measurement of the Chest

1) "The distance is 9 *cun* from the supraclavicular fossa to the sternocostal angle." (*Ling Shu*)

2) Xuanji (RN 21) is 1 *cun* below Tiantu (RN 22); Huagai (RN 20) is 1 *cun* below Xuanji (RN 21); Zigong (RN 19), Yutang (RN 18), Danzhong (RN 17) and Zhongting (RN 16) are

*The titles of the medical books here and elsewhere are abbreviated. For their full titles please see "Bibliography" in this book.

1.6 *cun* from each other respectively." (*Jia Yi*)

Note: *Ling Shu* defines the distance as 9 *cun* from Tiantu (RN 22), which is at the midpoint between bilateral supraclavicular fossa, to the sternocostal angle." *Jia Yi* defines it as 8.4 *cun* from Tiantu (RN 22) to Zhongting (RN 16). *Da Cheng* changes the distance between Xuanji (RN 21) and Huagai (RN 20) from 1 *cun* to 1.6 *cun*, then the distance results in 9 *cun*. The xiphoid process was named "Bigu" in ancient times. Because of the individual variation, it is difficult to take the xiphoid process as a landmark for point location. Therefore, the xiphosternal synchondrosis may serve as a landmark (named "Qigu" by the ancients).

4. Longitudinal Measurement of the Upper Abdomen

1) "The distance between the sternocostal angle and Tianshu (ST 25) is 8 *cun*." (*Ling Shu*)

2) "Jiuwei (RN 15) is 0.5 *cun* below the xiphoid process; Juque (RN 14) is 1 *cun* below Jiuwei (RN 15); Shangwan (RN 13) is 1.5 *cun* below Juque (RN 14); Zhongwang (RN 12), Jianli (RN 11), Xiawan (RN 10), Shuifen (RN 9) and the umbilicus are 1 *cun* from each other respectively."

Note: *Ling Shu* says Tianshu (ST 25) is on the level of the umbilicus. *Jia Yi* points out the summary of the distances between those points from the xiphoid process to the centre of the umbilicus is equal to 8 *cun*. Now Juque (RN 14) is located 6 *cun* above the umbilicus and Jiuwei (RN 15) 7 *cun* above the umbilicus, 1 *cun* below the sternocostal angle. It is stated in *Zi Sheng Jing* that "If the xiphoid process is absent, the measurement should be taken from the sternocostal angle, by adding 1 *cun*." This is the way to locate points on the upper abdomen.

5. Longitudinal Measurement of the Lower Abdomen

1) "It is 6.5 *cun* from Tianshu (ST 25) to the upper border of the pubic symphysis." (*Ling Shu*)

2) "Zhongji (RN 3) is 4 *cun* below the umbilicus; Qugu (RN 2) is on the upper border of the pubic symphysis, 1 *cun* below Zhongji (RN 3) and in the depression above the pubic hair." (*Jia Yi*)

Note: *Ling Shu* determines the distance between the centre of the umbilicus and the upper border of the pubic symphysis as 6.5 *cun*. But *Jia Yi* says it is 5 *cun*. In the later ages all follow the definition in *Jia Yi*.

6. Transverse Measurement of the Chest and Abdomen

1) "It is 9.5 *cun* between the nipples." (*Ling Shu*)

2) "On the chest, the line connecting Shufu (KI 27) and Bulang (KI 22) is 2 *cun* from the Ren Meridian; the line connecting Qihu (ST 13) and Rugen (ST 18) is 2 *cun* from Shufu (KI 27); and the line connecting Yunmen (LU 2) and Shidou (SP 17) is 2 *cun* from Qihu (ST 13)." (*Jia Yi*)

3) "8 *cun* between the nipples is used for the transverse measurement of the abdomen." (*Sheng Ying*)

Note: *Ling Shu* says the distance between the nipples is 9.5 *cun*, but *Jia Yi* treats it as 8 *cun*, because Shufu (KI 27) is 2 *cun* lateral to the Ren Meridian and Qihu (ST 13), which is directly above Ruzhong (ST 17) and Rugen (ST 18), is 2 *cun* lateral to Shufu (KI 27), so it is 8 *cun* bilaterally in all. *Da Cheng* takes the transverse measurement of the chest and abdomen as 8 *cun*. The distance between the nipples is 8 *cun*, same as that between Qihu (ST 13) bilaterally, to which 2 *cun* lateral is Yunmen (LU 2). It is 12 *cun* between bilateral Yunmen (LU 2), and used as the criterion for locating points on the chest. It is 8 *cun* between two Quepen (ST 12) or the two nipples, and used as the criterion for point location on the abdomen.

7. Longitudinal Measurement of the Hypochondrium

"It is 12 *cun* from the end of the axillary fold to the free tip of the 11th rib." (*Ling Shu*)

Note: It is used for point location on the hypochondrium.

8. Transverse Measurement of the Back

1) "On the back from the 2nd to 21st vertebrae, the distance between Jiaji and the spinous process is 3 *cun*." (*Jia Yi*)

2) "It is 17 *cun* from the shoulder to the elbow." (*Ling Shu*)

3) "Jianzhen (SI 9) is inferior to the shoulder joint, about 8 *cun* lateral to the spinous process, directly above the posterior end of the axillary fold." (*Ji Cheng*)

Note: *Ling Shu* says the length of the human body is 75 *cun*. When the arms are horizontally abducted, the length is also 75 *cun*. It is 17 *cun* from the shoulder, namely Dazhui (DU 14), to the elbow; 12.5 *cun* from the elbow to the wrist; 4 *cun* from the wrist to the metacarpophalangeal joint to the middle finger, another 4.5 *cun* to its tip. Bilaterally, the distance in all is 76 *cun*. (If the forearm is 12 *cun*, it should be 75 *cun* altogether.)

Practically, it is 17 *cun* from the spinous process on the level of Dazhui (DU 14) to the elbow, the distance between Dazhui (DU 14) and the acromion is 8 *cun*, and 9 *cun* from the shoulder (axilla) to the elbow. The measurement in *Ji Cheng* is in accordance with it.

Jianjing (GB 21) is midway between Dazhui (DU 14) and the acromion, anteriorly facing Quepen (ST 12) and Ruzhong (ST 17) and posteriorly facing Tianliao (SJ 15) and Quyuan (SI 13). It is exactly 4 *cun* lateral to the midline of the back.

The medial border of the scapula is just 3 *cun* lateral to the midline of the back, so half of it is 1.5 *cun*.

9. Longitudinal Measurement of the Upper Extremities

1) "It is 17 *cun* from the shoulder to the elbow." (*Ling Shu*)

2) "Tianfu (LU 3) is 3 *cun* below the end of the axillary fold; Xiabai (LU 4) is 1 *cun* below Tianfu (LU 3) and 5 *cun* from the elbow." (*Xun Jing*)

3) "It is 12.5 *cun* from the elbow to the wrist." (*Ling Shu*)

Note: As mentioned above it is 17 *cun* from the shoulder to the elbow, hence the distance from the spinous process on the level of Dazhui(DU 14) to the acromion is 8 *cun* and from the acromion to the elbow is 9 *cun*. *Ling Shu* suggests to locate points with arms horizontally abducted, but in clinical practice the arm is usually adducted, therefore the end of the axillary fold is used as a landmark. *Xun Jing* says it is 9 *cun*, in accordance with the bone proportional measurement.

It is said the distance from the elbow to the wrist is 12.5 *cun*, but for clinical practice it is 12 *cun*. The total length is in conformity with the total length of the human body—75 *cun*.

10. Longitudinal Measurement of the Lower Extremities

1) "It is 18 *cun* from the upper border of the pubic symphysis to the upper border of the medial epicondyle of the femur"; and "it is 13 *cun* from the lower border of the medial condyle of the tibia to the tip of the medial malleolus." (*Ling Shu*)

2) "It is 19 *cun* from the prominence of the great trochanter to the centre of the patella; and "it is 16 *cun* from the knee to the lateral malleolus." (*Ling Shu*)

Note: According to *Ling Shu*, it is 18 *cun* from the upper border of the pubic symphysis to the medial epicondyle of the femur, which is used as the criterion for point location on the medial side of the thigh; it is 13 *cun* between the lower border of the medial condyle of the tibia and the tip of the medial malleolus, which is used as the criterion for point location on the medial side of the leg.

It is 19 *cun* from the prominence of the great trochanter to the centre of the patella (Dubi ST 35, Weizhong BL 40); and 16 *cun* from the knee to the tip of the lateral malleolus, which is used as the criterion for point location on the three yang meridians of the lower extremities.

Finger Measurement

1. "When the four fingers (index, middle, ring and little fingers) of the patient are kept close together, their width is called 1 *fu*." (*Zhou Hou*)

2. "The length of the first segment of the middle finger is taken as 1 *cun*. The width of the interphalangeal joint of the thumb is also taken as 1 *cun*. When the index, middle, ring and little fingers are extended and kept close together, their width on the level of the proximal interphalangeal joint of the middle finger is 1 *fu*." (*Qian Jin*)

3. "The distance between the two medial ends of the interphalangeal joint creases is taken as 1 *cun* when the patient's middle finger (the left hand of males and the right hand of females) is flexed."

Note: There are three methods of finger measurement mentioned in *Qian Jin*:

1) The last segment of the middle finger is 1 *cun*;

2) The width of the last segment of the thumb is 1 *cun*;

3) The width of the index, middle, ring and little fingers, when they are kept close together, is 1 *fu* and equals to 3 *cun*. In ancient times the width of the four fingers was considered as 4 *cun*. *Sheng Hui* points out that the distance between the two medial ends of the creases of the interphalangeal joints of the middle finger is 1 *cun*, known as "middle finger *cun* for the whole body."

2. 1 Points of the Lung Meridian of Hand-Taiyin, LU

手太陰肺經穴

Shǒutàiyīn Fèijīng Xué

2. 1. 1 LU 1 Zhōngfǔ 中府

Name: Seen in *Mai Jing*; named as "Yingzhongshu" in *Shu Wen* (as a substitute name of Zhongfu in *Jia Yi*).

Location:

1) "1 *cun* below Yunmen (LU 2), in the depression 3 intercostal spaces above the nipple, where the pulsation is palpable." (*Jia Yi*, etc.)

2) "In the depression 2 intercostal spaces above the nipple." (*Qian Jin*, etc.)

3) "1.6 *cun* below Yunmen (LU 2), 3 intercostal spaces above the nipple, where the pulsation is palpable." (*Sheng Hui*, etc.)

Note: Yunmen (LU 2) is located at the infraclavicular fossa. 1 or 1.6 *cun* indicates the width of the intercostal space. On the upper part of the chest, the space between the ribs is narrower and equals to 1 *cun*. The nipple is at the 4th intercostal space and "3 intercostal spaces above the nipple" suggests the 1st intercostal space. The location defined at the 2nd intercostal space in *Qian Jin* is not correct. Therefore, the location of the point should be based on *Jia Yi*.

2. 1. 2 LU 2 Yúnmén 雲門

Name: Seen in *Su Wen*.

Location:

"Below the large bone (clavicle), in the depression 2 *cun* lateral to Qihu (ST 13), where the pulsation is palpable. It can be located with the arm raised."

Note: Medical literature through the ages holds the same view on the location of this point. Qihu (ST 13) is 2 *cun* lateral to Shufu (KI 27), which is 2 *cun* lateral to Xuanji (RN 21). Yunmen (LU 2) now is 6 *cun* lateral to the anterior midline. The point is situated in the depression in the infraclavicular fossa and between the greater pectoral and deltoid muscles. It can be accurately located when the arm is raised forward to the level of the shoulder.

2. 1. 3 LU 3 Tiānfǔ 天府

Name: Seen in *Ling Shu* and *Su Wen*.

Location:

1) "On the medial side of the upper arm, 3 *cun* below the end of the axillary fold, where the pulsation is palpable. (*Jia Yi*, etc.)

2) "3 *cun* below the end of the axillary fold, where the pulsation is palpable. It can be located with the tip of the nose touching the arm." (*Tong Ren*, etc.)

3) "3 *cun* below the end of the axillary fold, 5 *cun* above the cubital crease, where the pulsation is palpable. It can be located with the tip of the nose touching the arm." (*Da Cheng*, etc.)

Note: It is stated in *Ji Cheng* that the point "is located on the medial side of the upper arm, directly above Chize (LU 5)." Because the Lung Meridian runs along the medial aspect of the arm, the point is located at the radial side of the biceps muscle of the arm, 3 *cun* below the anterior end of the axillary fold. But, according to *Da Cheng* and other classics, "It is 3 *cun* below the end of the axillary fold and 5 *cun* above th cubital crease." If so, the distance from the end of the axillary fold to the cubital crease is only 8 *cun*, not in keeping with the rule of 9 *cun*. "To locate the point with the tip of the nose touching the arm" is only one of the ways to know where it is, and it cannot be taken as the basis for locating the point.

2. 1. 4 LU 4 Xiábái 俠白

Name: Seen in *Jia Yi*.

Location:

1) "Below Tianfu (LU 3), 5 *cun* from the cubital crease, where the pulsation is palpable." (*Jia Yi*, etc.)

2) "1 *cun* below Tianfu (LU 3), 5 *cun* from the cubital crease, a little away from where the pulsation is palpable." (*Xun Jing*, etc.)

Note: *Jia Yi* only indicates that the point is located 5 *cun* above the cubital crease; but according to *Xun Jing* it is located 1 *cun* farther below Tianfu (LU 3), i. e. on the radial side of the biceps muscle of the arm, 4 *cun* below the anterior end of the axillary fold. 4 and 5 *cun* makes 9 *cun*, which is in conformity with the distance from the end of the axillary fold to the cubital crease.

2. 1. 5 LU 5 Chǐzé 尺澤

Name: Seen in *Ling Shu*.

Location:

1) "In the cubital crease, near the artery." (*Jia Yi*, etc.)

2) "In the cubital crease, in the depression lateral to the big tendon." (*Annotations to "Yu Long Jing"*)

Note: It is stated in the *Annotations to "Yu Long Jing"* that the point is located in the cubital crease, in the depression on the radial side of the tendon of the biceps muscle of the arm when the arm is slightly flexed. Now this is the basis for location of the point.

2. 1. 6 LU 6 Kǒngzuì 孔最

Name: Seen in *Jia Yi*.

Location:

1) "7 *cun* above the crease of the wrist." (*Jia Yi*, etc.)

2) "Below Chize (LU 5) and 7 *cun* above the crease of the wrist, in the depression between the upper and lower bones (radius and ulna)." (*Jin Jian*, etc.)

Note: Medical literature through the ages holds similar views on the location of this point. The point is on the line connecting Chize (LU 5) and Taiyuan (LU 9), and 7 *cun* above the crease of the wrist. Because the Lung Meridian runs along the radial side of the arm, the point cannot be considered to be located in the depression between the radius and ulna.

2. 1. 7 LU 7 Lièquē 列缺

Name: Seen in *Ling Shu*.

Location:

1) "0.5 *cun* above the crease of the wrist." (*Ling Shu*, etc.)

2) "1.5 *cun* above the crease of the wrist." (*Jia Yi*, etc.)

3) "1.5 *cun* above the crease of the wrist, on the lateral side." (*Sheng Hui*, etc.)

4) "According to Zhen Quan, it is 3 *cun* superior to the wrist on the lateral side of the forearm, in the depression between two tendons, right under the tip of the index finger when the index fingers and thumbs of both hands are crossed." (*Wai Tai*)

Note:

1) *Ling Shu* says the point is 0.5 *cun* above the crease of the wrist, but *Jia Yi* takes it as 1.5 *cun*. Here the definition in *Jia Yi* is followed.

2) This is a Luo-Connecting point, located at the place deviating to the Hand-Yangming Meridian from the line connecting Chize (LU 5) and Taiyuan (LU 9). That is why *Sheng Hui* says "it is located at the lateral side, 1.5 *cun* above the wrist." Now it is located proximal to the styloid process of the radius, 1.5 *cun* above the crease of the wrist, between the tendons of the brachioradial and long abductor muscles of the thumb. When the index fingers and thumbs of both hands are crossed, the index finger of one hand is placed on the styloid process of the radius of the other. The point is in the depression right under the tip of the index finger, same as the description in *Da Cheng*.

2. 1. 8. LU 8 Jīngqú 經渠

Name: Seen in *Ling Shu*.

Location:

1) "At *cunkou*, with pulsation." (*Ling Shu*, etc.)

2) "In the depression of *cunkou*." (*Jia Yi*, etc.)

Note: "*cunkou*" is the place 1 *cun* posterior to the crease of the wrist, and the "depression" is between the styloid process of the radius and the radial artery.

2. 1. 9 LU 9 Tàiyuān 太淵

Name: Seen in *Ling Shu*.

Location:

1) "In the depression on the crease of the wrist." (*Jia Yi*, etc.)

2) "In the depression at the radial end of the crease of the wrist." (*Sheng Hui*, etc.)

3) "At the radial end of the crease of the wrist, where the pulsation is palpable." (*Da Cheng*, etc.)

Note: Although the above descriptions are more or less different, the location defined is the same. They all agree that the point is at the radial end of the crease of the wrist where the pulsation of the radial artery is palpable. This is the accurate location of today.

2. 1. 10 LU 10 Yújì 魚際

Name: Seen in *Ling Shu*.

Location:

1) "On the posterior (proximal) medial side of the metacarpophalangeal joint of the thumb, where are present many capillaries." (*Jia Yi*, etc.)

2) "On the junction of the red and white skin, posterior and medial to the metacarpophalangeal joint of the thumb." (*Da Cheng*, etc.)

3) "About 1 *cun* posterior to the crease of the wrist." (*Xun Jing*)

Note: According to *Jia Yi*, *Da Cheng*, etc., the point is on the border of the 1st metacarpal bone. In terms of position, the border of the thenal muscle may well be called "Yuji," but the point should be located posterior to the metacarpophalangeal joint, on the radial side of the midpoint of the 1st metacarpal bone, and on the junction of the red and white skin.

2. 1. 11 LU 11 Shàoshāng 少商

Name: Seen in *Ling Shu*.

Location:

1) "On the medial (radial) side of the thumb, about the width of a chive leaf from the nail." (*Jia Yi*, etc.)

2) "On the medial side of the thumb, about the width of a chive leaf from the corner of the nail." (*Qian Jin*, etc.)

3) "On the lateral (radial) side of the nail of the thumb, about the width of a chive leaf from the corner of the nail, in the depression on the border of the white skin." (*Wai Tai*, etc.)

4) "On the medial side of the thumb, about the width of a chive leaf from the nail, on the level of the nail root, in the depression on the border of the white skin." (*Yu Long Jing*, etc.)

Note: Medical literature through the ages holds the same view on the location of this point. It is located at the radial side of the last (distal) segment of the thumb, posterior to the nail. "The width of a chive leaf from the nail" is an indication of a distance from the corner of the nail, and "on the level of the nail root" is to define the location. Accordingly, the point should be located on the radial side of the distal segment of the thumb, 0.1 *cun* from the corner of the nail.

2. 2 Points of the Large Intestine Meridian of Hand-Yangming, LI
手陽明大腸經穴
Shŏuyángmíng Dàchángjīng Xué

2. 2. 1 LI 1 Shāngyáng 商陽

Name: Seen in *Ling Shu*.

Location:

1) "At the tip of the index finger." (*Ling Shu*, etc.)

2) "On the medial (radial) side of the index finger, about the width of a chive leaf from the nail." (*Jia Yi*, etc.)

3) "On the medial side of the index finger, about the width of a chive leaf from the corner of the nail." (*Qian Jin*, etc.)

Note: Medical literature through the ages holds similar views on the location of this point. Now it is located on the radial side of the distal segment of the index finger, 0.1 *cun* from the corner of the nail.

2. 2. 2 LI 2 Èrjiān 二間

Name: Seen in *Ling Shu*.

Location:

1) "Anterior (distal) to the metacarpophalangeal joint." (*Ling Shu*, etc.)

2) "In the depression on the radial side and anterior to the 2nd metacarpophalangeal joint." (*Jia Yi*, etc.)

3) "On the medial (radial) side and anterior to the 2nd metacarpophalangeal joint, in the depression at the end of the crease between the metacarpal bone and phalanx." (*Xun Jing*)

Note: The point is in the depression on the radial side of and distal to the 2nd metacarpophalangeal joint. "The end of the crease" indicates that it is between the metacarpal bone and phalanx." It cannot be taken as an evidence to locate the point because it is ambiguous and vague.

2. 2. 3 LI 3 Sānjiān 三間

Name: Seen in *Ling Shu*.

Location:

1) "Posterior (proximal) to the 2nd metacarpophalangeal joint." (*Ling Shu*)

2) "In the depression on the medial (radial) side and posterior to the 2nd metacarpophalangeal joint." (*Jia Yi*)

3) "Between the 1st and 2nd metacarpal bones, 1 *cun* below the root of the 2nd metacarpal bone." (*Qian Jin Yi*)

4) "On the medial side and proximal to the 3rd (proximal) segment of the index finger, at the end of the crease when a loose fist is made." (*Annotations to "Yu Long Jing"*)

5) "In the depression on the medial side and posterior to the 2nd metacarpophalangeal joint, in the depression about 0.2 *cun* from that joint." (*Jun Jing*)

Note: When the index finger is slightly flexed, a depression emerges. So we cannot only take the end of the crease as an evidence to locate the point. "1 *cun* below the root of the 2nd metacarpal bone" described in *Qian Jin Yi* implies that the distance between both ends of the 2nd metacarpophalangeal joint is 1 *cun*, therefore the location defined in *Qian Jin Yi* is the same as that mentioned in other books.

2. 2. 4 LI 4 Hégŭ 合谷

Name: Seen in *Ling Shu*.

Location:

1) "Between the 1st and 2nd metacarpal bones." (*Ling Shu*)

2) "Between the thumb and index finger." (*Jia Yi*, etc.)

3) "At the end of the longitudinal crease between the thumb and index finger, in the depression when the thumb is tilted upward." (*Qian Jin Yi*)

4) "In the depression of the bone cleft between the thumb and index finger." (*Sheng Hui*)

5) "In the depression between the 1st and 2nd metacarpal bones"; "To keep the two fingers close to each other and to needle the highest part at the end of the crease." (*Xun Jing*)

Note: *Sheng Hui*'s location of the point "in the bone cleft" seems too close to the joining part of the two bones. *Qian Jin Yi* and *Xun Jing* both suggest the point is located at the end of the crease between the 1st and 2nd metacarpal bones and at the highest part when the thumb and index finger are kept close to each other. The highest part is approximately at the midpoint of the radial border of the 2nd metacarpal bone.

2. 2. 5 LI 5 Yángxī 陽谿

Name: Seen in *Ling Shu*.

Location:

1) "In the depression between the two tendons." (*Ling Shu*)

2) "In the depression between the two tendons above the wrist." (*Jia Yi*)

3) "Posterior (proximal) to the interosseous space between the 1st and 2nd metacarpal bones, between the two tendons on the radial side of the wrist, on the level of Taiyuan (LU 9), directly above the 2nd metacarpophalangeal joint, where the pulsation is palpable." (*Xun Jing*)

Note: Medical literature through the ages holds similar views on the location of the point. When the thumb is tilted upward, the point is in the depression between the tendons of the short and long extensor muscles of the thumb, on the radial side of the wrist. Yangxi (LI 5) and Taiyuan (LU 9) are both on the wrist joint.

2. 2. 6 LI 6 Piānlì 偏歷

Name: Seen in *Ling Shu*.

Location:

1) "3 *cun* from the wrist." (*Ling Shu*, etc.)

2) "3 *cun* above the wrist, on the radial side of the forearm, obliquely above Yangxi (LI 4), or 1.5 *cun* above Lieque (LI 7)." (*Xun Jing*)

Note: Medical literature through the ages holds similar views on the location of the point. It is on the line connecting Yangxi (LI 5) and Quchi (LI 11), 3 *cun* above the crease of the wrist.

2. 2. 7 LI 7 Wēnliū 温溜

Name: Seen in *Jia Yi*.

Location:

1) "5 *cun* posterior (proximal) to the wrist in short persons and 6 *cun* posterior to the wrist in tall persons," or "5 *cun* posterior to the wrist." (*Jia Yi*, etc.)

2) "6 *cun* posterior to the wrist." (*Qian Jin*)

3) "Between 5 and 6 *cun* posterior to the wrist, where the pulsation is palpable." (*Sheng Hui*, etc.)

4) "5 *cun* posterior to the wrist in short persons and 6 *cun* posterior to the wrist in tall persons." (*Tong Ren*, etc.)

5) "5 *cun* posterior to the wrist," (*Da Quan*, etc.)

Note: According to *Jia Yi*, it is "5 *cun* posterior to the wrist." Now the point is located on the line connecting Yangxi (LI 5) and Quchi (LI 11) and 5 *cun* above the crease of the wrist.

2. 2. 8 LI 8 Xiàlián 下廉

Name: Seen in *Jia Yi*.

Location:

1) "Below the (upper end of) radius, 1 *cun* from Shanglian (LI 9) and in the oblique cleft lateral to the prominent muscle." (*Jia Yi*, etc.)

2) "Below the (upper end of) radius, 1 *cun* from Shanglian (LI 9) and in the oblique cleft lateral to the prominent muscle." (*Wai Tai*, etc.)

3) "4 *cun* below Quchi (LI 5) when the elbow is flexed, and 5 *cun* below Quchi (LI 5) when the elbow is extended." (*Xun Jing*, etc.)

4) "2.5 *cun* above Wenliu (LI 7), in the oblique cleft lateral to the prominent muscle." (*Jin Jian*, etc.)

Note: Medical literature through the ages holds similar views on the location of the point. But *Jin Jian* says "it is 2.5 *cun* above Wenliu (LI 7)," which is 5 *cun* above the wrist. Then Xialian (LI 8) must be 7.5 *cun* above the wrist. With another 4 *cun* between this point and Quchi (LI 11), the distance from the elbow to the wrist is 11.5 *cun* in all, which is not conformable to the bone proportional measurement. Therefore the location of the point should be basad on *Jia Yi*, i.e. on the line connecting Yangxi (LI 5) and Quchi (LI 11), 4 *cun* below the cubital crease.

2. 2. 9 LI 9 Shànglián 上廉

Name: Seen in *Jia Yi*.

Location:

1) "1 *cun* below Shousanli (LI 10)." (*Jia Yi*, etc.)

2) "3 *cun* below Quchi (LI 11) when the elbow is flexed, but 4 *cun* below Quchi (LI 11) when the elbow is extended." (*Xun Jing*)

Note: All scholars through the ages follow the location of this point described in *Jia Yi*.

2. 2. 10 LI 10 Shŏusānlĭ 手三裏

Name: Seen in *Jia Yi*.

Location:

1) "2 *cun* below Quchi (LI 11) when a fist is made." (*Jia Yi*, etc.)

2) "3 *cun* below Quchi (LI 11), where the prominence of the muscle (radial long extensor muscle of the wrist) appears when a fist is made." (*Zi Sheng*)

3) "3 *cun* below Quchi (LI 11) on location of it when the elbow is flexed -- annotated by

Guang." (*Xun Jing*)

Note: Medical literature through the ages has followed the description in *Jia Yi*. By quoting *Tong Ren*, *Zi Sheng* says it is 3 *cun* below Quchi (LI 11). But the extant copies of *Tong Ren* all take it as 2 *cun* below Quchi (LI 11). Now the location of the point follows *Jia Yi*.

2. 2. 11 LI 11 Qūchí 曲池

Name: Seen in *Ling Shu*.

Location:

1) "Between the humerus and radius when the elbow is flexed and the hand is put on the chest." (*Jia Yi*, etc.)

2) "Between the bones when the elbow is flexed." (*Qian Jin*, etc.)

3) "On the radius, lateral to the elbow, in the depression at the end of the cubital crease when the elbow is flexed." (*Sheng Hui*, etc.)

4) "On the radius, lateral to the elbow when the elbow is flexed and the hand is put on the chest." (*Tong Ren*, etc.)

Note: Medical literature through the ages holds similar views on the location of the point. The location of the point, based on *Sheng Hui*, is in the depression at the end of the cubital crease when the elbow is flexed, and according to *Xun Jing* it is "on the radius near the elbow joint." It is on the lateral end of the cubital crease and at the midpoint of the line connecting Chize (LU 5) and the external humeral epicondyle, when the elbow is flexed.

2. 2. 12 LI 12 Zhǒuliáo 肘髎

Name: Seen in *Jia Yi*.

Location:

1) "In the depression on the lateral (radial) side of the humerus." (*Jia Yi*, etc.)

2) "2 *cun* superior and lateral to Quchi (LI 11), in the depression on the radial side of the humerus when the elbow is flexed and the hand is put on the chest." (*Liu Ji*)

3) "In the depression on the radial side of the humerus, on the level of and 1.4 *cun* from Tianjing (SJ 10)." (*Tu Yi*)

4) "In the depression on the radial side, about 0.1-0.2 *cun* above the bone. Or in the depression 1 *cun* lateral to Quchi (LI 11)." (*Xun Jing*)

Note: The point is on the radial side of the humerus. According to *Liu Ji* the distance from the elbow is 2 *cun*, while based on *Tu Yi* it is on the level of Tianjing (SJ 10). Now following the latter it is 1 *cun* above Quchi (LI 11), and on the border of the humerus.

2. 2. 13 LI 13 Shǒuwǔlǐ 手五裏

Name: Seen in *Jia Yi*. Also named as "Wuli" in *Ling Shu*.

Location:

1) "3 *cun* above the elbow, medial to Zhouliao (LI 12) and on the big vessel (probably the cephalic vein), when the elbow is flexed." (*Jia Yi*, etc.)

2) "2 *cun* above the elbow, medial to Zhouliao (LI 12) and on the big vessel, when the elbow is flexed." (*Fa Hui*)

3) "2.5 *cun* obliquely above Zhouliao (LI 12), when the elbow is flexed and the hand is put on the chest." (*Xun Jing*)

Note: Medical literature through the ages follows the description in *Jia Yi*, i.e. 3 *cun* directly above Quchi (LI 11). The Wuxi edition of *Fa Hui* locates it as 2 *cun* above the elbow, which is a slip of the pen. The Wanli and Dongxitang editions both take it as 3 *cun* above the elbow.

Xun Jing says it is 2.5 *cun* above the elbow, which has not been accepted by later practitioners. Now according to the majority, the point is located 3 *cun* above Quchi (LI 11), on the line connecting Quchi (LI 11) and Jianyu (LI 15) and on the lateral side of the upper arm.

2. 2. 14 LI 14 Bìnào 臂臑

Name: Seen in *Jia Yi*.

Location:

1) "7 *cun* above the elbow, at the lower end of the deltoid muscle." (*Jia Yi*, etc.)

2) "1 *fu* (3 *cun*) below Jianyu (LI 15), in the depression between the two tendons and two bones." (*Sheng Hui*, etc.)

3) "1 *cun* below Jianyu (LI 15), in the depression between the two tendons when the arm is raised to the shoulder level." (*Ju Ying*)

Note: The lower end of the deltoid muscles is the landmark of its location. *Ju Ying* says the point is 1 *cun* below Jianyu (LI 15). "1 *cun*" may be a mistake of "1 *fu*"; it should be 3 *cun*.

2. 2. 15 LI 15 Jiānyú 肩髃

Name: Seen in *Jia Yi*.

Location:

1) "Between two bones (the acromion and the greater tubercle of the humerus) on the shoulder." (*Jia Yi*, etc.)

2) "Between two bones (the acromion and the greater tubercle of the humerus) on the shoulder, in the depression which appears when the arm is raised to the level of the shoulder (or slightly anterior to the depression), directly above the radial end of the cubital crease with the arms hanging down freely or akimbo." (*Xun Jing*)

Note: Medical literature through the ages holds similar views on the location of the point. It is on the shoulder, in the depression anterior and inferior to the acromion when the arm is abducted or raised forward to the level of the shoulder, directly above Quchi (LI 11).

2. 2. 16 LI 16 Jùgǔ 巨骨

Name: Seen in *Su Wen*.

Location:

"In the depression at the junction of two bones (acromial extremity of the clavicle and scapular spine) on the shoulder." (*Jia Yi*)

Note: Medical literature through the ages holds the same view on the location of the point. The point is located on the shoulder, in the depression between the acromial extremity of the clavicle and the scapular spine.

2. 2. 17 LI 17 Tiāndǐng 天鼎

Name: Seen in *Jia Yi*.

Location:

1) "In the supraclavicular fossa, directly below Futu (LI 18) and 1.5 *cun* lateral to Qishe (ST 11)." (*Jia Yi*)

2) "In the supraclavicular fossa, below Futu (LI 18), 1 *cun* below the angle of the mandible and posterior to Renying (ST 9)." (*Qian Jin*)

3) "In the supraclavicular fossa, directly below Futu (LU 18) and 0.5 *cun* posterior to Qishe (ST 11)." (*Su Wen*, annotated by Wang)

4) "In the supraclavicular fossa, below Futu (LI 18), in the depression 1 *cun* posterior to

Qishe (ST 11)." (*Sheng Hui*)

5) "On the course of the meridian that runs from Jugu (LI 16) along the neck, directly above Quepen (ST 12) and 1 *cun* below Futu (LI 18)." (*Jin Jian*)

Note: Medical literature through the ages says that it is on the neck, above Quepen (ST 12) and below Futu (LI 18). In general, Qishe (ST 11) is taken as the landmark. The point is said to be 1.5, 1.0 or 0.5 *cun* lateral to Qishe (ST 11), but Tianding (LI 17) is not level with Qishe (ST 11), and it is hard to take Qishe (ST 11) as the landmark for location. *Qian Jin* says it is 1 *cun* below the angle of the mandible, which seems too high, not conformable to the fact "directly below Futu (LI 18)." Now according to *Jin Jian*, the point is on the posterior border of the sternocleidomastoid muscle, between Futu (LI 18) and Quepen (ST 12).

2. 2. 18 LI 18 Fútū 扶突

Name: Seen in *Ling Shu* and *Su Wen*.

Location:

1) "1.5 *cun* posterior to Renying (ST 9)." (*Jia Yi*, etc.)

2) "1.5 *cun* posterior to Qishe (ST 11)." (*Qian Jin*, etc.)

3) "1 *cun* below the angle of the mandible and posterior to Renying (ST 9)." (*Wai Tai*, etc.)

4) "1 *cun* below the angle of the mandible and 1.5 *cun* posterior to Renying (ST 9)." (*Tong Ren*)

Note: Medical literature through the ages holds similar views on the location of the point. The majority says it is 1 *cun* below the angle of the mandible and 1.5 *cun* posterior to Renying (ST 9). The former is just at the midpoint of the sternocleidomastoid muscle, on the level of and posterior to Renying (ST 9). As to the description of 1.5 *cun* posterior to Qishe (ST 11) in the current edition of *Qian Jin*, Qishe (ST 11) may be a mistake of Renying (ST 9).

2. 2. 19 LI 19 Kǒuhéliáo 口禾髎

Name: Seen in *Jia Yi* as "heliao," the word "kou" being added later.

Location:

"Directly below the nostril, 0.5 *cun* lateral to Shuigou (DU 26)." (*Jia Yi* -- hand-written copies of the Ming Dynasty)

Note: All medical literature follows the description in *Jia Yi* and now the point is located directly below the lateral border of the nostril, on the level of Shuigou (DU 26).

2. 2. 20 LI 20 Yíngxiāng 迎香

Name: Seen in *Jia Yi*.

Location:

1) "Above Kouheliao (LI 19), lateral to the lower border of the nostril." (*Jia Yi*, etc.)

2) "1 *cun* above Kouheliao (LI 19), lateral to the nostril." (*Qian Jin*)

3) "1 *cun* above Kouheliao (LI 19) and 0.5 *cun* lateral to the nostril." (*Tong Ren*)

4) "1 *cun* above Kouheliao (LI 19), in the nasolabial groove, 0.5 *cun* from the nostril." (*Xun Jing*)

Note: All medical literature locates it as 1 *cun* above Kouheliao (LI 19). But the distance to the nostril varies: 1) Lateral to the lower border of the nostril; 2) 0.5 *cun* lateral to the nostril; and 3) in the nasolabial groove, 0.5 *cun* from the nostril and 1 *cun* above Kouheliao (LI 19). Now it is located in the nasolabial groove, beside the midpoint of the lateral border of the nasal ala.

2. 3. Points of the Stomach Meridian of Foot-Yangming, ST
足陽明胃經穴
Zúyángmíng Wèijīng Xué

2. 3. 1 ST 1 Chéngqì 承泣

Name: Seen in *Jia Yi*.

Location:

1) "0.7 *cun* directly below the eye when the eyes look straight forward." (*Jia Yi*, etc.)

2) "0.7 *cun* directly below the eye, in the orbit, in the depression directly below the pupil." (*Qian Jin Yi*)

Note: Medical literature through the ages holds similar views on the location of the point. It is below the pupil, and between the eyeball and the infraorbital ridge.

2. 3. 2 ST 2 Sìbái 四白

Name: Seen in *Jia Yi*.

Location:

1) "1 *cun* below the eye, at the foramen of the zygomatic bone." (*Jia Yi*, etc.)

2) "1 *cun* below the eye when the eyes look straight forward." (*Tong Ren*, etc.)

Note: Medical literature through the ages holds similar views on the location of the point. Now it is located directly below the pupil, in the depression of the infraorbital foramen.

2. 3. 3 ST 3 Jùliáo 巨髎

Name: Seen in *Jia Yi*.

Location:

1) "0.8 *cun* lateral to the nostril, directly below the pupil when the eyes look straight forward." (*Jia Yi*, etc.)

2) "0.8 *cun* lateral to the nostril, directly below the pupil when the eyes look straight forward, on the level of Shuigou (DU 26)." (*Ju Ying*, etc.)

Note: Medical literature through the ages holds similar views on the location of the point. It is directly below the pupil and on the level of the lower border of the nostril. *Ju Ying* says "it is level with Shuigou (DU 26)," which seems too low, because Shuigou (DU 26) is below the nostril.

2. 3. 4 ST 4 Dìcāng 地倉

Name: Seen in *Jia Yi*.

Location:

1) "0.4 *cun* lateral to the corner of the mouth." (*Jia Yi*, etc.)

2) "0.4 *cun* lateral to the corner of the mouth, where the pulsation is palpable." (*Sheng Hui*, etc.)

3) "0.4 *cun* lateral to the corner of the mouth, in the nasolabial groove." (*Liu Ji*)

Note: Medical literature through the ages holds the same view. It is 0.4 *cun* lateral to the corner of the mouth. Now it is located beside the mouth angle, directly below the pupil.

2. 3. 5 ST 5 Dàyíng 大迎

Name: Seen in *Ling Shu*.

Location:

1) "In the depression, 1.3 *cun* anterior to the angle of the mandible, where the pulsation

is palpable." (*Jia Yi*, etc.)

2) "In the depression, 1.2 *cun* anterior to the angle of the mandible, where the pulsation is palpable." (*Qian Jin*, etc.)

3) "In the depression, 1.3 *cun* anterior to the angle of the mandible, where the pulsation is apparently palpable and similar to that at Renying (ST 9), or anterior to the angle of the mandible, 1.5 *cun* below the ear." (*Xun Jing*)

Note: Medical literature through the ages holds similar views on the location of the point. It is at the place where the pulsation is palpable, which is an evidence in locating the point. Now it is located anterior to the angle of the mandible and on the anterior border of the masseter muscle, where the pulsation of the facial artery is palpable.

2. 3. 6 ST 6 Jiáchē 頰車

Name: Seen in *Ling Shu*.

Location:

1) "In the depression of the angle of the mandible, below the ear with the mouth open." (*Jia Yi*, etc.)

2) "0.8 *cun* below the ear, slightly anterior to the angle of the mandible." (*Qian Jin*, etc.)

3) "In the depression below the ear and anterior to the angle of the mandible with the mouth open." (*Ju Ying*, etc.)

4) "0.3 *cun* below the lobe of the ear." (*Liu Ji*)

Note: Medical literature dated after *Ju Ying* points out that it is in the depression slightly anterior to the angle of the mandible, but not on its (posterior) border. The distance from the point of the lobe of the ear is said to be 0.3 or 0.8 *cun*. Generally, 0.8, about one finger breadth, is accepted. The point is just at the attachment of the masseter muscle. When the teeth are clenched, a prominence of this muscle appears and a depression can be found when the mouth is open.

2. 3. 7 ST 7 Xiàguān 下關

Name: Seen in *Ling Shu* and *Su Wen*.

Location:

"Below Shangguan (GB 3), in the depression below the anterior auricular artery, which appears when the mouth is closed and disappears when the mouth is open." (*Jia Yi*, etc.)

Note: Medical literature through the ages follows the description in *Jia Yi*. Now it is located in the depression between the zygomatic arch and the mandibular notch.

2. 3. 8 ST 8 Tóuwéi 頭維

Name: Seen in *Jia Yi*.

Location:

1) "On the anterior hairline, at the corner of the forehead, 1.5 *cun* lateral to Benshen (GB 13)." (*Jia Yi*, etc.)

2) "Above the anterior hairline, at the corner of the forehead, 1.5 *cun* lateral to Benshen (GB 13)." (*Tong Ren*, etc.)

Note: According to *Jia Yi*, it is on the anterior hairline, at the corner of the forehead, and according to *Tong Ren*, it is 0.5 *cun* above the anterior hairline, 4.5 *cun* from Shenting (DU 24). Benshen (GB 13) is "3 *cun* lateral to Shenting (DU 24) and 0.5 *cun* above the anterior hairline." Therefore, Touwei (ST 8) is also 0.5 *cun* above the anterior hairline, at the corner of the forehead, and 4.5 *cun* lateral to the midline of the head.

2. 3. 9 ST 9 Rényíng 人迎

Name: Seen in *Ling Shu* and *Su Wen*.

Location:

1) "Anterior to the sternocleidomastoid muscle." (*Ling Shu*)

2) "On the common carotid artery, where the pulsation is palpable, on the level of the tip of Adam's apple." (*Jia Yi*, etc.)

3) "On the common carotid artery, where the pulsation is palpable, 1.5 *cun* lateral to the tip of Adam's apple." (*Tong Ren*, etc.)

Note: The point is lateral to the tip of Adam's apple, at the place where the pulsation of the common cartoid artery is palpable. From what is described in *Jia Yi* and *Tong Ren*, the location of the point is clear enough, i.e. on the level of the tip of Adam's apple, on the anterior border of the sternocleidomastoid muscle, on the place where the pulsation of the common carotid artery is palpable.

2. 3. 10 ST 10 Shuǐtū 水突

Name: Seen in *Jia Yi*.

Location:

1) "On the anterior border of the sternocleidomastoid muscle, directly below Renying (ST 9) and above Qishe (ST 11)." (*Jia Yi*, etc.)

2) "Directly below Renying (ST 9), anterior to the sternocleidomastoid muscle and lateral to the trachea." (*Jin Jian*, etc.)

Note: Medical literature through the ages holds similar views on the location of the point. *Ru Men* states that it is "between two points," while *Jin Jian* points out that it is lateral to the trachea. Therefore, the location of the point is quite clear, i.e. at the midpoint of the line connecting Renying (ST 9) and Qishe (ST 11), between the anterior border of the sternocleidomastoid muscle and the trachea.

2. 3. 11 ST 11 Qìshè 氣舍

Name: Seen in *Jia Yi*.

Location:

1) "On the neck, directly below Renying (ST 9), in the depression beside Tiantu (RN 22)." (*Jia Yi*, etc.)

2) "On the neck, directly below Renying (ST 9), in the depression 1.5 *cun* lateral to Tiantu (RN 22)." (*Liu Ji*, etc.)

3) "Directly below Shuitu (ST 10), in the depression about 1 *cun* below Adam's apple and anterior to the sternocleidomastoid muscle, close to the superior border of the medial end of the clavicle." (*Jin Jian*, etc.)

Note: According to *Jia Yi*, the location is clear. Now the point is located lateral to Tiantu (RN 22), on the upper border of the medial end of the clavicle, between the sternal and clavicular heads of the sternocleidomastoid muscle.

2. 3. 12 ST 12 Quēpén 缺盆

Name: Seen in *Su Wen*.

Location:

1) "In the centre of the supraclavicular fossa." (*Jia Yi*, etc.)

2) "In the centre of the infraclavicular fossa." (*Tong Ren*, etc.)

3) "In the centre of the supraclavicular fossa, 4 *cun* lateral to Tiantu (RN 22)." (*Liu Ji*)

Note: No transverse distance is pointed out in *Su Wen* and *Jia Yi*. In *Liu Ji*, it is said to be 4 *cun* lateral to Tiantu (RN 22). Then the location of the point becomes clear, i.e. 4 *cun* lateral to the anterior midline, at the centre of the supraclavicular fossa. Because of a slip of the pen, *Tong Ren* describes it "in the infraclavicular fossa."

2. 3. 13 ST 13 Qìhù 氣户

Name: Seen in *Jia Yi*.

Location:

1) "Below the big bone (clavicle), in the depression 2 *cun* lateral to Shufu (KI 27)." (*Jia Yi*, etc.)

2) "Down from Quepen (ST 12) to 1 *cun* below the big bone, in the depression 4 *cun* lateral to the anterior midline. Make the patient lie in a supine position and locate it." (*Jin Jian*)

Note: Medical literature through the ages holds the same view. It is below the midpoint of the lower border of the clavicle, 4 *cun* lateral to the anterior midline.

2. 3. 14 ST 14 Kùfáng 庫房

Name: Seen in *Jia Yi*.

Location:

1) "In the depression 1.6 *cun* below Qihu (ST 13)." (*Jia Yi*, etc.)

2) "In the depression 1.6 *cun* below Qihu (ST 13), 4 *cun* lateral to the anterior midline." (*Ju Ying*, etc.)

Note: Medical literature through the ages holds similar views on the location of the point. Now it is located in the 1st intercostal space, 4 *cun* lateral to the anterior midline.

2. 3. 15 ST 15 Wūyì 屋翳

Name: Seen in *Jia Yi*.

Location:

"1.6 *cun* below Kufang (ST 14)." (*Jia Yi*, etc.)

Note: Medical literature through the ages holds similar views on the location of the point. Now it is located in the 2nd intercostal space, 4 *cun* lateral to the anterior midline.

2. 3. 16 ST 16 Yīngchuāng 膺窗

Name: Seen in *Jia Yi*.

Location:

"1.6 *cun* below Wuyi (ST 15)." (*Jia Yi*, etc.)

Note: Medical literature through the ages holds similar views on the location of the point. Now it is located in the 3rd intercostal space, 4 *cun* lateral to the anterior midline.

2. 3. 17 ST 17 Rǔzhōng 乳中

Name: Seen in *Jia Yi*.

Location:

1) "In the centre of the nipple." (*Tong Ren*, etc.)

2) "On the nipple." (*Liu Ji*, etc.)

Note: Medical literature through the ages holds the same view on the location of the point. It is at the centre of the nipple.

2. 3. 18 ST 18 Rǔgēn 乳根

Name: Seen in *Jia Yi*.

Location:

1) "In the depression 1.6 *cun* below the nipple." (*Jia Yi*, etc.)

2) "In the depression 1.6 *cun* below Ruzhong (ST 17), 4 *cun* lateral to the anterior midline. It can be located with the patient in a supine position." (*Ju Ying*, etc.)

Note: Medical literature through the ages holds similar views on the location of the point. Now it is located in the 5th intercostal space, 4 *cun* lateral to the anterior midline.

2. 3. 19 ST 19 Bùróng 不容

Name: Seen in *Jia Yi*.

Location:

1) "1.5 *cun* lateral to Youmen (KI 21), 3 *cun* from the Ren Meridian and 2 *cun* from the anterior end of the rib." (*Jia Yi*)

2) "1.5 *cun* lateral to Youmen (KI 21), 2 *cun* from the Ren Meridian and 2 *cun* from the anterior end of the rib." (*Qian Jin*, etc.)

3) "1 *cun* lateral to Shangwan (RN 13)." (*Sheng Hui*)

4) "1.5 *cun* lateral to Youmen (KI 21), 3 *cun* lateral to the Ren Meridian, 1 *cun* lateral to Shangwan (RN 13), on the level of the 4th intercostal space." (*Ju Ying*)

5) "1.5 *cun* lateral to Youmen (KI 21) and 3 *cun* lateral to the anterior midline." (*Da Cheng*, etc.)

6) "1.5 *cun* lateral to Youmen (KI 21) and 2 *cun* lateral to the Ren Meridian, on the level of the 4th intercostal space." (*Liu Ji*).

7) "At the anterior end of the 4th rib, on the level of Rugen (ST 18), 2 *cun* lateral to the midline." (*Jin Jian*)

Note: In medical literature the views on the location of the point vary markedly, but most agree that it is "1.5 *cun* lateral to Youmen (KI 21)." It indicates that the point is 6 *cun* above and 2 *cun* lateral to the umbilicus (Juque, RN 14). The difference only lies in the transverse distance, which may be 3, 2 or 2.5 *cun* lateral to the Ren Meridian in different books. This is caused by the difference of distance from Youmen (KI 21) to the Ren Meridian, which may be 0.5 *cun* or 1 *cun*. *Jia Yi* points out that according to the Ming edition and the newly revised edition of *Su Wen*, "3 *cun* lateral to the Ren Meridian" defined in the current edition of *Jia Yi* may be a slip of the pen. The description in *Ju Ying* is self-contradictory, so it is not acceptable. In a word, according to *Jia Yi* and *Qian Jin* the point is located 6 *cun* above the umbilicus, and 2 *cun* lateral to the anterior midline.

2. 3. 20 ST 20 Chéngmǎn 承满

Name: Seen in *Jia Yi*.

Location:

1) "1 *cun* below Burong (ST 19)." (*Jia Yi*, etc.)

2) "1 *cun* below Burong (ST 19), 2.5 *cun* lateral to the Ren Meridian." (*Liu Ji*)

Note: All medical literature says it is 1 *cun* below Burong (ST 19), but the transverse distance is different (see Youmen, KI 21). Now according to *Jia Yi*, the point is located 5 *cun* above the centre of the umbilicus and 2 *cun* lateral to the anterior midline.

2. 3. 21 ST 21 Liángmén 梁門

Name: Seen in *Jia Yi*.

Location:

1) "1 *cun* below Chengman (ST 20)." (*Jia Yi*, etc.)

2) "1 *cun* below Chengman (ST 20), 2.5 *cun* lateral to the Ren Meridian." (*Liu Ji*)

Note: All medical literature locates it as 1 *cun* below Chengman (ST 20), but the transverse distance is different (see Youmen, KI 20). Now according to *Jia Yi*, it is located 4 *cun* above the centre of the umbilicus and 2 *cun* lateral to the midline.

2. 3. 22 ST 22 Guānmén 關門

Name: Seen in *Jia Yi*.

Location:

1) "Below Liangmen (ST 21), and above Taiyi (ST 3)." (*Jia Yi*)

2) "0.5 *cun* or 1 *cun* below Liangmen (ST 21), above Taiyi (ST 23)." (*Wai Tai*)

3) "1 *cun* below Liangmen (ST 21), 1 *cun* above Taiyi (ST 23), slightly lateral to the course of the meridian." (*Liu Ji*)

Note: All medical literature says it is 1 *cun* below Liangmen (ST 21) and 1 *cun* above Taiyi (ST 23). *Wai Tai* says it is 0.5 *cun* below Liangmen (ST 21). The transverse distance also varies (see Youmen KI 21). Now according to *Jia Yi*, it is located 3 *cun* above the centre of the umbilicus, 2 *cun* lateral to the midline.

2. 3. 23 ST 23 Tàiyí 太乙

Name: Seen in *Jia Yi*.

Location:

1) "1 *cun* below Guanmen (ST 22)." (*Jia Yi*, etc.)

2) "1 *cun* below Guanmen (ST 22), 2.5 *cun* lateral to the Ren Meridian." (*Liu Ji*)

Note: All medical literature locates it as 1 *cun* below Guanmen (ST 22). The transverse distance varies (see Youmen, KI 21). Now it is located as 2 *cun* above the centre of the umbilicus and 2 *cun* lateral to the midline.

2. 3. 24 ST 24 Huáròumén 滑肉門

Name: Seen in *Jia Yi*.

Location:

1) "1 *cun* below Taiyi (ST 23)." (*Jia Yi*, etc.)

2) "1 *cun* below Taiyi (ST 23), 2.5 *cun* lateral to the Ren Meridian." (*Liu Ji*)

Note: All medical literature locates it as 1 *cun* below Taiyi (ST 23). The transverse distance varies (see Youmen, KI 21). Now according to *Jia Yi* it is located 1 *cun* above the centre of the umbilicus and 2 *cun* lateral to the midline.

2. 3. 25 ST 25 Tiānshū 天樞

Name: Seen in *Ling Shu*.

Location:

1) "1.5 *cun* from Huangshu (KI 16), in the depression 2 *cun* lateral to the umbilicus." (*Jia Yi*, etc.)

2) "0.5 *cun* from Huangshu (KI 16), in the depression 2 *cun* lateral to the centre of the umbilicus." (*Ju Ying*)

3) "1 *cun* from Huangshu (KI 16), in the depression 2 *cun* lateral to the centre of the umbilicus." (*Da Cheng*)

Note: All medical literature locates it as lateral to Huangshu (KI 16), although it is said to be 0.5, 1.0, or 1.5 *cun* from Huangshu (KI 16). "In the depression 2 *cun* lateral to the centre of the umbilicus" is widely accepted to locate the point. Various schools hold different views about the distance from Tianshu (ST 25) to Huangshu (KI 16) and from Qichong (ST 30) to Henggu (KI 11), because their opinion differs on the distance between the Ren and Kidney meridians (see Henggu, KI 11).

2. 3. 26 ST 26 Wàilíng 外陵

Name: Seen in *Jia Yi*.

Location:

1) "Below Tianshu (ST 25) and above Daju (ST 27)." (*Jia Yi*)

2) "0.5 *cun* below Tianshu (ST 25) and above Daju (ST 27)." (*Qian Jin*)

3) "1 *cun* below Tianshu (ST 25)." (*Su Wen*, annotated by Wang)

Note: The point is located at the midpoint between Tianshu (ST 25) and Daju (ST 27), and it is 1 *cun* below Tianshu (ST 25), because Daju (ST 27) is 2 *cun* below Tianshu (ST 25). Now it is located 1 *cun* below the centre of the umbilicus and 2 *cun* lateral to the anterior midline. *Qian Jin* says "Daju (ST 27) is 1 *cun* below the umbilicus," so Wailing (ST 26) is 0.5 *cun* below Tianshu (ST 25). But it also points out that Daju (ST 27) is 2 *cun* below Tianshu (ST 25), which is adopted as the basis for the present location. It is not correct to say Wailing (ST 26) is 0.5 *cun* below Tianshu (ST 25).

2. 3. 27 ST 27 Dàjù 大巨

Name: Seen in *Jia Yi*.

Location:

1) "2 *cun* below Tianshu (ST 25)." (*Jia Yi*, etc.)

2) "1 *cun* below and 2 *cun* lateral to the umbilicus, 2 *cun* below Tianshu (ST 25)." (*Qian Jin*)

Note: Medical literature through the ages holds similar views on the location of the point. It is located 2 *cun* below the centre of the umbilicus and 2 *cun* lateral to the anterior midline. *Qian Jin* says it is "1 *cun* below the umbilicus," and "2 *cun* below Tianshu (ST 25)," which is self-contradictory. Now 2 *cun* below Tianshu (ST 25) is accepted.

2. 3. 28 ST 28 Shǔidào 水道

Name: Seen in *Jia Yi*.

Location:

1) "3 *cun* below Daju (ST 27)." (*Jia Yi*, etc.)

2) "2 *cun* below Daju (ST 27); 3 *cun* below Daju (ST 27) and 2 *cun* lateral to the anterior midline in the "Annotation to *Su Wen*." (*Ju Ying*)

3) "1 *cun* below Daju (ST 27), 2 *cun* lateral to Guanyuan (RN 4)." (*Xun Jing*, etc.)

Note: The above-mentioned points all take Tianshu (ST 25) as the basis for location, so should Shuidao (ST 28). Therefore, Daju (ST 27) may be a mistake of Tianshu (ST 25) in the first quotation. If Shuidao (ST 28) is 3 *cun* below Tianshu (ST 25), it is just 1 *cun* below Daju (ST 27), on the level of Guanyuan (RN 4). *Ju Ying* says it is "2 *cun* below Daju (ST 27)." Although it is only 1 *cun* in deviation, it still violates the principle of the bone proportional measurement of the lower abdomen, i.e. 6.5 *cun* between Tianshu (ST 25) and the pubis. If we follow the location of the point defined in *Xun Jing*, etc., it should be 1 *cun* below Daju (ST 27).

2. 3. 29 ST 29 Guīlái 歸來

Name: Seen in *Jia Yi*.

Location:

1) "2 *cun* below Shuidao (ST 28)." (*Jia Yi*, etc.)

2) "3 *cun* below Shuidao (ST 28)." (*Wai Tai*)

3) "2 *cun* below Shuidao (ST 28), on the level of Qugu (RN 2), 5 *cun* below the

umbilicus." (*Xun Jing*)

4) "1 *cun* below Shuidao (ST 28) (or 2 *cun* in the old edition), 2 *cun* lateral to the midline." (*Feng Yuan*)

Note: Most of the medical literature through the ages follow the definition in *Jia Yi*, i.e. "2 *cun* below Shuidao (ST 28). *Xun Jing* adds that "it is on the level of Qugu (RN 2), about 5 *cun* below the umbilicus." *Feng Yuan* locates it as 1 *cun* below Shuidao (ST 28), thus the point may be level with the points of other meridians on the lower abdomen. Now, this is the basis for the location of this point.

2. 3. 30 ST 30 Qìchōng 氣衝

Name: Seen in *Jia Yi* (also named "Qijie" in *Su Wen*).

Location:

1) "Below Guilai (ST 29) and 1 *cun* above the groin, where the pulsation is palpable." (*Jia Yi*, etc.)

2) "1 *cun* below Guilai (ST 29) and 1 *cun* above the groin." (*Qian Jin*, etc.)

3) "1 *cun* below Guilai (ST 29) and 2 *cun* lateral to the midline, in the depression where the pulsation is palpable." (*Da Cheng*)

Note: Medical literature holds similar views on the location of the point. The difference lies in the distances between the points above it. Now the location defined in *Feng Yuan* serves as the basis, i.e. the point is 5 *cun* below the centre of the umbilicus and 2 *cun* lateral to the anterior midline.

2. 3. 31 ST 31 Bìguān 髀關

Name: Seen in *Ling Shu*.

Location:

1) "Above the knee, posterior to the prominent muscle belly of the thigh (rectus muscle of the thigh), in the intermuscular groove (between the sartorius muscle and the tensor muscle of the fascia lata)." (*Jia Yi*, etc.)

2) "Posterior to the prominent muscle belly of the thigh and in the intermuscular groove, about 1 *cun* posterior to the muscle belly." (*Xun Jing*)

3) "About 12 *cun* above the knee." (*Tu Yi*, etc.)

Note: The description in *Jia Yi* does not show the particular location of the point. *Tu Yi* says it is 12 *cun* above the knee, which does not correspond to the bone proportional measurement of the thigh. As far as the running course of the meridian is concerned, this point is directly above Futu (ST 32) and Dubi (ST 35), on the line connecting the anterior superior iliac spine and the superior lateral corner of the patella. On the level of the perineum and in the depression lateral to the sartorius muscle, when the thigh is flexed. The position mentioned in *Xun Jing*, about 1 *cun* posterior to the muscle belly, is too low and not conformable to the original location.

2. 3. 32 ST 32 Fútù 伏兔

Name: Seen in *Ling Shu* and *Su Wen*.

Location:

1) "6 *cun* above the knee, on the anterior prominent muscle (quadriceps muscle) of the thigh." (*Jia Yi*, etc.)

2) "7 *cun* above the patella." (*Tong Ren*, etc.)

Note: Medical literature through the ages holds similar views on the location of the points, i.e. "6 *cun* above the knee and on the anterior prominent muscle of the thigh (quadriceps muscle of the thigh). Since the meridian runs on the anterior lateral side of the thigh, the point is located on the line connecting the anterior superior iliac spine and the superior lateral corner of the patella, 6 *cun* above this corner. The description in *Jia Yi* is the basis for the location of the point in later ages, although "7 *cun* above the patella" is proposed in *Tong Ren*.

2. 3. 33 ST 33 Yīnshì 陰市

Name: Seen in *Jia Yi*.

Location: "3 *cun* above the knee, below Futu (ST 32)." (*Jia Yi*, etc.)

Note: Medical literature through the ages holds similar views on the location of the point. Now it is located on the line connecting the anterior superior iliac spine and the superior lateral corner of the patella, 3 *cun* above this corner.

2. 3. 34 ST 34 Liángqiū 梁丘

Name: Seen in *Jia Yi*.

Location:

1) "2 *cun* above the knee." (*Jia Yi*, etc.) ("2 *cun* above the knee and between the two muscles" as mentioned in *Qian Jin*)

2) "3 *cun* above the knee, between the two muscles." (*Sheng Hui*)

3) "With the knee flexed it is in the depression above the patella." (*Xun Jing*)

Note: Medical literature holds similar views on the location of the point, i.e. "2 *cun* above the knee, between the rectus and lateral vastus muscles of the thigh," namely, on the line connecting the anterior superior iliac spine and the superior lateral corner of the patella, 2 *cun* above this corner. The description in *Sheng Hui* is not correct, which is confused with the location of Yinshi (ST 33). The location mentioned in *Xun Jing* seems too low, not conformable to a distance of "2 *cun*."

2. 3. 35 ST 35 Dúbí 犢鼻

Name: Seen in *Ling Shu* and *Su Wen*.

Location:

1) "On the lower border of the patella, in the depression beside the large ligament (patellar ligament)." (*Jia Yi*, etc.)

2) "In the depression lateral to the large ligament." (*Ru Men*)

Note: Medical literature holds similar views on the location of the point, i.e. on the lower border of the patella, in the depression lateral to the patella and its ligament. The view is widely accepted.

2. 3. 36 ST 36 Zúsānlǐ 足三裏

Name: Seen in *Sheng Ji Zong Lu* (also named "Sanli" in *Ling Shu* and *Nei Jing*).

Location:

1) "3 *cun* below the knee." (*Su Wen*)

2) "3 *cun* below the knee, on the lateral side of the tibia." (*Jia Yi*, etc.)

3) "3 *cun* below the knee, on the lateral side of the tibia, between the two muscles." (*Tong Ren*, etc.)

4) "3 *cun* below Dubi (ST 35), in the depression lateral to the tibia and medial to the big muscle." (*Fa Hui*)

5) "Again, 3 *cun* below Dubi (ST 35)." (*Ju Ying*)

Note: Medical literature through the ages holds similar views on the location of the point.

The definition in *Jia Yi*, inherited from *Shu Wen*, is more accurate, i.e. 3 *cun* directly below Dubi (ST 35), one finger-breadth from the anterior crest of the tibia, or in the anterior tibia muscle. The location mentioned in *Tong Ren* is slightly deviated to the lateral side, not directly below Dubi (ST 35). Now all accept the location defined in *Jia Yi*.

2. 3. 37 ST 37 Shàngjùxū 上巨虚

Name: Seen in *Qian Jin Yi*. Also named "Juxushanglian" in *Ling Shu* and *Su Wen*.

Location:

1) "3 *cun* below Zusanli (ST 36)." (*Ling Shu*)

2) "4 *cun* below the knee." (*Da Quan*)

Note: Medical literature through the ages holds similar views on the location of the point. Now it is accepted to locate it 6 *cun* below Dubi (ST 35) and one finger-breadth from the anterior crest of the tibia. The description in *Da Quan* is not in line with those found in other medical books.

2. 3. 38 ST 38 Tiáokǒu 條口

Name: Seen in *Jia Yi*.

Location:

1) "1 *cun* above Xiajuxu (ST 39)." (*Jia Yi*, etc.)

2) "1 *cun* below Shangjuxu (ST 37)." (*Sheng Hui*)

3) "About 5 *cun* below the knee." (*Da Quan*)

Note: Most of the medical literature follow the definition in *Jia Yi*. Now it is located 8 *cun* below Dubi (ST 35), one finger-breadth from the anterior crest of the tibia. The description in *Sheng Hui* and *Da Quan* is not the same as that in *Jia Yi*, and should therefore be rejected.

2. 3. 39 ST 39 Xiàjùxū 下巨虚

Name: Seen in *Qian Jin*. Also named "Juxuxialian" in *Ling Shu* and *Su Wen*.

Location:

1) "3 *cun* below Shangjuxu (ST 37)." (*Ling Shu*)

2) "3 *cun* below Shangjuxu (ST 37)." (*Jia Yi*, etc.)

3) "3 *cun* above Fenglong (ST 40)." (*Xun Jing*)

Note: Most of the medical literature follow the definition found in *Ling Shu* and *Jia Yi*, to which is conformable the present location. From the descriptions of Fenglong (ST 40) and Shangjuxu (ST 37) in *Xun Jing*, it is not difficult to find the mistake about the location of Xiajuxu (ST 39) in those books.

2. 3. 40 ST 40 Fēnglóng 豐隆

Name: Seen in *Ling Shu*.

Location:

1) "8 *cun* from the malleolus." (*Ling Shu*)

2) "8 *cun* above the external malleolus, in the depression on the lateral side of the tibia." (*Jia Yi*, etc.)

3) "Obliquely superior and posterior to Xiajuxu (ST 39), 8 *cun* above the external malleolus, in the depression on the lateral side of the tibia." (*Jin Jian*, etc.)

Note: Medical literature holds similar views on the location of the point, which is defined as 8 *cun* above the external malleolus and in the depression on the lateral side of the tibia. However, it is easily confused with Tiaokou (ST 38). Fenglong (ST 40) is a Luo-Connecting point, laterally deviated, two finger-breadths from the anterior crest of the tibia, 8 *cun* directly above the external malleolus, while Tiaokou (ST 38) is on the line from Zusanli (ST 36) to Xiajuxu (ST 39), conformable to the definition in *Jin Jian*.

2. 3. 41 ST 41 Jiěxī 解谿

Name: Seen in *Ling Shu*.

Location:

1) "In the depression 1.5 *cun* above Chongyang (ST 42)." (*Ling Shu*)

2) "1.5 *cun* posterior to Chongyang (ST 42), in the depression of the crease of the ankle." (*Jia Yi*, etc.)

3) "3.5 *cun* posterior to Chongyang (ST 42), in the depression of the crease of the ankle," or "2.5 *cun* posterior to Chongyang (ST 42)." (*Su Wen*, annotated by Wang)

Note: Most of the medical literature accord with *Ling Shu* and *Jia Yi*. The annotations to *Su Wen* by Wang are self-contradictory. The newly revised edition says the suggestion in *Jia Yi* should be followed, that it is "in the depression at the ankle"; thus the point is located at the midpoint of the dorsal crease of the ankle joint, between the tendons of the long extensor muscle of the great toe and the long extensor muscle of the toes.

2. 3. 42 ST 42 Chōngyáng 衝陽

Name: Seen in *Ling Shu*.

Location:

1) "In the depression on the instep of the foot, 5 *cun* proximal to Neiting (ST 44)." (*Ling Shu*)

2) "On the instep of the foot, 5 *cun* proximal to Neiting (ST 44), between the bones where the pulsation is palpable and 3 *cun* from Xiangu (ST 43)." (*Jia Yi*, etc.)

3) "On the instep of the foot, 5 *cun* proximal to Neiting (ST 44) and between the bones, 3 *cun* (or 2 *cun*) from Xiangu (ST 43)." (*Qian Jin*, etc.)

4) "5 *cun* from Neiting (ST 44)." (*Da Quan*)

Note: Most of the medical literature locate it as "5 *cun* proximal to Neiting (ST 44), between the bones where the pulsation is palpable and 3 *cun* from Xiangu (ST 43)." Neiting (ST 44) is 2 *cun* from Xiangu (ST 43) and Xiangu (ST 43) is 3 *cun* from Chongyang (ST 42), which conforms to 5 *cun* from Neiting (ST 44) as recorded in *Da Quan*. In line with the above definition, it is located on the dome of the instep of the foot, between the tendons of the long extensor muscle of the great toe and the long extensor muscle of the toes, where the pulsation of the dorsal artery of the foot is palpable. By a comparison of the location of Neiting (ST 44) with that of Xiangu (ST 43) in *Qian Jin*, it is easy to find the mistake, for it says Xiangu (ST 43) is 2 *cun* proximal to Neiting (ST 44), and Chongyang (ST 42) is 5 *cun* proximal to Neiting (ST 44). Thus the distance between Xiangu (ST 43) and Chongyang (ST 42) should be 3 *cun* instead of 2 *cun*.

2. 3. 43 ST 43 Xiàngǔ 陷谷

Name: Seen in *Ling Shu*.

Location:

1) "On the medial side of the 3rd metatarsal bone, in the depression 2 *cun* above Neiting (ST 44)." (*Ling Shu*)

2) "Between the 1st and 2nd toes, in the depression proximal to the metatarsophalangeal joint and 2 *cun* from Neiting (ST 44)." (*Jia Yi*, etc.)

3) "On the lateral side of the 2nd toe, proximal to the metatarsophalangeal joint and 2 *cun*

from Neiting (ST 44)." (*Qian Jin*, etc.)

4) "2 *cun* distal to Chongyang (ST 42), in the depression proximal to the 2nd metatarsophalangeal joint." (*Jin Jian*)

Note: The records in *Ling Shu* and *Jia Yi* are actually the same. The scholars of the later ages all follow this definition. The current edition of *Jia Yi* says "it is between the 1st and 2nd toes." But the Ming Dynasty edition says "it is on the lateral side of the 2nd toe," in light of which, it should be located 2 *cun* proximal to Neiting (ST 44), namely, in the depression between the 2nd and 3rd metatarsal bones of the instep of the foot. The description in *Jin Jian* is hard to be clarified, because there is no rigid measurement set for the location of Chongyang (ST 42) in that book.

2. 3. 44 ST 44 Nèitíng 内庭

Name: Seen in *Ling Shu*.

Location:

1) "On the lateral side of the 2nd toe." (*Ling Shu*)

2) "In the depression on the lateral side of the 2nd toe." (*Jia Yi*, etc.)

3) "In the web between the 2nd and 3rd toes." (*Xun Jing*)

Note: Medical literature holds the same view on the location of the point. Now it is located between the 2nd and 3rd toes, at the junction of the white and red skin, proximal to the margin of the web.

2. 3. 45 ST 45 Lìduì 厲兑

Name: Seen in *Ling Shu*.

Location:

1) "On the 2nd toe, about the width of a chive leaf from the corner of the nail." (*Jia Yi*, etc.)

2) "On the lateral side of the 2nd toe, about the width of a chive leaf from the nail." (*Liu Ji*, etc.)

Note: The descriptions in medical literature through the ages are conformable to that in *Jia Yi*, locating it as near the corner of the nail. It must be on the lateral side on the running course of the meridian concerned, although no mention has been made whether it is "on the medial side" or "on the lateral side." Then, precisely the point is located on the lateral side of the distal segment of the 2nd toe, and 0.1 *cun* from the corner of the toe nail.

2. 4. Points of the Spleen Meridian of Foot-Taiyin, SP
足太陰脾經穴
Zútàiyīn Píjīng Xué

2. 4. 1 SP 1 Yǐnbái 隱白

Name: Seen in *Ling Shu* and *Su Wen*.

Location:

1) "On the medial side of the distal segment of the great toe." (*Ling Shu*)

2) "On the medial side of the distal segment of the great toe, about the width of a chive leaf from the nail." (*Jia Yi*, etc.)

3) "On the medial side of the distal segment of the great toe, about the width of a chive

leaf from the corner of the nail." (*Wai Tai*, etc.)

Note: Medical literature through the ages holds the same view on the location of the point, and "most Jing-Well points are located at the place where it is the width of a chive leaf from the (corner of the) nail." This point is on the medial side of the distant segment of the great toe and 0.1 *cun* from the corner of the toenail.

2. 4. 2 SP 2 Dàdū 大都

Name: Seen in *Ling Shu*.

Location:

1) "In the depression proximal to the 1st metatarsophalangeal joint." (*Ling Shu*)

2) "In the depression proximal to the 1st metatarsophalangeal joint." (*Jia Yi*, etc.)

3) "On the medial side of the great toe, at the junction of the red and white skin, proximal to the 1st metatarsophalangeal joint." (*Qian Jin*)

4) "On the medial side of the great toe, at the junction of the red and white skin, 1 *cun* from the 1st metatarsophalangeal joint." (*Wai Tai*)

5) "In the depression on the medial side of the great toe, proximal to the 1st metatarsophalangeal joint, in the bony cleft at the junction of the red and white skin. (*Ju Ying*, etc.)

6) "On the medial side of and proximal to the 2nd segment of the great toe, distal to the metatarsophalangeal joint, in the depression of the bony cleft, at the junction of the red and white skin." (*Ji Cheng*)

Note: Most of the medical literature locate it proximal to the metatarsophalangeal joint, quite different from the present location -- distal to the metatarsophalangeal joint, at the junction of the red and white skin. But *Ling Shu* and other medical books all say that Gongsun (SP 4) is 1 *cun* proximal to the metatarsophalangeal joint. Dadu (SP 2) and Taibai (SP 3) must be within the space from the point Yinbai (SP 1) posterior to the corner of the toenail of the great toe to the point 1 *cun* proximal to the metatarsophalangeal joint. Now, according to *Ji Cheng*, Dadu (SP 2) is located distal, and Taibai (SP 3) proximal, to the metatarsophalangeal joint, both at the junction of the red and white skin.

2. 4. 3 SP 3 Tàibái 太白

Name: Seen in *Ling Shu*.

Location:

1) "Proximal to the metatarsophalangeal joint of the great toe." (*Ling Shu*)

2) "On the medial border of the foot, in the depression, proximal to the metatarsophalangeal joint of the great toe." (*Jia Yi*, etc.)

3) "On the medial side of the great toe, 1 *cun* proximal and inferior to Dadu (SP 2)." (*Sheng Ying*)

4) "Posterior (proximal) to the metatarsophalangeal joint of the great toe, closely medial to the bony depression, at the junction of the red and white skin." (*Xun Jing*)

Note: According to medical literature, it is located proximal and inferior to the 1st metatarsophalangeal joint, at the junction of the red and white skin.

2. 4. 4 SP 4 Gōngsūn 公孫

Name: Seen in *Ling Shu*.

Location:

1) "1 *cun* posterior (proximal) to the metatarsophalangeal joint." (*Ling Shu*, etc.)

2) "1 *cun* posterior to the metatarsophalangeal joint." (*Jia Yi*, etc.)

3) "1 *cun* posterior to the metatarsophalangeal joint of the great toe, anterior to the medial malleolus." (*Da Cheng*)

Note: Medical literature through the ages holds similar views on the location of the point. Now it is located proximal to the metatarsophalangeal joint, distal and inferior to the base of the 1st metatarsal bone.

2. 4. 5 SP 5 Shāngqiū 商丘

Name: Seen in *Ling Shu*.

Location:

1) "In the depression below the medial malleolus." (*Ling Shu*)

2) "In the depression inferior and slightly anterior to the medial malleolus." (*Jia Yi*, etc.)

3) "In the depression inferior and slightly anterior to the medial malleolus, anterior and posterior to which there locate Zhongfeng (LR 4) and Zhaohai (KI 6) respectively." (*Da Cheng*)

Note: Medical literature through the ages holds similar views on the location of the point. It is located at the midpoint of the line connecting the tuberosity of the navicular bone and the tip of the medial malleolus.

2. 4. 6 SP 6 Sānyīnjiāo 三陰交

Name: Seen in *Jia Yi*.

Location:

1) "3 *cun* above the medial malleolus, in the depression posterior to the tibia." (*Jia Yi*, etc.)

2) "8 *cun* above the medial malleolus, in the depression posterior to the tibia." (*Qian Jin*, etc.)

3) "3 *cun* above the medial malleolus, in the depression posterior to the tibia." (*Jin Jian*)

Note: Medical literature through the ages says it is "3 *cun* above the medial malleolus." The point is now located posterior to the medial border of the tibia, 3 *cun* above the tip of the medial malleolus. The assertion "8 *cun* above the medial malleolus" in *Qian Jin* has not been followed after the Song Dynasty.

2. 4. 7 SP 7 Lòugŭ 漏谷

Name: Seen in *Jia Yi*.

Location:

1) "6 *cun* above the medial malleolus, in the depression posterior to the tibia." (*Jia Yi*, etc.)

2) "6 *cun* above the medial malleolus, in the depression posterior to the tibia." (*Ju Ying*, etc.)

Note: Medical literature through the ages holds similar views on the location of the point. It is located 6 *cun* above the tip of the medial malleolus, posterior to the medial border of the tibia.

2. 4. 8 SP 8 Dìjī 地機

Name: Seen in *Jia Yi*.

Location:

1) "5 *cun* below the knee." (*Jia Yi*, etc.)

2) "In the depression below the medial bony tuberosity of the knee (the medial condyle of the tibia) when the leg is stretched." (*Sheng Hui*, etc.)

3) "5 *cun* below the knee, in the depression below the medial bony tuberosity of the knee

when the leg is stretched." (*Ju Ying*, etc.)

4) "In the depression below the bony tuberosity of the knee; or 5 *cun* below Yinlingquan (SP 9), medial to the bone and lateral to the big muscle, opposite to Juxu (ST 37), when the leg is stretched; or 1 *cun* obliquely anterior to and 8 *cun* above the tip of the medial malleolus when the leg is stretched." (*Ju Ying*, etc.)

5) "5 *cun* below Lougu (SP 7), in the depression 5 *cun* below the knee, medial to the tibia, when the leg is stretched." (*Jin Jian*)

Note: "5 *cun* below the knee" is equal to 3 *cun* below Yinlingquan (SP 9). The location described in *Sheng Hui* is actually the location of Yinlingquan (SP 9). The point is said to be 8 *cun* above the tip of the medial malleolus in *Xun Jing*, which is incompatible with the bone proportional measurement and not an adequate basis of location. *Jin Jian* says it is "5 *cun* below the knee," then it should not be 5 *cun* above Lougu (SP 7), otherwise it will not correspond to the bone proportional measurement. Now according to *Jia Yi*, the point is located 3 *cun* below Yinlingquan (SP 9).

2. 4. 9 SP 9 Yīnlíngquán 陰陵泉

Name: Seen in *Ling Shu*.

Location:

1) "In the depression below the medial condyle of the tibia when the leg is stretched." (*Ling Shu*)

2) "On the medial side below the knee, in the depression below the medial condyle of the tibia when the leg is stretched." (*Jia Yi*, etc.)

3) "On the medial side below the knee, in the depression one finger-breadth below the medial condyle of the tibia when the leg is flexed." (*Liu Ji*)

Note: Medical literature through the ages holds similar views on the location of the point. The point is located in the depression posterior and inferior to the medial condyle of the tibia, to which the description in *Liu Jing* is almost conformable.

2. 4. 10 SP 10 Xuèhǎi 血海

Name: Seen in *Jia Yi*.

Location:

1) "2.5 *cun* above the patella, at the junction of the red and white skin on the medial side of the knee." (*Jia Yi*, etc.)

2) "2 *cun* above the patella, at the junction of the red and white skin on the medial side of the knee." (*Qian Jin Yi*, etc.)

3) "1 *cun* above the patella, in the depression at the junction of the red and white skin on the medial side of the knee, or above the medial bony tuberosity of the knee (epicondyle of the femur), but 0.5 *cun* deviated to the medial side." (*Tu Yi*)

4) "1 *cun* above the patella, in the depression at the junction of the red and white skin, on the medial side of the knee." (*Jin Jian*, etc.)

Note: Books of various medical schools accept that the point is "on the medial side of and above the patella," or "above the medial bony tuberosity of the knee." All refer to the medial side of the thigh above the superior medial corner of the patella, or above the medial tuberosity of the femur. But there is divergence on the distance between the point and the base of the patella, such as 1 *cun*, 2 *cun* and 2.5 *cun*. The distance of 2.5 *cun* mentioned in the current edition of *Jia Yi* may be a slip of the pen. Now the point is located 2 *cun* above the superior medial corner of the patella when the knee is flexed, on the prominence of the medial head of the quadriceps muscle of the thigh.

2. 4. 11 SP 11 Jīmén 箕門

Name: Seen in *Jia Yi*.

Location:

1) "In the groove between two muscles (sartorius and gracilis muscles), where the pulsation is palpable." (*Jia Yi*)

2) "In the groove between two muscles (sartorius and gracilis muscles), where the pulsation is palpable, and medial to Yinshi (ST 33)." (*Qian Jin*, etc.)

3) "In the groove between two muscles (sartorius and gracilis muscles), and on the pulsating vessel of the medial side of the thigh." (*Tong Ren*, etc.)

4) "6 *cun* above Xuehai (SP 10), between two muscles (sartorius and gracilis muscles), where the pulsation is palpable." (*Zhen Jiu Wen Da*, etc.)

Note: The position of the point is clear, i.e. between the two muscles on the medial side of the thigh, where the muscles bulge. Now according to *Zhen Jiu Wen Da* it is on the line connecting Xuehai (SP 10) and Chongmen (SP 12), and 6 *cun* above Xuehai (SP 10).

2. 4. 12 SP 12 Chōngmén 衝門

Name: Seen in *Jia Yi*.

Location:

1) "5 *cun* below Daheng (SP 15), below Fushe (SP 13), on both ends of the pubes, in the groin where the pulsation is palpable." (*Jia Yi*, etc.)

2) "5 *cun* below Daheng (SP 15), below Fushe (SP 13), on both ends of the pubes where the pulsation is palpable." (*Wai Tai*)

3) "5 *cun* below Daheng (SP 15), below Fushe (SP 13), on the end of the pubis where the pulsation is palpable, ... 4.5 *cun* lateral to the anterior midline." (*Zi Sheng*, etc)

4) "Directly below the nipples, 5 *cun* from Daheng (SP 15), below Fushe (SP 13), on both ends of the pubes, in the groin where the pulsation is palpable, 4 *cun* lateral to the Ren Meridian." (*Liu Ji*)

5) "0.7 *cun* below Fushe (SP 13) (*Da Cheng* wrongly takes it as 1 *cun*), 5 *cun* below Daheng (SP 15), on both ends of the pubes, in the groin where the pulsation is palpable, and 3.5 *cun* lateral to the anterior midline." (*Feng Yuan*)

Note: *Jia Yi* and other medical books all hold that the point is "5 *cun* from Daheng (SP 15)," i.e. 5 *cun* below the umbilicus, on the level of the upper border of the pubic symphysis. However, there is disagreement on its transverse distance to the anterior midline. It is said to be 3 *cun* in *Jia Yi*, 4 *cun* in *Liu Ji* and 4.5 *cun* in *Zi Sheng*. The point described in *Jia Yi* is directly below Qimen (LI 14) and 3.5 *cun* lateral to the Ren Meridian. Therefore, it is located 3.5 *cun* lateral to the midpoint of the upper border of the pubic symphysis, and lateral to the pulsating external iliac artery.

2. 4. 13 SP 13 Fǔshè 府舍

Name: Seen in *Jia Yi*.

Location:

1) "3 *cun* below Fujie (SP 14)" (3.5 *cun* from the anterior midline). (*Jia Yi*, etc.)

2) "3 *cun* below Fujie (SP 14)" (4.5 *cun* from the anterior midline). (*Zi Sheng*, etc.)

3) "2 *cun* below Fujie (SP 14) and 4.5 *cun* from the anterior midline." (*Da Cheng*)

4) "3 *cun* below Fujie (SP 14), directly below the nipples, and 4 *cun* lateral to the Ren Meridian." (*Liu Ji*)

5) "0.7 *cun* above Chongmen (SP 12) and 3.5 *cun* lateral to the anterior midline." (*Jin Jian*)

Note: The interspaces between Fushe (SP 13), Fujie (SP 14), Daheng (SP 15) and Fu'ai (SP 16) have been unanimous since ancient times, i.e. Fushe (SP 13) is 3 *cun* below Fujie (SP 14), which is 1.3 *cun* below Daheng (SP 15), which is on the level of the umbilicus, and Fu'ai (SP 16) is 1.5 *cun* below Riyue (GB 24). But there is divergence of opinions on the distance from the anterior midline.

At present, medical books in this country all follow the definition made in *Liu Ji*, i.e. 4 *cun* lateral to the anterior midline. *Jia Yi* describes Jimen (SP 11) "directly below the nipples." The distance between the nipples and the anterior midline is 4 *cun* and all the above-mentioned points are on the vertical line through Jimen (SP 11). So all the points of this meridian on the abdomen are 4 *cun* lateral to the midline except Chongmen (SP 12), which is 3.5 *cun* lateral to the midline, because the lower abdomen is narrower. It is not correct to define the point as 4.5 *cun* from the midline. *Da Cheng* says it is "2 *cun* below Fujie (SP 14)." "Two" may be a slip of the pen; it should be "three."

2. 4. 14 SP 14 Fùjié 腹結

Name: Seen in *Jia Yi*.

Location:

1) "1.3 *cun* below Daheng (SP 15)." (3.5 *cun* from the anterior midline.) (*Jia Yi*, etc.)

2) "0.3 *cun* below Daheng (SP 15)." (*Tong Ren*)

3) "1.3 *cun* below Daheng (SP 15) ... 4.5 *cun* from the anterior midline." (*Fa Hui*, etc.)

4) "Directly below the nipples, 1.3 *cun* below Daheng (SP 15), and 4 *cun* lateral to the Ren Meridian." (*Liu Ji*)

5) "1.8 *cun* below Daheng (SP 15), 3.5 *cun* from the anterior midline, and lateral to the umbilicus." (*Ji Cheng*)

Note: Concerning the distance of this point to Daheng (SP 15), most of the medical literature take "1.3 *cun*" defined by *Jia Yi*, which is the basis for the present location. The descriptions in *Tong Ren* and *Ji Cheng* are wrong. As to the difference on the transverse distance to the anterior midline, please see the Note in Fushe (SP 13).

2. 4. 15 SP 15 Dàhéng 大横

Name: Seen in *Jia Yi*.

Location:

1) "3 *cun* below Fu'ai (SP 16) and directly lateral to the umbilicus" (3.5 *cun* lateral to the anterior midline). (*Jia Yi*, etc.)

2) "2 *cun* below Fu'ai (SP 16) and directly lateral to the umbilicus." (*Qian Jin*)

3) "3.5 *cun* below Fu'ai (SP 16) and directly lateral to the umbilicus." (*Tong Ren*, etc.)

4) "3.5 *cun* below Fu'ai (SP 16), 2.5 *cun* directly lateral to the umbilicus and 4.5 *cun* from the anterior midline." (*Ju Ying*)

5) "3 *cun* below Fu'ai (SP 16), directly lateral to the umbilicus, in the large crease directly below the nipples and 4 *cun* lateral to the Ren Meridian." (*Liu Ji*, etc.)

6) "6.5 *cun* below Fu'ai (SP 16) [3.5 *cun* below Fu'ai (SP 16) is an old wrong definition], on the level of the umbilicus and 3.5 *cun* lateral to the anterior midline." (*Feng Yuan*).

7) "1.8 *cun* above Fujie (SP 14), lateral to the midpoint between Shuifen (RN 9) and Xiawan (RN 10)." (*Ji Cheng*)

Note: The emphasis in the location of this point is on "directly lateral to the umbilicus," but the distance varies from 3.5 *cun* to 4 *cun*. The latter is adopted, because it is "directly below the nipples."

2. 4. 16 SP 16 Fù'āi 腹哀

Name: Seen in *Jia Yi*.

Location:

1) "1.5 *cun* below Riyue (GB 24) (3.5 *cun* from the anterior midline)." (*Jia Yi*, etc.)

2) "On the end of the 3rd rib, 2.5 *cun* lateral to the xiphoid process, and directly below the nipples." (*Su Wen*, annotated by Wang)

3) "1.5 *cun* below Riyue (GB 24), directly below the nipples, and 4 *cun* lateral to the Ren Meridian." (*Liu Ji*)

4) "1 *cun* below Riyue (GB 24)." (*Ru Men*)

Note: In ancient times Riyue (GB 24) was taken as a landmark for location of points below it on the abdomen. It is described in *Jia Yi* that Qimen (LI 14) is on the level of Juque (RN 14) (6 *cun* above the umbilicus). Riyue (GB 24) is 1.5 *cun* below Qimen (LI 14) (4.5 *cun* above the umbilicus), while Fu'ai (SP 16) is 1.5 *cun* below Riyue (GB 24), thus it is 3 *cun* above the umbilicus. Therefore, *Jia Yi* defines the location of Daheng (SP 15), as 3 *cun* below Fu'ai (SP 16) and lateral to the umbilicus. Now, this definition in *Jia Yi* is followed, that the point is located 3 *cun* above the centre of the umbilicus and 4 *cun* lateral to the anterior midline.

2. 4. 17 SP 17 Shídòu 食竇

Name: Seen in *Jia Yi*.

Location:

1) "In the depression 1.6 *cun* below Tianxi (SP 18), in the supine position." (6 *cun* from the anterior midline.) (*Jia Yi*)

2) "6 *cun* from the anterior midline, or 1.6 *cun* below and 1 *cun* lateral to the nipples, and on the level of Zhongting (RN 16)." (*Xun Jing*)

3) "1.5 *cun* lateral to the vertical line through the nipples when the arm is raised." (*Liu Ji*)

Note: "1.6 *cun*" is the intercostal distance. Tianxi (SP 18) is located in the 4th intercostal space, so this point is in the 5th intercostal space and 6 *cun* lateral to the anterior midline. The locations described in *Xun Jing* and *Liu Ji* are not acceptable.

2. 4. 18 SP 18 Tiánxī 天谿

Name: Seen in *Jia Yi*.

Location:

1) "In the depression 1.6 *cun* below Xiongxiang (SP 19), in a supine position." (6 *cun* from the anterior midline.) (*Jia Yi*, etc.)

2) "6 *cun* from the anterior midline; or 6 *cun* lateral to Xuanji (RN 21), and then 5.8 *cun* downward, on the level of Danzhong (RN 17)." (*Xun Jing*)

3) "2 *cun* lateral to the nipples." (*Ji Cheng*)

Note: Medical literature through the ages holds similar views on the location of the point. It is 2 *cun* lateral to the nipples, and in the 4th intercostal space.

2. 4. 19 SP 19 Xiōngxiāng 胸鄉

Name: Seen in *Jia Yi*.

Location:

"In the depression 1.6 *cun* below Zhourong (SP 20), in the supine position." (6 *cun* from the anterior midline.) (*Jia Yi*)

Note: Medical literature through the ages holds similar views on the location of the point. It is in the 3rd intercostal space, 6 *cun* lateral to the anterior midline.

2. 4. 20 SP 20 Zhōuróng 周榮

Name: Seen in *Jia Yi*.

Location:

1) "In the depression 1.6 *cun* below Zhongfu (LU 1), in the supine position." (6 *cun* from the anterior midline.) (*Jia Yi*, etc.)

Note: Medical literature holds similar views on the location of the point. It is in the 2nd intercostal space, 6 *cun* lateral to the anterior midline.

2. 4. 21 SP 21 Dàbāo 大包

Name: Seen in *Ling Shu*.

Location:

1) "3 *cun* below Yuanye (GB 22)." (*Ling Shu*, etc.)

2) "3 *cun* below Yuanye (GB 22), in the 9th intercostal space and in the hypochondrium." (*Jia Yi*, etc.)

3) "6 *cun* below the axilla, in the 9th intercostal space, on the level of Juque (RN 14)." (*Xun Jing*)

Note: Medical literature through the ages describes the location of the point as 3 *cun* below Yuanye (GB 22), which is on the mid-axillary line and in the 4th intercostal space. In the old days, the distance between the intercostal spaces was defined as 1.6 *cun*. Three *cun* here equals to two intercostal spaces. Therefore, this point now is located on the mid-axillary line, and in the 6th intercostal space.

2. 5. Points of the Heart Meridian of Hand-Shaoyin, HT

手少陰心經穴

Shǒushàoyīn Xīnjīng Xué

2. 5. 1 HT 1 Jíquán 極泉

Name: Seen in *Jia Yi*.

Location:

1) "Between the muscles under the axilla where the artery enters the chest." (*Jia Yi*, etc.)

2) "Inside the axillary hair, where the artery enters the chest." (*Liu Ji*)

Note: Medical literature through the ages holds similar views on the location of the point. "Between the muscles under the axilla" refers to the part between the anterior and posterior axillary folds. The point is located at the apex of the axillary fossa where the pulsation of the axillary artery is palpable.

2. 5. 2 HT 2 Qīnglíng 青靈

Name: Seen in *Sheng Hui*.

Location:

"3 *cun* above the elbow when the arm is raised and the elbow extended." (*Sheng Hui*, etc.)

Note: Medical literature through the ages holds the same view on the location of the point. It is on the line connecting Jiquan (HT 1) and Shaohai (HT 3), 3 *cun* above the cubital crease and in the groove medial to the biceps muscle of the arm.

2. 5. 3 HT 3 Shàohaǐ 少海

Name: Seen in *Ling Shu*.

Location:

1) "In the depression posterior (proximal) and medial to the elbow, where the pulsation is palpable." (*Jia Yi*, etc.)

2) "In the depression of the medial end of the cubital crease when the elbow is flexed with the hand towards the head, defined by Zhen Quan." (*Wai Tai*)

3) "In the depression 0.5 *cun* from the tip of the elbow, lateral to the big bone (medial epicondyle of the humerus) on the medial side of the elbow, when the elbow is flexed." (*Su Wen*, annotated by Wang)

4) "2 *cun* below the elbow on the medial side, and directly below Qingling (HT 2)."

Note: Medical literature through the ages holds similar views on the location of the point. The description by Wang Bing in *Su Wen* is confused with Xiaohai (SI 8); while *Ji Cheng* also makes a wrong definition. Now the point is located at the midpoint of the line connecting the medial end of the cubital crease and the medial epicondyle of the humerus.

2. 5. 4 HT 4 Língdào 靈道

Name: Seen in *Jia Yi*.

Location:

1) "1.5 *cun*, or 1 *cun* posterior (proximal) to the wrist." (*Jia Yi*, etc.)

2) "1.5 *cun* posterior to the wrist." (*Qian Jin*, etc.)

3) "1.5 *cun* from the wrist or 1 *cun* posterior to Yanggu (SI 5), under the pisiform bone and on the big tendon (tendon of the ulnar flexor muscle of the wrist)." (*Xun Jing*)

Note: Medical literature through the ages holds similar views on the location of the point. It is located 1.5 *cun* proximal to the crease of the wrist, on the radial side of the tendon of the ulnar flexor muscle of the wrist. The description in *Xun Jing* is not correct and should not be followed, because Yanggu (SI 5), a point of the Hand-Taiyang Meridian, is not on the meridian of this point.

2. 5. 5 HT 5 Tōnglǐ 通裏

Name: Seen in *Ling Shu*.

Location:

1) "1.5 *cun* from the wrist, ... and 1 *cun* posterior (proximal) to the palm." (*Ling Shu*)

2) "1 *cun* posterior to the wrist." (*Jia Yi*, etc.)

3) "1 *cun* posterior to the wrist, on the palmar side." (*Liu Ji*)

Note: According to *Tai Su* the description of "1.5 *cun* from the wrist" in *Ling Shu* is a slip of the pen. This point is located 1 *cun* proximal to the crease of the wrist and on the radial side of the tendon of the ulnar flexor muscle of the wrist.

2. 5. 6 HT 6 Yīnxì 陰郄

Name: Seen in *Jia Yi*.

Location:

"0.5 *cun* from the wrist, and on the vessel (ulnar artery) posterior (proximal) to the palm."

(*Jia Yi*, etc.)

Note: Medical literature through the ages holds similar views on the location of the point. The point now is located 0.5 *cun* proximal to the crease of the wrist and on the radial side of the tendon of the ulnar flexor muscle of the wrist.

2. 5. 7 HT 7 Shénmén 神門

Name: Seen in *Jia Yi*.

Location:

1) "At the tip of the pisiform bone." (*Ling Shu*, etc.)

2) "In the depression posterior (proximal) to the tip of the pisiform bone." (*Jia Yi*, etc.)

Note: This point is in the depression proximal to the pisiform bone. Now the point is located at the ulnar end of the crease of the wrist, and in the depression on the radial side of the tendon of the ulnar flexor muscle of the wrist.

2. 5. 8 HT 8 Shàofǔ 少府

Name: Seen in *Jia Yi*.

Location:

1) "In the depression posterior (proximal) to the 5th metacarpophalangeal joint, on the level of Laogong (PC 8)." (*Jia Yi*, etc.)

2) "In the depression between the bones (4th and 5th metacarpal bones), posterior to the 5th metacarpophalangeal joint on the level of Laogong (PC 8)." (*Ju Ying*, etc.)

3) "In the depression between the bones and lateral to the line from Shenmen (HT 7) to the 5th metacarpophalangeal joint." (*Jin Jian*, etc.)

Note: When a fist is made, the point is at the part of the arm where the tip of the little finger touches, on the level of Laogong (PC 8).

2. 5. 9 HT 9 Shàochōng 少衝

Name: Seen in *Jia Yi*.

Location:

1) "On the radial side of the little finger, and the width of a chive leaf from the nail." (*Jia Yi*, etc.)

2) "On the radial side of the little finger, and the width of a chive leaf from the corner of the nail." (*Qian Jin*, etc.)

Note: Medical literature through the ages holds similar views on the location of the point. The width of a chive leaf is about 0.1 *cun*. The point is located at the radial side of the distal segment of the little finger, 0.1 *cun* from the corner of the nail.

2. 6. Points of the Small Intestine Meridian of Hand-Taiyang, SI
手太陽小腸經穴
Shǒutàiyáng Xiǎochángjīng Xué

2. 6. 1 SI 1 Shàozé 少澤

Name: Seen in *Ling Shu*.

Location:

1) "On the distal segment of the little finger." (*Ling Shu*)

2) "On the distal segment of the little finger, in the depression 0.1 *cun* from the nail." (*Jia*

Yi, etc.)

3) "On the ulnar side of the distal segment of the little finger, in the depression 0.1 *cun* from the nail." (*Qian Jin*, etc.)

Note: *Ling Shu* locates the points "on the distal segment of the little finger." *Jia Yi* says "it is in the depression 0.1 *cun* from the nail." Since the Small Intestine Meridian runs along the ulnar side of the little finger, *Qian Jin* points out it is "on the lateral (ulnar) side of the distal segment of the little finger." Afterwards, *Ju Ying* says it is "in the depression 0.1 *cun* from the corner of the nail." These descriptions have been followed by various medical books, so this point is now located on the ulnar side of the distal segment of the little finger 0.1 *cun* from the corner of the nail.

2. 6. 2 SI 2 Qiángǔ 前谷

Name: Seen in *Ling Shu*.

Location:

1) "In the depression anterior (distal) to the 5th metacarpophalangeal joint, on the lateral (ulnar) side." (*Ling Shu*)

2) "In the depression anterior to the 5th metacarpophalangeal joint, on the lateral side." (*Jia Yi*, etc.)

3) "On the lateral side of the little finger, anterior to the 5th metacarpophalangeal joint, in the depression on the crease." (*Liu Ji*)

Note: According to the descriptions in *Ling Shu* and *Jia Yi*, the location of the point is quite clear. *Liu Ji* adds that it is on the ulnar end of the crease of the 5th metacarpophalangeal joint, when a loose fist is made.

2. 6. 3 SI 3 Hòuxī 後谿

Name: Seen in *Ling Shu*.

Location:

1) "On the lateral (ulnar) side of the hand and posterior (proximal) to the 5th metacarpophalangeal joint." (*Ling Shu*, etc.)

2) "In the depression posterior to the 5th metacarpophalangeal joint and on the lateral side of the little finger." (*Jia Yi*, etc.)

3) "In the depression under the prominent bone anterior (distal) to the wrist, on the lateral side of the hand." (*Sheng Hui*, etc.)

4) "On the lateral side of the little finger, at the end of the crease of the 5th metacarpophalangeal joint, when a fist is made." (*Ru Men*, etc.)

Note: Medical literature holds similar views on the location of the point. All agree that it is in the depression proximal to the 5th metacarpophalangeal joint of the little finger. *Ru Men* described it as "at the end of the crease of the 5th metacarpophalangeal joint," implying the ulnar end of the distal palmar crease. The assertion in *Sheng Hui* is quite confused with the location of Wangu (SI 4). Now it is at the ulnar end of the distal palmar crease and proximal to the 5th metacarpophalangeal joint, at the junction of the red and white skin.

2. 6. 4 SI 4 Wàngǔ 腕骨

Name: Seen in *Ling Shu*.

Location:

1) "On the lateral side of the hand and anterior (distal) to the wrist." (*Ling Shu*).

2) "On the lateral side of the hand, in the depression under the prominent bone (base of

the 5th metacarpal bone) anterior to the wrist." (*Jia Yi*, etc.)

3) "On the lateral side of the hand and in the cleft of the prominent bone anterior to the wrist, which appears when the hand is supinated." (*Liu Ji*)

Note: The point is located in the depression between the base of the 5th metacarpal bone and the triangular bone. According to the above descriptions the point is on the ulnar border of the hand, in the depression between the proximal end of the 5th metacarpal bone and the hamate bone, and at the junction of the red and white skin.

2. 6. 5 SI 5 Yánggǔ 陽谷

Name: Seen in *Ling Shu*.

Location:

1) "In the depression below the sharp bone (styloid process of the ulnar)." (*Ling Shu*)

2) "On the lateral side of the wrist, in the depression below the sharp bone." (*Jia Yi*, etc.)

3) "On the lateral side of the wrist, in the depression 0.2 *cun* below the sharp bone." (*Liu Ji*)

Note: Most of the medical literature follow the definition made in *Jia Yi*. The point is located on the ulnar border of the wrist and in the depression between the styloid process of the ulna and the triangular bone.

2. 6. 6 SI 6 Yǎnglǎo 養老

Name: Seen in *Jia Yi*.

Location:

1) "In the cleft above the head of the ulna, in the depression 1 *cun* posterior (proximal) to the wrist." (*Jia Yi*, etc.)

2) "Anterior (distal) to the head of the ulna, or in the depression 1 *cun* posterior to the wrist. (*Ju Ying*, etc.)

3) "1.5 *cun* posterior to Yanggu (SI 5)." (*Xun Jing*)

4) "1.2 *cun* from Yanggu (SI 5) and on the lateral (ulnar) side." (*Ji Cheng*)

Note: A cleft above the head of the ulna can be felt when the forearm is supinated. The cleft is about 1 *cun* proximal to the wrist, or 1.2 to 1.5 *cun* to Yanggu (SI 5). Now the point is located in the depression proximal to and on the radial side of the head of the ulna. The description in *Ju Ying* is wrong.

2. 6. 7 SI 7 Zhīzhèng 支正

Name: Seen in *Ling Shu*.

Location:

1) "5 *cun* above the wrist." (*Ling Shu*)

2) "5 *cun* posterior (proximal) to the wrist." (*Jia Yi*, etc.)

3) "5 *cun* posterior to the wrist, in the muscular groove on the bone." (*Su Wen*, annotated by Wang)

4) "5 *cun* posterior to the wrist and in the depression 4 *cun* from Yanglao (SI 6)." (*Sheng Hui*, etc.)

5) "At the midpoint between the wrist and the elbow." (*Liu Ji*)

Note: *Jia Yi* and other works locate it "5 *cun* posterior (proximal) to the wrist" and "4 *cun* from Yanglao (SI 6)." Only *Liu Ji* is an exception, arguing that it is located "at the midpoint between the wrist and elbow." In this case, the forearm is measured 10 *cun*, but according to present bone proportional measurement it is 12 *cun*. The Heart Meridian runs "on the posterior side of the forearm," so the point is located on the line connecting Yanggu (SI 5) and Xiaohai (SI 8), 5 *cun* proximal to the dorsal crease of the wrist.

2. 6. 8 SI 8 Xiǎohǎi 小海

Name: Seen in *Ling Shu*.

Location:

1) "Lateral to the big bone on the medial side of the elbow, in the depression 0.5 *cun* from the tip of the elbow." (*Ling Shu*)

2) "Lateral to the big bone on the medial side of the elbow, in the depression 0.5 *cun* from the tip of the elbow when the elbow is flexed." (*Jia Yi*, etc.)

3) "On the posterior side of the elbow and 1.5 *cun* lateral to the tip of the elbow." (*Ji Cheng*)

Note: Medical literature through the ages follows the description of *Ling Shu*. "The big bone on the medial side of the elbow" refers to the medial epicondyle of the humerus. The point now is located in the depression between the olecranon of the ulna and the medial epicondyle of the humerus, and 0.5 *cun* from the tip of the elbow. The description "1.5 *cun* lateral to the tip of the elbow" in *Ji Cheng* must be a slip of the pen; it should be 0.5 *cun*.

2. 6. 9 SI 9 Jiānzhēn 肩貞

Name: Seen in *Su Wen*.

Location:

1) "In the cleft between the two bones (scapula and humerus) below the scapula, in the depression posterior to Jianyu (LI 15)." (*Jia Yi*, etc.)

2) "Below the scapula, lateral to the big bone (scapular spine) and in the cleft between the two bones, in the depression posterior to the acromion." (*Jin Jian*)

3) "Below the scapula, lateral to the big bone, and in the cleft between the two bones, in the depression posterior to Jianyu (LI 15)." (*Feng Yuan*).

4) "Directly below Jugu (LI 16) and 6 *cun* from it, 8 *cun* lateral to the spinal column, and slightly above the axillary fold." (*Ji Cheng*)

Note: Most medical literature follows the description in *Jia Yi*. "Posterior to Jianyu (LI 15)" means posterior to the shoulder joint. The description "posterior to the acromion in *Jin Jian* carries the same meaning. The point is located posterior and inferior to the shoulder joint, 1 *cun* above the posterior end of the axillary fold.

2. 6. 10 SI 10 Nàoshū 臑俞

Name: Seen in *Jia Yi*.

Location:

1) "Below the big bone (scapular spine) posterior to Jianliao (SJ 14), and in the depression at the upper part of the scapula." (*Jia Yi*, etc.)

2) "Below the big bone posterior to Jianliao (SJ 14), and in the depression at the upper part of the scapula." (*Qian Jin*, etc.)

3) "1.5 *cun* below Jianzhen (SI 9)." (*Xun Jing*)

4) "1 *cun* above and 0.8 *cun* lateral to Jianzhen (SI 9)." (*Ji Cheng*)

Note: Most of the medical literature follow the description in *Qian Jin*. The point is posterior to Jianliao (SJ 14) and in the depression inferior to the scapular spine. *Xun Jing* and *Ji Cheng* say that the point is on the straight line through Jianzhen (SI 9), but the distance between them is varied. The natural landmark should be taken as the basis for the location. *Xun*

Jing says it is "below Jianzhen (SI 9)," but it should be "above Jianzhen (SI 9)." Now the point is located directly above Jianzhen (SI 9), in the depression below the lower border of the scapular spine.

2. 6. 11 SI 11 Tiānzōng 天宗

Name: Seen in *Jia Yi*.

Location:

1) "Behind Bingfeng (SI 12), and in the depression below the big bone (scapular spine)." (*Jia Yi*, etc.)

2) "In the depression below the scapular spine." (*Xun Jing*)

Note: Most of the medical literature follow the description in *Jia Yi*. Here "the depression" means the infrascapular fossa. Now, the point is in the depression at the centre of the infrascapular fossa and directly below Bingfeng (SI 12).

2. 6. 12 SI 12 Bǐngfēng 秉風

Name: Seen in *Jia Yi*.

Location:

1) "Lateral to Tianliao (SJ 15), posterior to the small tubercle of the bone (acromial end of the clavicle), in the depression when the arm is raised." (*Jia Yi*, etc.)

2) "1 *cun* anterior to Tianzong (SI 11), lateral to Jianliao (TE 14) and in the depression when the arm is raised." (*Xun Jing*)

Note: Most of the medical literature are in conformity with the description in *Jia Yi*, but *Xun Jing* supplements that it is 1 *cun* anterior to Tianzong (SI 11), indicating that the point is directly above Tianzong (SI 11), in the centre of the suprascapular fossa. Now, the point is located accordingly.

2. 6. 13 SI 13 Qūyuán 曲垣

Name: Seen in *Jia Yi*.

Location:

1) "Midway (between the spinal column and the acromion) of the shoulder and in the depression on the curved bone (medial corner of the suprascapular fossa)." (*Jia Yi*, etc.)

2) "Below the high bone." (*Xun Jing*)

3) "1.5 *cun* above Tianzong (SI 11) and slightly less than 3 *cun* below Jianjing (GB 21), between the two points but slightly deviated to the lateral side." (*Ji Cheng*)

Note: About the location of this point most books follow the description in *Jia Yi*. "The curved bone" refers to the medial corner of the suprascapular fossa, and it is roughly midway between the spinal column and the acromion. *Xun Jing* expresses the same meaning, but the description in *Ji Cheng* is not correct.

2. 6. 14 SI 14 Jiānwàishū 肩外俞

Name: Seen in *Jia Yi*.

Location:

1) "On the upper part of the scapula and in the depression 3 *cun* lateral to the spinal column." (*Jia Yi*, etc.)

2) "Below the shoulder process, above the scapula, close to Tianliao (SJ 15), and 3 *cun* lateral to Dazhui (DU 14)." (*Xun Jing*)

3) "On the upper part of the scapula, in the depression 3 *cun* lateral to the spinal column, on the level of Dazhu (BL 11)." (*Feng Yuan*)

Note: Medical literature through the ages all follows the description in *Jia Yi*. Accurate location of the point is given in *Feng Yuan*. The assertion in *Xun Jing* is not in conformity with that in *Jia Yi*, and should not be adopted.

2. 6. 15 SI 15 Jiānzhōngshū 肩中俞

Name: Seen in *Jia Yi*.

Location:

1) "On the medial side of the scapula, and in the depression 2 *cun* from the spinal column." (*Jia Yi*, etc.)

2) "2 *cun* lateral to Dazhui (DU 14)." (*Xun Jing*, etc.)

Note: Most medical books through the ages follow the description in *Jia Yi*. The present location of the point follows *Xun Jing*, which defines it as "2 *cun* lateral to Dazhui (DU 14)."

2. 6. 16 SI 16 Tiānchuāng 天窗

Name: Seen in *Ling Shu* and *Su Wen*.

Location:

1) "Below the angle of the mandible, posterior to Futu (LI 18), in the depression where the pulsation is palpable." (*Jia Yi*, etc.)

2) "Anterior to the big muscle on the neck, below the angle of the mandible, posterior to Futu (LI 18) and in the depression where the pulsation is palpable." (*Tong Ren*, etc.)

3) "Below the mastoid process, above the hairline, on the big muscle of the neck, and in the depression where the pulsation is palpable." (*Ru Men*, etc.)

4) "2 *cun* right below the ear." (*Ji Cheng*)

Note: Most of the medical literature follow the description in *Jia Yi*. The description in *Tong Ren* cannot be considered as the basis of location. According to *Jia Yi*, the point is located at the posterior border of the sternocleidomastoid muscle, posterior to Futu (LI 18), on the level of the laryngeal protuberance.

2. 6. 17 SI 17 Tiānróng 天容

Name: Seen in *Ling Shu*.

Location:

1) "Posterior to the ear and the mandibular angle." (*Jia Yi*, etc.)

2) "Below the ear and posterior to the mandibular angle." (*Qian Jin*, etc.)

3) "Below the ear and in the depression posterior to Jiache (ST 6)." (*Ru Men*)

Note: Medical literature through the ages holds the same view on the location of the point, which is posterior to the mandibular angle and in the depression on the anterior border of the sternocleidomastoid muscle.

2. 6. 18 SI 18 Quánliáo 顴髎

Name: Seen in *Jia Yi*.

Location:

1) "In the depression below the zygomatic bone." (*Jia Yi*, etc.)

2) "Below the zygomatic bone, and in the depression below the prominence of the bone." (*Tong Ren*, etc.)

3) "Directly below Tongziliao (GB 1)." (*Xun Jing*)

4) "About 2 *cun* directly below Tongziliao (GB 1) and inferior to the zygomatic bone." (*Ji Cheng*)

Note: Medical literature holds similar views on the location of the point, i.e. "in the depression below the zygomatic bone." *Tong Ren* also defines it as "below the prominence of the bone." Now, the point is directly below the outer canthus, and in the depression below the zygomatic bone.

2. 6. 19 SI 19 Tīnggōng 聽宮

Name: Seen in *Ling Shu*.

Location:

1) "Anterior to the tragus, which is like a piece of red bean." (*Jia Yi*, etc.)

2) "Anterior to the tragus." (*Jin Jian*, etc.)

3) "On the medial side of the muscle prominence anterior to the ear." (*Ji Cheng*)

Note: *Jia Yi* and other medical books all agree that this point is "anterior to the tragus." Now the point is located anterior to the tragus, posterior to the mandibular condyloid process and in the depression found when the mouth is open.

2. 7. Points of the Bladder Meridian of Foot-Taiyang, BL
足太陽膀胱經穴
Zútàiyáng Pángguāngjīng Xué

2. 7. 1 BL 1 Jīngmíng 睛明

Name: Seen in *Jia Yi*.

Location:

1) "Outside the inner canthus." (*Jia Yi*, etc.)

2) "At the inner canthus." (*Wai Tai*)

3) "In the depression outside the end of the inner canthus." (*Sheng Hui*)

4) "In the tear sac orifice at the inner canthus." (*Yu Long Jing*)

5) "In the depression 0.1 *cun* outside the inner canthus." (*Ju Ying*, etc.)

6) "In the depression in the red flesh of the inner canthus." (*Ru Men*)

Note: Medical literature through the ages holds similar views on the location of the point, and there are opinions such as "outside the inner canthus," "in the depression outside the inner canthus," and "0.1 *cun* outside the inner canthus." Therefore, the point is located on the face, in the depression slightly above the inner canthus. The locations recorded in *Yu Long Jing* and *Ru Men* are scarcely accepted.

2. 7. 2 BL 2 Cuánzhú 攢竹

Name: Seen in *Jia Yi*.

Location:

1) "In the depression on the medial end of the eyebrow." (*Jia Yi*, etc.)

2) "Directly above the inner canthus and in the depression of the medial end of the eyebrow." (*Xun Jing*)

Note: Medical literature through the ages is in conformity with the description in *Jia Yi*, thus the point is located on the face, in the depression of the medial end of the eyebrow, and at the supraorbital notch.

2. 7. 3 BL 3 Méichōng 眉衝

Name: Seen in *Mai Jing*.

Location:

1) "Directly above the medial end of the eyebrow and above the hairline." (*Sheng Hui*)

2) "Directly above the medial end of the eyebrow (0.5 *cun* above the hairline), and between Shenting (DU 24) and Qucha (BL 4)." (*Ru Men*)

Note: Originally the point had been located just on the hairline, but later *Ru Men* and others changed it to 0.5 *cun* above the hairline, which is accepted nowadays. Therefore the point is located on the head, directly above Cuanzhu (BL 2), 0.5 *cun* above the anterior hairline and on the line connecting Shenting (DU 24) and Qucha (BL 4).

2. 7. 4 BL 4 Qūchā 曲差

Name: Seen in *Jia Yi*.

Location:

1) "1.5 *cun* lateral to Shenting (DU 24) on both sides, and just on the hairline." (*Jia Yi*, etc.)

2) "1.5 *cun* lateral to Shenting (DU 24) and above the hairline." (*Tong Ren*)

3) "1 *cun* lateral to Shenting (DU 24)." (*Ji Cheng*)

Note: Originally *Jia Yi* located the point at 1.5 *cun* lateral to Shenting (DU 24) and just on the hairline, and later *Tong Ren* changed it to 0.5 *cun* above the anterior hairline. This opinion is adopted nowadays. Now, the point is located on the head, 0.5 *cun* directly above the midpoint of the anterior hairline and 1.5 *cun* lateral to the midline and at the junction of the medial third and middle third of the line connecting Shenting (DU 24) and Touwei (ST 8).

2. 7. 5 BL 5 Wǔchù 五處

Name: Seen in *Jia Yi*.

Location:

1) "Lateral to the Du Meridian, and 1.5 *cun* apart from Shangxing (DU 23) (1 *cun* apart from Qucha BL 4)." (*Jia Yi*)

2) "1.5 *cun* lateral to Shangxing (DU 23) (0.5 *cun* away from Qucha BL 4)." (*Tong Ren*)

Note: Medical literature through the ages is in conformity with the description in *Jia Yi*, locating the point as "lateral to the Du Meridian and 1.5 *cun* apart from Shangxing (DU 23)," but there are differing opinions concerning the distance between this point and Qucha (BL 4) —0.5 *cun* or 1 *cun*, because there are two locations of Qucha (BL 4), i.e. "just on the hairline" and "0.5 *cun* above the hairline." Now the point is located on the head, 1 *cun* directly above the midpoint of the anterior hairline and 1.5 *cun* lateral to the midline.

2. 7. 6 BL 6 Chéngguāng 承光

Name: Seen in *Jia Yi*.

Location:

1) "2 *cun* posterior to Wuchu (BL 5)." (*Jia Yi*, etc.)

2) "1 *cun* posterior to Wuchu (BL 5)." (*Qian Jin*, etc.)

3) "1.5 *cun* posterior to Wuchu (BL 5)." (*Tong Ren*)

Note: All the ancient medical literature regards Wuchu (BL 5) as the basis for locating Chengguang (BL 6), but there is a divergence of opinions on how far it is posterior to Wuchu (BI 5). Some propose 2 *cun* (such as *Jia Yi*, *Wai Tai*, *Su Wen*, annotated by Wang Bing, and *Sheng Hui*, etc.), some 1 *cun* (such as *Qian Jin* and *Ju Ying*) and some 1.5 *cun* (such as *Qian Jin*, *Tong Ren* and most of the medical literature since the Song Dynasty). Nowadays, the last one is adopted, thus the point is located on the head, 2.5 *cun* directly above the midpoint of the anterior hairline and 1.5 *cun* lateral to the midline.

2. 7. 7 BL 7 Tōngtiān 通天

Name: Seen in *Jia Yi*.

Location:

1) "1.5 *cun* posterior to Chengguang (BL 6)." (*Jia Yi*, etc.)

2) "1.5 *cun* lateral to Baihui (DU 20)." (*Tu Yi*)

Note: Medical literature through the ages says it is 1.5 *cun* posterior to Chengguang (BL 6), but there are differing opinions on the distance between the points of this meridian on the vertex. For instance, *Jia Yi* describes that Wuchu (BL 5) is 1 *cun* above the hairline and 2 *cun* posterior to Chengguang (BL 6), and Tongtian (BL 7) is 1.5 *cun* posterior to Chengguang (BL 6), amounting to 4.5 *cun* above the hairline. *Tong Ren* illustrates the same location of Wuchu (BL 5) as *Jia Yi*, but locates Chengguang (BL 6) 1.5 *cun* posterior to Wuchu (BL 5), and Tongtian (BL 7) 1.5 *cun* posterior to Chengguang (BL 6), thus amounting to 4 *cun* above the hairline. This opinion has been adopted nowadays. So the point is located on the head, 4 *cun* directly above the midpoint of the anterior hairline and 1.5 *cun* lateral to the midline.

2. 7. 8 BL 8 Luòquè 絡卻

Name: Seen in *Jia Yi*.

Location:

1) "1.3 *cun* posterior to Tongtian (BL 7)." (*Jia Yi*)

2) "1.5 *cun* posterior to Tongtian (BL 7)." (*Qian Jin*, etc.)

Note: Medical literature after the Tang Dynasty all locates it 1.5 *cun* posterior to Tongtian (BL 7). This opinion is accepted today. Now, the point is located on the head, 5.5 *cun* directly above the midpoint of the anterior hairline and 1.5 *cun* lateral to the midline.

2. 7. 9 BL 9 Yùzhěn 玉枕

Name: Seen in *Jia Yi*.

Location:

1) "0.7 *cun* posterior to Luoque (BL 8), 1.3 *cun* lateral to Naohu (DU 17), on the muscular prominence of the occiput and 3 *cun* above the hairline." (*Jia Yi*, etc.)

2) "0.75 *cun* posterior to Luoque (BL 8), 1.3 *cun* lateral to Naohu (DU 17), on the muscular prominence of the occiput and 3 *cun* above the hairline." (*Qian Jin*, etc.)

3) "1.5 *cun* posterior to Luoque (BL 8), 1.3 *cun* lateral to Naohu (DU 17), on the muscular prominence of the occiput and 3 *cun* above the hairline." (*Tong Ren*, etc.)

4) "1.5 *cun* or 0.7 *cun* posterior to Luoque (BL 8), 1.3 *cun* lateral to Naohu (DU 17), on the muscular prominence of the occiput and 2 *cun* above the hairline." (*Ju Ying*, etc.)

5) "1.5 *cun* posterior to Luoque (BL 8), 1.5 *cun* lateral to Naohu (DU 17), on the muscular prominence of the occiput, and 2 *cun* above the hairline; or, to measure from the anterior hairline to which Naohu (DU 17) is located 9.5 *cun* posteriorly, and Yuzhen (BL 9) is 1.5 *cun* lateral to it on both sides." (*Xun Jing*)

6) "1.8 *cun* posterior to Luoque (BL 8)." (*Ji Cheng*)

Note: Medical literature through the ages all says the location of this point is "posterior to Luoque (BL 8)" and "lateral to Naohu (DU 17)," although there is wide divergence of opinions on the distance between these points. However, the natural landmark is quite distinguishable, i.e., the location should be on the level of the superior border of the external occipital protuberance (where Naohu, DU 17, is located). Concerning the transverse distance from this point to the midline, most medical books are in conformity with the description in *Jia Yi*. Therefore, the point is located on the occiput, 2.5 *cun* directly above the midpoint of the posterior hairline, 1.3 *cun* lateral to the midline, and in the depression of the level with the upper border of the external occipital protuberance.

2. 7. 10 BL 10 Tiānzhù 天柱

Name: Seen in *Ling Shu* and *Su Wen*.

Location:

1) "On the border of the posterior hairline, and in the depression lateral to the big muscle." (*Jia Yi*, etc.)

2) "In the posterior hairline, 0.5 *cun* lateral to the midline, in the depression lateral to the big muscle, 1.5 *cun* below Fengchi (GB 20)." (*Xun Jing*)

3) "Nearly 2 *cun* posterior to Yuzhen (BL 9), 0.7 *cun* apart from Fengfu (DU 16) and 0.6 *cun* from Fengchi (GB 20)." (*Ji Cheng*)

Note: Most of the medical literature follow the definition in *Jia Yi*, i.e. on the posterior hairline lateral to the big muscle (m. trapezius). This opinion is also adopted today. The distance from this point to the Du Meridian and to Fengchi (GB 20) described in *Xun Jing* and *Ji Cheng* can be only taken as reference, and the anatomical landmark should be regarded as the basis. Now, the point is located on the nape, in the depression on the lateral border of the trapezius muscle and 1.3 *cun* lateral to the midpoint of the posterior hairline.

2. 7. 11 BL 11 Dàzhù 大杼

Name: Seen in *Ling Shu* and *Su Wen*.

Location:

1) "Below the 1st vertebra on the nape, and in the depression 1.5 *cun* lateral to the midline." (*Jia Yi*, etc.)

2) "1.5 *cun* lateral to the midline." (*Zi Sheng*)

3) "Below the 1st vertebra on the nape, and in the depression 2 *cun* lateral to the midline." (*Tu Yi*, etc.)

Note: All the points on the back and low back below Dazhu (BL 11) are longitudinally measured with the spinous process as the basis, and this measurement has been recorded unanimously in various medical books. Now, the distance between the medial border of the scapula and the posterior midline is measured as 3 *cun*, and the middle is 1.5 *cun*. The points on the back are located longitudinally on the middle between the medial border of the scapula and the posterior midline, and transversely on the same level with the lower border of the corresponding spinous process. So Dazhu (BL 11) is located on the back, below the spinous process of the 1st thoracic vertebra, and 1.5 *cun* lateral to the posterior midline.

2. 7. 12 BL 12 Fēngmén 風門

Name: Seen in *Jia Yi*.

Location:

1) "1.5 *cun* lateral to the lower border of the 2nd vertebra on both sides." (*Jia Yi*, etc.)

2) "Below the 2nd vertebra, 2 *cun* lateral to the midline of the spine on both sides. To be located with the patient sitting upright." (*Tu Yi*, etc.)

Note: Medical literature through the ages holds similar views on the location of the point. Fengmen (BL 12) is located on the back, below the spinous process of the 2nd thoracic vertebra, and 1.5 *cun* lateral to the posterior midline.

2. 7. 13 BL 13 Fèishū 肺俞

Name: Seen in *Ling Shu* and *Su Wen*.

Location:

1) "On both sides of the 3rd vertebra, and 3 *cun* apart from each other." (*Ling Shu*)

2) "Below the 3rd vertebra and 1.5 *cun* lateral to the midline." (*Jia Yi*, etc.)

3) "Below the 3rd vertebra and 2 *cun* lateral to the spine." (*Shen Ying*, etc.)

Note: The statement "3 *cun* apart from each other" includes the spine, so the points are 1.5 *cun* lateral to the posterior midline on each side. Feishu (BL 13) is located on the back, below the spinous process of the 3rd thoracic vertebra, and 1.5 *cun* lateral to the posterior midline.

2. 7. 14 BL 14 Juéyīnshū 厥陰俞

Name: Seen in *Qian Jin*.

Location:

1) "1.5 *cun* lateral to the 4th vertebra." (*Qian Jin*, etc.)

2) "Below the 4th vertebra and 2 *cun* lateral to the midline of the spine. To be located with the patient sitting upright." (*Tu Yi*, etc.)

Note: Medical literature through the ages holds similar views on the location of the point, and the opinion in *Qian Jin* is adopted nowadays. So Jueyinshu (BL 14) is located on the back, below the spinous process of the 4th thoracic vertebra, and 1.5 *cun* lateral to the posterior midline.

2. 7. 15 BL 15 Xīnshū 心俞

Name: Seen in *Ling Shu* and *Su Wen*.

Location:

1) "On both sides of the 5th vertebra, and 3 *cun* apart from each other." (*Ling Shu*)

2) "Below the 5th vertebra and 1.5 *cun* lateral to the midline." (*Jia Yi*, etc.)

3) "Below the 5th vertebra and 2 *cun* lateral to the spine. To be located with the patient sitting upright." (*Tu Yi*, etc.)

Note: Medical literature through the ages holds similar views on the location of the point, and the opinion in *Jia Yi* is adopted nowadays. So Xinshu (BL 15) is located on the back, below the spinous process of the 5th thoracic vertebra, and 1.5 *cun* lateral to the posterior midline.

2. 7. 16 BL 16 Dūshū 督俞

Name: Seen in *Sheng Hui*.

Location:

1) "Below and 1.5 *cun* lateral to the 6th vertebra." (*Sheng Hui*)

2) "Below the 6th vertebra, down from Xinshu (BL 15), 2 *cun* lateral to the midline of the spine. To be located with the patient sitting upright." (*Jin Jian*, etc.)

Note: Medical literature through the ages holds similar views on the location of the point, and the location in *Sheng Hui* is adopted nowadays. So Dushu (BL 16) is located on the back, below the spinous process of the 6th thoracic vertebra and 1.5 *cun* lateral to the posterior midline.

2. 7. 17 BL 17 Géshū 膈俞

Name: Seen in *Ling Shu*.

Location:

1) "On the level of the 7th vertebra, ... and 3 *cun* apart from each other." (*Ling Shu*)

2) "Below the 7th vertebra and 1.5 *cun* lateral on both sides." (*Jia Yi*, etc.)

3) "Below and 2 *cun* lateral to the 7th vertebra." (*Shen Ying*, etc.)

Note: Medical literature through the ages holds similar views on the location of the point, and the location in *Jia Yi* is adopted nowadays. So Geshu (BL 17) is located on the back below the spinous process of the 7th thoracic vertebra and 1.5 *cun* lateral to the posterior midline.

2. 7. 18 BL 18 Gānshū 肝俞

Name: Seen in *Ling Shu* and *Su Wen*.

Location:

1) "On the level of the 9th vertebra, ... and 3 *cun* apart from each other." (*Ling Shu*)

2) "Below and 1.5 *cun* lateral to the 9th vertebra." (*Jia Yi*, etc.)

3) "Below and 2 *cun* lateral to the 9th vertebra." (*Shen Ying*, etc.)

Note: Medical literature through the ages holds similar views on the location of the point, and the location in *Jia Yi* is adopted nowadays. So Ganshu (BL 18) is located on the back, below the spinous process of the 9th thoracic vertebra and 1.5 *cun* lateral to the posterior midline.

2. 7. 19 BL 19 Dǎnshū 膽俞

Name: Seen in *Mai Jing*.

Location:

1) "Below and 1.5 *cun* lateral to the 10th vertebra." (*Jia Yi*, etc.)

2) "Below the 10th vertebra and 2 *cun* lateral to the midline of the spine. To be located with the patient sitting upright." (*Tu Yi*, etc.)

Note: Medical literature through the ages holds similar views on the location of the point, and the location in *Jia Yi* is adopted nowadays. So Danshu (BL 19) is located on the back, below the spinous process of the 10th thoracic vertebra and 1.5 *cun* lateral to the posterior midline.

2. 7. 20 BL 20 Píshū 脾俞

Name: Seen in *Ling Shu* and *Su Wen*.

Location:

1) "On the level of the 11th vertebra, ... and 3 *cun* apart from each other." (*Ling Shu*)

2) "Below and 1.5 *cun* lateral to the 11th vertebra." (*Jia Yi*, etc.)

3) "Below the 11th vertebra and 2 *cun* lateral to the midline of the spine. To be located with the patient sitting upright." (*Tu Yi*, etc.)

Note: Medical literature through the ages holds similar views on the location of the point, and the location in *Jia Yi* is adopted nowadays. So Pishu (BL 20) is located on the back, below the spinous process of the 11th thoracic vertebra and 1.5 *cun* lateral to the posterior midline.

2. 7. 21 BL 21 Wèishū 胃俞

Name: Seen in *Mai Jing*.

Location:

1) "Below and 1.5 *cun* lateral to the 12th vertebra." (*Jia Yi*, etc.)

2) "Below the 12th vertebra and 2 *cun* lateral to the midline of the spine. To be located with the patient sitting upright." (*Tu Yi*, etc.)

Note: Medical literature through the ages holds similar views on the location of the point, and the location in *Jia Yi* is adopted nowadays. So Weishu (BL 21) is located on the back, below the spinous process of the 12th thoracic vertebra, and 1.5 *cun* lateral to the posterior midline.

2. 7. 22 BL 22 Sānjiāoshū 三焦俞

Name: Seen in *Jia Yi*.

Location:

1) "Below and 1.5 *cun* lateral to the 13th vertebra." (*Jia Yi*, etc.)

2) "Below the 13th vertebra and 2 *cun* lateral to the midline of the spine. To be located with the patient sitting upright." (*Tu Yi*, etc.)

Note: Medical literature through the ages holds similar views on the location of the point, and the location in *Jia Yi* is adopted nowadays. So Sanjiaoshu (BL 22) is located on the low back, below the spinous process of the 1st lumbar vertebra and 1.5 *cun* lateral to the posterior midline.

2. 7. 23 BL 23 Shènshū 腎俞

Name: Seen in *Ling Shu* and *Su Wen*.

Location:

1) "On the level of the 14th vertebra and 3 *cun* apart from each other." (*Ling Shu*)

2) "Below and 1.5 *cun* lateral to the 14th vertebra." (*Jia Yi*, etc.)

3) "Below the 14th vertebra, on the level of the umbilicus, and 2 *cun* lateral to the posterior midline." (*Shen Ying*, etc.)

Note: Medical literature through the ages holds similar views on the location of the point, and the location in *Jia Yi* is adopted nowadays. So Shenshu (BL 23) is located on the low back, below the spinous process of the 2nd lumbar vertebra and 1.5 *cun* lateral to the posterior midline.

2. 7. 24 BL 24 Qìhǎishū 氣海俞

Name: Seen in *Sheng Hui*.

Location:

1) "Below and 2 *cun* lateral to the 15th vertebra." (*Sheng Hui*, etc.)

2) "Below the 15th vertebra down from Shenshu (BL 23) and 2 *cun* lateral to the midline of the spine. To be located with the patient sitting upright. (*Jin Jian*, etc.)

Note: Medical literature through the ages holds similar views on the location of the point, and the location in *Sheng Hui* is adopted nowadays. So Qihaishu (BL 24) is located on the low back below the spinous process of the 3rd lumbar vertebra, and 1.5 *cun* lateral to the posterior midline.

2. 7. 25 BL 25 Dàchángshū 大腸俞

Name: Seen in *Mai Jing*.

Location:

1) "On the level of the 16th vertebra." (*Mai Jing*)

2) "Below and 1.5 *cun* lateral to the 16th vertebra." (*Jia Yi*, etc.)

3) "Below the 16th vertebra and 2 *cun* lateral to the midline of the spine. To be located with the patient in a prone position." (*Tu Yi*, etc.)

Note: Medical literature through the ages holds similar views on the location of the point, and the location in *Jia Yi* is adopted nowadays. So Dachangshu (BL 25) is located on the low back below the spinous process of the 4th lumbar vertebra, and 1.5 *cun* lateral to the posterior midline.

2. 7. 26 BL 26 Guānyuánshū 關元俞

Name: Seen in *Sheng Hui*.

Location:

1) "Below and 1.5 *cun* lateral to the 17th vertebra." (*Sheng Hui*)

2) "Down from Dachangshu (BL 25), below the 17th vertebra and 2 *cun* lateral to the midline of the spine. To be located with the patient in a prone position." (*Jin Jian*, etc.)

Note: Medical literature through the ages holds similar views on the location of the point, and the location in *Jia Yi* is followed. So Guanyuanshu (BL 26) is located on the low back, below the spinous process of the 5th lumbar vertebra, and 1.5 *cun* lateral to the posterior midline.

2. 7. 27 BL 27 Xiǎochángshū 小腸俞

Name: Seen in *Mai Jing*.

Location:

1) "On the back and on the level of the 18th vertebra." (*Mai Jing*)

2) "Below and 1.5 *cun* lateral to the 18th vertebra." (*Jia Yi*, etc.)

3) "Below the 18th vertebra and 2 *cun* lateral to the midline of the spine. To be located with the patient in a prone position." (*Tu Yi*, etc.)

Note: Medical literature through the ages holds similar views on the location of the point, and the location in *Jia Yi* is accepted. So Xiaochangshu (BL 23) is located on the sacrum on the level of the 1st posterior sacral foramen, and 1.5 *cun* lateral to the median sacral crest.

2. 7. 28 BL 28 Pángguāngshū 膀胱俞

Name: Seen in *Mai Jing*.

Location:

1) "On the level of the 19th vertebra." (*Mai Jing*)

2) "Below and 1.5 *cun* lateral to the 19th vertebra." (*Jia Yi*, etc.)

3) "Below the 19th vertebra and 2 *cun* lateral to the midline. To be located with the patient in a prone position." (*Tu Yi*, etc.)

Note: Medical literature through the ages holds similar views on the location of the point, and the location in *Jia Yi* is followed. So Pangguangshu (BL 28) is located on the sacrum on the level of the 2nd posterior sacral foramen, and 1.5 *cun* lateral to the median sacral crest.

2. 7. 29 BL 29 Zhōnglǚshū 中膂俞

Name: Seen in *Ling Shu*.

Location:

1) "Below and 1.5 *cun* lateral to the 20th vertebra." (*Jia Yi*, etc.)

2) "Below the 20th vertebra, 2 *cun* lateral to the midline of the spine, in the paravertebral muscle. To be located with the patient in a prone position." (*Tu Yi*, etc.)

Note: Medical literature through the ages holds similar views on the location of the point, and the location in *Jia Yi* is followed. So Zhonglushu (BL 29) is located on the sacrum on the level of the 3rd posterior sacral foramen, and 1.5 *cun* lateral to the median sacral crest.

2. 7. 30 BL 30 Báihuánshū 白環俞

Name: Seen in *Jia Yi*.

Location:

1) "Below and 1.5 *cun* lateral to the 21st vertebra." (*Jia Yi*, etc.)

2) "Below the 21st vertebra and 2 *cun* lateral to the midline of the spine. To be located with the patient sitting upright." (*Tu Yi*, etc.)

Note: Medical literature through the ages holds similar views on the location of the point, and the location in *Jia Yi* is followed. So Baihuanshu (BL 30) is located on the sacrum on the level of the 4th posterior sacral foramen, and 1.5 *cun* lateral to the median sacral crest.

2. 7. 31 BL 31 Shàngliáo 上髎

Name: Seen in *Jia Yi*.

Location:

1) "In the 1st hole, 1 *cun* below the ilium and in the depression lateral to the spine." (*Jia*

Yi, etc.)

2) "In the iliac region with four holes in the bone on each side, ... in the depression below the ilium." (*Su Wen*, annotated by Wang)

3) "0.5 *cun* lateral to the 17th vertebra." (*Xun Jing*)

4) "1 *cun* below the ilium, lateral to the lower border of the 18th vertebra, and in the 1st depression beside the spine." (*Feng Yuan*)

5) "0.5 *cun* below Yaoyangguan (DU 3), 1 *cun* lateral to the posterior midline, and medial to Xiaochangshu (BL 27)." (*Ji Cheng*)

Note: The location of this point is quite clear, i.e. in the 1st posterior sacral foramen of the lumbosacral region. The assertion in *Xun Jing*, or "0.5 *cun* lateral to the lower border of the spinous process of the 5th lumbar vertebra," cannot be followed because it is not in the 1st sacral foramen. The opinion in *Ji Cheng* and *Feng Yuan* is not in conformity with the illustration in *Jia Yi*, but the distance of "1 *cun* lateral to the posterior midline" can be used as a reference in finding the anatomical landmark. Now, the point is located on the sacrum, at the midpoint between the posterior superior iliac spine and the posterior midline, just at the 1st posterior sacral foramen.

2. 7. 32 BL 32 Cìliáo 次髎

Name: Seen in *Jia Yi*.

Location:

1) "In the 2nd hole, and in the depression lateral to the spine." (*Jia Yi*)

2) "0.5 *cun* lateral to the 18th vertebra." (*Xun Jing*)

3) "Below the 19th vertebra and in the 2nd depression beside the spine." (*Feng Yuan*)

4) "Below Shangliao (BL 31), and medial to Pangguangshu (BL 28)." (*Ji Cheng*)

Note: This point is located at the 2nd sacral foramen, but *Xun Jing* illustrates the point as "0.5 *cun* lateral to the lower border of the 18th vertebra," which is evidently not in the 2nd posterior sacral foramen. The descriptions in *Ji Cheng* and *Feng Yuan* are unanimous with that in *Jia Yi*. So the point is located on the sacrum, medial and inferior to the posterior superior iliac spine, just at the 2nd posterior sacral foramen.

2. 7. 33 BL 33 Zhōngliáo 中髎

Name: Seen in *Jia Yi*.

Location:

1) "In the 3rd hole, and in the depression lateral to the spine." (*Jia Yi*, etc.)

2) "0.5 *cun* lateral to the 19th vertebra." (*Xun Jing*)

3) "Below the 20th vertebra and in the 3rd depression beside the spine." (*Feng Yuan*)

4) "Below Ciliao (BL 32) and medial to Zhonglushu (BL 29)." (*Ji Cheng*)

Note: *Xun Jing* locates the point 0.5 *cun* lateral to the lower border of the 19th vertebra, so it is not in the 3rd sacral foramen. The opinion in *Ji Cheng* and *Feng Yuan* are in accord with that in *Jia Yi*. Now, the point is located on the sacrum, medial and inferior to Ciliao (BL 32), just at the 3rd posterior sacral foramen.

2. 7. 34 BL 34 Xiàliáo 下髎

Name: Seen in *Jia Yi*.

Location:

1) "In the 4th hole and in the depression lateral to the spine." (*Jia Yi*, etc.)

2) "0.5 *cun* lateral to the 20th vertebra." (*Xun Jing*)

3) "Below the 21st vertebra and in the 4th depression beside the spine." (*Feng Yuan*)

4) "1.2 *cun* below Zhongliao (BL 33)." (*Ji Cheng*)

Note: This point is located in the 4th posterior sacral foramen, but *Xun Jing* locates it 0.5 *cun* lateral to the lower border of the 20th vertebra, so it is not in the 4th sacral foramen. *Ji Cheng* and *Xun Jing* illustrate the same location as *Jia Yi*. Now, the point is located on the sacrum, medial and inferior to Zhongliao (BL 33), just at the 3rd posterior sacral foramen.

2. 7. 35 BL 35 Huìyáng 會陽

Name: Seen in *Jia Yi*.

Location:

1) "On both sides of the coccyx." (*Jia Yi*, etc.)

2) "1.5 *cun* lateral to the coccyx." (*Ru Men*)

3) "On both sides of Changqiang (DU 1) and 1.5 *cun* lateral to the spine." (*Xun Jing*)

4) "Below Xialiao (BL 34), 0.5 *cun* lateral to the coccyx." (*Jin Jian*, etc.)

Note: This point is beside the coccyx. The location in *Xun Jing* is too low and lateral, and cannot be accepted. The description of "0.5 *cun* lateral to the coccyx" in *Jin Jian* is in conformity with that in *Jia Yi* and is accepted today. Therefore, Huiyang (BL 35) is located on the sacrum, 0.5 *cun* lateral to the tip of the coccyx.

2. 7. 36 BL 36 Chéngfú 承扶

Name: Seen in *Jia Yi*.

Location:

1) "Below the buttock on the posterior aspect of the thigh, and in the middle of the crease." (*Jia Yi*, etc.)

2) "Below the buttock on the posterior aspect of the thigh, and in the middle of the crease." (*Qian Jin*, etc.)

3) "In the middle of the transverse crease below the buttock." (*Sheng Hui*, etc.)

Note: Medical literature through the ages holds similar views on the location of the point, that is, in the middle of the crease below the buttock. Now the point is located on the posterior side of the thigh, and at the midpoint of the inferior gluteal crease.

2. 7. 37 BL 37 Yīnmén 殷門

Name: Seen in *Jia Yi*.

Location:

1) "6 *cun* below Chengfu (BL 36)." (*Jia Yi*, etc.)

2) "3 *cun* below Fuxi (BL 38)." (*Da Cheng*, etc.)

3) "1 *cun* below Fuxi (BL 38) and 2.5 *cun* above Weizhong (BL 40)." (*Xun Jing*, etc.)

Note: Most medical books follow the opinion in *Jia Yi*, locating the point 6 *cun* directly below Chengfu (BL 36). *Da Cheng* and *Xun Jing* are wrong by determining the point as below Fuxi (BL 38), because Fuxi (BL 38) is located 1 *cun* above Weiyang (BL 39). If Yinmen (BL 37) is 3 *cun* below Fuxi (BL 38), it should be situated on the leg, and if it is 1 *cun* below, it would overlap with Weiyang (BL 39). Now, the point is located on the posterior side of the thigh and on the line connecting Chengfu (BL 36) and Weizhong (BL 40), and 6 *cun* below Chengfu (BL 36).

2. 7. 38 BL 38 Fúxì 浮郄

Name: Seen in *Jia Yi*.

Location:

1) "1 *cun* above Weiyang (BL 39), and to be located with the patient's knees flexed." (*Jia Yi*, etc.)

2) "1 *cun* above Weiyang (BL 39), and to be located with the patient's knees extended." (*Qian Jin*, etc.)

3) "2.5 *cun* above Weizhong (BL 40)." (*Xun Jing*)

4) "1 *cun* obliquely laterosuperior to Yinmen (BL 37) and can be located with the patient's knees flexed. Hence it is 1 *cun* above Weiyang (BL 39)." (*Jin Jian*)

5) "1.3 *cun* below Yinmen (BL 37)." (*Ji Cheng*)

Note: Most of the medical literature agree the point is "1 *cun* above Weiyang (BL 39)," and this location is adopted nowadays. *Xun Jing* wrongly locates this point, as well as Yinmen (BL 37), as "2.5 *cun* above Weizhong (BL 40)." The location described in *Ji Cheng* is too high. The opinion in *Jin Jian* is wrong too because "1 *cun* obliquely laterosuperior to Yinmen (BL 37)" cannot coincide with "1 *cun* above Weiyang (BL 39)." Now, the point is located at the lateral end of the popliteal crease, 1 *cun* above Weiyang (BL 39), medial to the tendon of the biceps muscle of the thigh.

2. 7. 39 BL 39 Wěiyáng 委陽

Name: Seen in *Ling Shu* and *Su Wen*.

Location:

1) "On the lateral side of the popliteal fossa." (*Ling Shu*, etc.)

2) "On the lateral side of the popliteal fossa, between the two tendons, and 6 *cun* below Chengfu (BL 36)." (*Jia Yi*, etc.)

3) "1.6 *cun* below Chengfu (BL 36)." (*Ju Ying*)

4) "On the lateral side of the popliteal crease, between the two tendons, 2 *cun* lateral to Weizhong (BL 40). To be located with the patient's body bent." (*Ru Men*)

5) "1.5 *cun* above Weizhong (BL 40), slightly oblique to the posterior aspect, on the level of Yinmen (BL 37)." (*Xun Jing*)

Note: Most medical books are in conformity with *Jia Yi*, locating the point on the lateral side of the popliteal fossa and between the two tendons, which refer to the tendon of the biceps muscle of the thigh and the lateral head of the gastrocnemius muscle. The major landmarks are the popliteal crease and the two tendons, thus the point is located at the lateral end of the popliteal crease, medial to the tendon of the biceps muscle of the thigh, 1 *cun* above Weiyang (BL 39).

2. 7. 40 BL 40 Wěizhōng 委中

Name: Seen in *Ling Shu* and *Su Wen*.

Location:

1) "In the centre of the popliteal fossa." (*Ling Shu*, etc.)

2) "In the centre of the popliteal fossa, at the midpoint of the crease where the pulsation is palpable." (*Jia Yi*, etc.)

3) "In the popliteal crease, and in the depression between the two tendons and two bones —Zhen Quan." (*Sheng Hui*)

Note: Medical literature through the ages holds similar views on the location of the point, i.e. the point is at the midpoint of the transverse crease of the popliteal fossa. The "two tendons" mentioned by Zhen Quan refer to the median and lateral heads of the gastrocnemius muscle, while the "two bones" to the knee joint. The current location is the same as that in *Jia Yi*. Now, the point is located at the midpoint of the popliteal crease, between the tendons of the biceps muscle of the thigh and the semitendinous muscle.

2. 7. 41 BL 41 Fùfēn 附分

Name: Seen in *Jia Yi*.

Location:

1) "Below the 2nd vertebra, 2 *cun* lateral to the medial border of the nape." (*Jia Yi*, etc.)

2) "Below the 2nd vertebra and 3.5 *cun* lateral to the midline of the spine. To be located with the patient sitting upright." (*Tu Yi*, etc.)

Note: Medical literature through the ages holds similar views on the location of the point, but there is a slight difference on the transverse distance from the point to the spine. Now Fufen (BL 41) is located on the back, below the spinous process of the 2nd thoracic vertebra and 3 *cun* lateral to the posterior midline.

2. 7. 42 BL 42 Pòhù 魄户

Name: Seen in *Jia Yi*.

Location:

1) "Below and 3 *cun* lateral to the 3rd vertebra." (*Jia Yi*, etc.)

2) "Below the 3rd vertebra and 3.5 *cun* lateral to the midline of the spine. To be located with the patient sitting upright." (*Tu Yi*, etc.)

Note: Medical literature through the ages holds similar views on the location of the point, though there is a slight difference on the transverse distance from the point to the spine. Now Pohu (BL 42) is located on the back, below the spinous process of the 3rd thoracic vertebra and 3 *cun* lateral to the posterior midline.

2. 7. 43 BL 43 Gāohuāng 膏肓

Name: Seen in *Qian Jin*.

Location:

1) "Below and 3 *cun* lateral to the 4th vertebra and above the 5th vertebra." (*Tong Ren*, etc.)

2) "Below and 3.5 *cun* lateral to the 4th vertebra, in the 4th intercostal space and one finger-breadth apart from the scapula." (*Shen Ying*, etc.)

Note: Medical literature through the ages holds similar views on the location of the point, though there is a slight difference on the transverse distance from the point to the spine. Now Gaohuang (BL 43) is located on the back, below the spinous process of the 4th thoracic vertebra and 3 *cun* lateral to the posterior midline.

2. 7. 44 BL 44 Shéntáng 神堂

Name: Seen in *Jia Yi*.

Location:

1) "Below the 5th vertebra, in the depression 3 *cun* lateral to the spine." (*Jia Yi*, etc.)

2) "Below the 5th vertebra and in the depression 3.5 *cun* lateral to the midline of the spine. To be located with the patient sitting upright," (*Tu Yi*, etc.)

Note: Medical literature through the ages holds similar views on the location of the point, though there is a slight difference on the transverse distance from the point to the spine. Now Shentang (BL 44) is located on the back, below the spinous process of the 5th thoracic vertebra and 3 *cun* lateral to the posterior midline.

2. 7. 45 BL 45 Yìxǐ 譩譆

Name: Seen in *Su Wen*.

Location:

1) "On the back, 3 *cun* lateral to the spine." (*Su Wen*)

2) "On the medial border of the scapula, below and 3 *cun* lateral to the 6th vertebra." (*Jia Yi*, etc.)

3) "On the medial border of the scapula, below the 6th vertebra and 3.5 *cun* lateral to the midline of the spine. To be located with the patient sitting upright." (*Tu Yi*, etc.)

Note: Most of the medical literature are in conformity with *Jia Yi*, though there is a slight difference on the transverse distance from the point to the spine. Now Yixi (BL 45) is located on the back, below the spinous process of the 6th thoracic vertebra and 3 *cun* lateral to the posterior midline.

2. 7. 46 BL 46 Géguān 膈關

Name: Seen in *Jia Yi*.

Location:

1) "In the depression, below and 3 *cun* lateral to the 7th vertebra." (*Jia Yi*, etc.)

2) "In the depression, below the 7th vertebra and 3.5 *cun* lateral to the midline of the spine. To be located with the patient sitting upright and the shoulders thrown back." (*Tu Yi*, etc.)

Note: Medical literature through the ages holds similar views on the location of the point, though there is a slight difference on the transverse distance from the point to the spine. Now Geguan (BL 46) is located on the back, below the spinous process of the 7th thoracic vertebra and 3 *cun* lateral to the posterior midline.

2. 7. 47 BL 47 Húnmén 魂門

Name: Seen in *Jia Yi*.

Location:

1) "In the depression, below and 3 *cun* lateral to the 9th vertebra." (*Jia Yi*, etc.)

2) "Below the 10th vertebra—*Wai Tai*." (*Qian Jin*)

3) "In the depression, below the 9th vertebra and 3.5 *cun* lateral to the midline of the spine. To be located with the patient sitting upright." (*Tu Yi*, etc.)

Note: Medical literature through the ages holds similar views on the location of the point, though there is a slight difference on the transverse distance from the point to the spine. Now Hunmen (BL 47) is located on the back, below the spinous process of the 9th thoracic vertebra and 3 *cun* lateral to the posterior midline.

2. 7. 48 BL 48 Yánggāng 陽綱

Name: Seen in *Jia Yi*.

Location:

1) "In the depression, below and 3 *cun* lateral to the 10th vertebra." (*Jia Yi*, etc.)

2) "In the depression, below the 10th vertebra and 3.5 *cun* lateral to the midline of the spine. To be located with the patient sitting upright." (*Tu Yi*, etc.)

Note: Medical literature through the ages holds similar views on the location of the point, though there is a slight difference on the transverse distance from the point to the spine. Now Yanggang (BL 48) is located on the back, below the spinous process of the 10th thoracic vertebra and 3 *cun* lateral to the posterior midline.

2. 7. 49 BL 49 Yìshè 意舍

Name: Seen in *Jia Yi*.

Location:

1) "In the depression, below and 3 *cun* lateral to the 11th vertebra." (*Jia Yi*, etc.)

2) "In the depression, below the 11th vertebra and 3.5 *cun* lateral to the midline of the spine. To be located with the patient sitting upright." (*Tu Yi*, etc.)

Note: Medical literature through the ages holds similar views on the location of the point, though there is a slight difference on the transverse distance from the point to the spine. Now Yishe (BL 49) is located on the back, below the spinous process of the 11th thoracic vertebra and 3 *cun* lateral to the posterior midline.

2. 7. 50 BL 50 Wèicāng 胃倉

Name: Seen in *Jia Yi*.

Location:

1) "In the depression, below and 3 *cun* lateral to the 12th vertebra." (*Jia Yi*, etc.)

2) "In the depression, below the 12th vertebra and 3.5 *cun* lateral to the midline of the spine. To be located with the patient sitting upright." (*Tu Yi*, etc.)

Note: Medical literature through the ages holds similar views on the location of the point, though there is a slight difference on the transverse distance from the point to the spine. Now Weicang (BL 45) is located on the back, below the spinous process of the 12th thoracic vertebra and 3 *cun* lateral to the posterior midline.

2. 7. 51 BL 51 Huāngmén 肓門

Name: Seen in *Jia Yi*.

Location:

1) "Below and 3 *cun* lateral to the 13th vertebra." (*Jia Yi*, etc.)

2) "Below the 13th vertebra, 3.5 *cun* lateral to the midline of the spine, in the depression between the ribs, on the level of Jiuwei (RN 15)." (*Tu Yi*, etc.)

Note: Medical literature through the ages holds similar views on the location of the point, though there is a slight difference on the transverse distance from the point to the spine. Now Huangmen (BL 51) is located on the low back, below the spinous process of the 1st lumbar vertebra and 3 *cun* lateral to the posterior midline.

2. 7. 52 BL 52 Zhìshì 志室

Name: Seen in *Jia Yi*.

Location:

1) "In the depression, below and 3 *cun* lateral to the 14th vertebra." (*Jia Yi*, etc.)

2) "In the depression, below and 3.5 *cun* lateral to the 14th vertebra. To be located with the patient sitting upright, torso bent slightly forward."(*Sheng Hui*, etc.)

Note: Medical literature through the ages holds similar views on the location of the point, though there is a slight difference on the transverse distance from the point to the spine. Now Zhishi (BL 52) is located on the low back, below the spinous process of the 2nd lumbar vertebra and 3 *cun* lateral to the posterior midline.

2. 7. 53 BL 53 Bāohuāng 胞肓

Name: Seen in *Jia Yi*.

Location:

1) "In the depression, below and 3 *cun* lateral to the 19th vertebra." (*Jia Yi*, etc.)

2) "In the depression, below the 19th vertebra and 3.5 *cun* lateral to the midline of the

spine. To be located with the patient in a prone position." (*Tu Yi*, etc.)

Note: Medical literature through the ages holds similar views on the location of the point, though there is a slight difference on the transverse distance from the point to the spine. Now Baohuang (BL 53) is located on the buttock, on the level of the 2nd posterior sacral foramen and 3 *cun* lateral to the median sacral crest.

2. 7. 54 BL 54 Zhìbiān 秩邊

Name: Seen in *Jia Yi*.

Location:

1) "In the depression, below and 3 *cun* lateral to the 21st vertebra." (*Jia Yi*, etc.)

2) "Below and 3 *cun* lateral to the 20th vertebra. To be located with the patient in a prone position." (*Sheng Hui*, etc.)

3) "In the depression, below the 21st vertebra and 3.5 *cun* lateral to the midline of the spine." (*Tu Yi*, etc.)

Note: There are differing opinions in locating this point. *Jia Yi* holds that the point is located below and 3 *cun* lateral to the 21st vertebra whereas *Qian Jin*, *Wai Tai*, *Su Wen* (annotated by Wang Bing), *Tong Ren*, and *Zi Sheng* agree that the point is located below and 3 *cun* lateral to the 20th vertebra, which is adopted by *Fa Hui*, *Ju Ying*, *Da Cheng*, *Liu Ji*, *Xun Jing*, etc. Now, the former is more commonly accepted, thus the point is located on the buttock, on the level of the 4th posterior sacral foramen, and 3 *cun* lateral to the median sacral crest.

2. 7. 55 BL 55 Héyáng 合陽

Name: Seen in *Jia Yi*.

Location:

1) "2 *cun* below the midpoint of the popliteal crease." (*Jia Yi*, etc.)

2) "3 *cun* below the midpoint of the popliteal crease." (*Qian Jin*, etc.)

Note: All medical literature holds that the point is located below the midpoint of the popliteal crease where Weizhong (BL 40) is situated. However, concerning the distance from the point to the crease, some of the books say it is 3 *cun* while others say it is 2 *cun*. At present, the illustration in *Jia Yi* is commonly accepted, thus the point is located on the posterior side of the leg, on the line connecting Weizhong (BL 40) and Chengshan (BL 57) 2 *cun* below Weizhong (BL 40).

2. 7. 56 BL 56 Chéngjīn 承筋

Name: Seen in *Jia Yi*.

Location:

1) "In the depression, at the centre of the belly of the gastrocnemius muscle." (*Jia Yi*, etc.)

2) "Posterior to the tibia, 7 *cun* above the heel, and in the depression, at the centre of the belly of the gastrocnemius muscle." (*Qian Jin*, etc.)

3) "In the depression, at the centre of the belly of the gastrocnemius muscle." (*Wai Tai*)

4) "5 *cun* below the popliteal crease, ... in the depression at the centre of the belly of the gastrocnemius muscle." (*Su Wen*, annotated by Wang)

5) "9 *cun* above Pucan (BL 61) or 1 *cun* above Chengshan (BL 57)." (*Xun Jing*)

6) "2 *cun* below Heyang (BL 55)." (*Ji Cheng*)

Note: This point is located on the posterior side of the leg, on the line connecting Weizhong (BL 40) and Chengshan (BL 57), at the centre of the gastrocnemius muscle belly, and 5 *cun* below Weizhong (BL 40). *Su Wen*, annotated by Wang Bing, implies the same location. The record in *Qian Jin* indicates a location inferior to Chengshan (BL 57). *Xun Jing* and *Ji Cheng* do not locate the point at the centre of the belly of the gastrocnemius muscle, so their opinion cannot be accepted.

2. 7. 57 BL 57 Chéngshān 承山

Name: Seen in *Ling Shu*.

Location:

1) "Below the belly of the gastrocnemius muscle, and in the depression at the junction of the muscles." (*Jia Yi*, etc.)

2) "At the junction of the muscles of the calf." (*Ju Ying*, etc.)

3) "Approximately 8 *cun* above Pucan (BL 61)." (*Xun Jing*)

4) "8.5 *cun* below Weizhong (BL 40)." (*Ji Cheng*)

Note: Most of the medical literature through the ages locate the point in conformity with the opinion in *Jia Yi*. "In the depression at the junction of the muscles" means that the point is below the top of the junction of the two bellies of the gastrocnemius muscle. The modern location is just the same. The bone-proportional *cun* measurement is not so definite as the muscular landmark. Now, this point is located on the posterior midline of the leg, between Weizhong (BL 40) and Kunlun (BL 60), in a pointed depression formed below the gastrocnemius muscle belly when the leg is stretched or the heel is lifted.

2. 7. 58 BL 58 Fēiyáng 飛揚

Name: Seen in *Ling Shu* and *Su Wen*.

Location:

1) "7 *cun* from the ankle." (*Ling Shu*, etc.)

2) "7 *cun* above the external malleolus." (*Jia Yi*, etc.)

3) "9 *cun* above the external malleolus." (*Zi Sheng*)

4) "1.5 *cun* below Chengshan (BL 57)." (*Xun Jing*)

5) "Obliquely inferior to Chengshan (BL 57) and in the depression 7 *cun* above the posterior border of the external malleolus." (*Jin Jian*)

Note: Most of the medical literature are in conformity with *Jia Yi*. *Jin Jian* points out definitely that the point is obliquely inferior to Chengshan (BL 57), and above the posterior border of the external malleolus, thus 7 *cun* directly above Kunlun (BL 60). Nowadays, the point is located on the posterior side of the leg, 7 *cun* directly above Kunlun (BL 60) and 1 *cun* lateral and inferior to Chengshan (BL 57). *Zi Sheng* illustrates the point 9 *cun* above the external malleolus and above Chengshan (BL 57), which is doubted as an incorrect description. The opinion in *Xun Jing* should be interpreted as the point being obliquely inferior to Chengshan (BL 57).

2. 7. 59 BL 59 Fūyáng 跗陽

Name: Seen in *Jia Yi*.

Location:

1) "3 *cun* above the external malleolus, anterior to the course of the Taiyang Meridian and posterior to that of the Shaoyang Meridian, and between the tendon and the bone." (*Jia Yi*, etc.)

2) "2 *cun* above the posterior border of the external malleolus, and in the depression between the tendon and the bone." (*Sheng Hui*)

3) "2 *cun* above Kunlun (BL 60)." (*Xun Jing*)

4) "3 *cun* above Kunlun (BL 60)." (*Ji Cheng*)

Note: Most of the medical literature through the ages follow the opinion in *Jia Yi*. The point is located on the posterior side of the leg, posterior to the lateral malleolus and 3 *cun* directly above Kunlun (BL 60).

2. 7. 60 BL 60 Kūnlún 昆侖

Name: Seen in *Ling Shu*.

Location:

1) "Posterior to the external malleolus and above the calcaneum." (*Ling Shu*, etc.)

2) "Posterior to the external malleolus and in the depression above the calcaneum, where the pulsation is palpable." (*Jia Yi*, etc.)

3) "0.5 *cun* posterior to the external malleolus, in the depression above the calcaneum, where the pulsation is palpable." (*Da Cheng*, etc.)

4) "On the level of the tip of the external malleolus and 1 *cun* posterior to it, where the artery is palpable, and opposite to Taixi (KI 3)." (*Xun Jing*)

Note: Medical literature through the ages holds similar views on the location of the point, all of which locate it "posterior to the external malleolus and above the calcaneum." Some illustrate it as "0.5 *cun* posterior to the external malleolus," which implies that the point is 0.5 *cun* posterior to the posterior border of the external malleolus. The detailed description in *Xun Jing* illustrates it as "on the level of the tip of the external malleolus" and "opposite to Taixi (KI 3)." Now, the point is located posterior to the lateral malleolus and in the depression between the tip of the external malleolus and the Achilles tendon.

2. 7. 61 BL 61 Púcān 僕参

Name: Seen in *Jia Yi*.

Location:

1) "In the depression of the calcaneum, and to be located with the patient's ankle extended." (*Jia Yi*, etc.)

2) "Below the eminent bone of the heel, at the junction of the red and white skin and in the depression of the wrinkled region. To be located with the patient's foot extended." (*Xun Jing*)

3) "More than 2 *cun* directly below Kunlun (BL 60), and on the border of the heel." (*Ji Cheng*)

Note: Most of the medical literature through the ages are in conformity with *Jia Yi*. The description "at the junction of the red and white skin" in *Xun Jing* is essentially the same as that of "on the border of the heel" in *Ji Cheng*. Now, this location is accepted, so Pucan (BL 61) is located on the lateral side of the foot, posterior and inferior to the external malleolus, directly below Kunlun (BL 60), lateral to the calcaneum and at the junction of the red and white skin.

2. 7. 62 BL 62 Shēnmài 申脈

Name: Seen in *Jia Yi*.

Location:

1) "0.5 *cun* below the external malleolus." (*Su Wen*)

2) "In the depression, a fingernail breadth below the external malleolus." (*Jia Yi*, etc.)

3) "In the depression, 1 *cun* anterior to the external malleolus." (*Sheng Hui*)

Note: *Su Wen* and *Jia Yi* locate the point in the depression directly below the tip of the external malleolus. Now the location of Shenmai (BL 62) follows that described in *Jia Yi*.

However, "1 *cun* anterior to the external malleolus" recorded in *Sheng Hui* is too low and anterior, which is discrepant with the location illustrated in *Jia Yi*. Now, the point is located on the lateral side of the foot and in the depression directly below the external malleolus.

2. 7. 63 BL 63 Jīnmén 金門

Name: Seen in *Jia Yi*.

Location:

1) "Below the external malleolus." (*Jia Yi*, etc.)

2) "Below the external malleolus, 1 *cun* below Shenmai (BL 62)." (*Ju Ying*, etc.)

3) "Posterior to Qiuxu (GB 40) and anterior to Shenmai (BL 62), in the depression below the external malleolus." (*Xun Jing*)

4) "1 *cun* below the external malleolus." (*Feng Yuan*)

Note: *Jia Yi* locates the point "below the external malleolus." *Ju Ying* describes it in detail, i.e. "1 *cun* below Shenmai (BL 62)" or "1 *cun* below the external malleolus," which shows the distance between this point and the external malleolus. *Xun Jing* locates it "posterior to Qiuxu (GB 40) and anterior to Shenmai (BL 62), in the depression below the external malleolus." After summarizing all these opinions, we can now conclude that Jinmen (BL 63) is located on the lateral side of the foot, directly below the anterior border of the external malleolus and on the lower border of the cuboid bone.

2. 7. 64 BL 64 Jīnggǔ 京骨

Name: Seen in *Ling Shu*.

Location:

1) "Below the big bone on the lateral side of the foot." (*Ling Shu*)

2) "Below the big bone on the lateral side of the foot, and in the depression at the junction of the red and white skin. It can be located by pressing." (*Jia Yi*, etc.)

Note: Medical literature through the ages holds similar views on the location of the point, i.e. below the big bone, at the junction of the red and white skin of the lateral side of the foot. The "big bone" is the tuberosity of the 5th metatarsal bone. Now, the point is located on the lateral side of the foot, below the tuberosity of the 5th metatarsal bone and at the junction of the red and white skin.

2. 7. 65 BL 65 Shùgǔ 束骨

Name: Seen in *Ling Shu*.

Location:

1) "In the depression posterior to the joint of the 5th toe." (*Ling Shu*)

2) "On the lateral side of the little toe, in the depression posterior to its joint." (*Mai Jing*, etc.)

3) "On the lateral side of the little toe, in the depression posterior to its joint, at the junction of the red and white skin." (*Su Wen*, annotated by Wang)

4) "2 *cun* anterior to Jinggu (BL 64), on the lateral side of the little toe, posterior to its joint." (*Ji Cheng*)

Note: Medical literature through the ages holds similar views on the location of the point, i.e. on the lateral side of the little toe, in the depression posterior to the joint of the little toe. In accordance with this opinion, now Shugu (BL 65) is located on the lateral side of the foot, posterior to the 5th metatarsophalangeal joint, and at the junction of the red and white skin.

2. 7. 66 BL 66 Zútōnggǔ 足通谷

Name: Seen in *Da Quan*, but known as Tonggu in *Ling Shu*.

Location:

1) "Anterolateral to the joint of the little toe." (*Ling Shu*)

2) "On the lateral side of the little toe, in the depression anterior to its joint." (*Jia Yi*, etc.)

3) "In the depression anterior to the joint of the little toe." (*Xun Jing*)

4) "Anterior to the lateral side of the proximal joint of the little toe, at the end of the crease of the joint." (*Ji Cheng*)

Note: Medical literature through the ages holds similar views on the location of the point, i.e. "on the lateral side of the little toe, in the depression anterior to its joint." Now Zutonggu (BL 66) is located on the lateral side of the foot, anterior to the 5th metatarsophalangeal joint and at the junction of the red and white skin.

2. 7. 67 BL 67 Zhiyin 至陰

Name: Seen in *Ling Shu*.

Location:

1) "At the top of the little toe." (*Ling Shu*)

2) "On the lateral side of the little toe, the width of a chive leaf from the nail." (*Jia Yi*)

3) "On the lateral side of the little toe, the width of a chive leaf from the corner of the nail." (*Qian Jin*, etc.)

Note: Medical literature through the ages holds similar views on the location of the point. Now it is located on the lateral side of the distal segment of the little toe, 0.1 *cun* from the corner of the toenail.

2. 8 Points of the Kidney Meridian of Foot-Shaoyin, KI
足少陰腎經穴
Zúshàoyin Shēnjīng Xué

2. 8. 1 KI 1 Yǒngquán 涌泉

Name: Seen in *Ling Shu* and *Su Wen*.

Location:

1) "In the centre of the sole." (*Ling Shu*)

2) "In the depression at the centre of the sole when the foot and toes are flexed." (*Jia Yi*, etc.)

3) "At the centre of the sole, on the margin of the white skin—Zhen Quan." (*Wai Tai*)

4) "In the 3rd crease of the foot, on the level of the 1st metatarsophalangeal joint, or at the midpoint of the line from the 3rd toe to the end of the heel." (*Liu Ji*)

Note: Medical literature through the ages holds similar views on the location of the point, i.e. in the centre of the sole, in the depression when the foot is in plantar flexion. The depression is not exactly in the centre of the sole, but a little anterior to it. In the bronze statue cast in the reign of Jiaqing, Yongquan (KI 1) is located in the depression of the anterior third of the sole. Now it is located on the sole in the depression appearing on the anterior part of the sole when the foot is in plantar flexion, approximately at the junction of the anterior third and the posterior two thirds of the line connecting the base of the 2nd and 3rd toes and the heel.

2. 8. 2 KI 2 Rángŭ 然谷

Name: Seen in *Ling Shu*.

Location:

1) "Below the navicular bone." (*Ling Shu*)

2) "In the depression below the big bone anterior to the medial malleolus." (*Jia Yi*, etc.)

3) "1 *cun* directly below the medial malleolus." (*Qian Jin*)

4) "In the depression below the navicular bone, 1 *cun* from Zhaohai (KI 6), at the junction of the red and white skin, on the opposite side of Jinggu (BL 64), slightly anterior to Yongquan (KI 1)." (*Xun Jing*)

5) "1 *cun* posterior to Gongsun (SP 4)." (*Ji Cheng*)

Note: Medical literature through the ages holds similar views on the location of the point. The "big bone anterior to the medial malleolus" refers to the navicular bone. The location in *Qian Jin* is not clear. *Xun Jing* locates this point "a little anterior" to Yongquan (KI 1), which is not consistent with the right situation. Now, the point is located on the medial border of the foot, below the tuberosity of the navicular bone and at the junction of the red and white skin.

2. 8. 3 KI 3 Tàixī 太谿

Name: Seen in *Ling Shu*.

Location:

1) "Posterior to the medial malleolus, in the depression above the calcaneus." (*Ling Shu*)

2) "Posterior to the medial malleolus, in the depression above the calcaneus, where the pulsation is palpable." (*Jia Yi*, etc.)

3) "0.5 *cun* posterior to the medial malleolus and above the calcaneus, where the pulsation is palpable." (*Shen Ying*)

4) "On the same level of the tip of the malleolus bone and 1 *cun* posterior to it, where the pulsation is palpable, and opposite to Kunlun (BL 60)." (*Xun Jing*)

Note: Medical literature through the ages holds similar views on the location of the point, i.e. posterior to the medial malleolus, above the calcaneus, and in the depression. Some say "0.5 *cun* posterior to the medial malleolus," or "0.1 *cun* posterior to the tip of the malleolus." According to their opinion, now Taixi (KI 3) is located on the medial side of the foot, posterior and inferior to the medial malleolus and in the depression between the tip of the medial malleolus and the Achilles tendon.

2. 8. 4 KI 4 Dàzhōng 大鐘

Name: Seen in *Ling Shu*.

Location:

1) "Posterior to the malleolus." (*Ling Shu*)

2) "In the depression of the heel." (*Jia Yi*, etc.)

3) "In the depression of the heel, on the big bone between two tendons." (*Ju Ying*)

4) "In the depression of the heel, approximately 0.5 *cun* posterior to Taixi (LI 3), at the junction of the red and white skin." (*Xun Jing*)

5) "1.5 *cun* posterior to Zhaohai (KI 6)." (*Ji Cheng*)

Note: In *Ling Shu*, *Jia Yi*, etc., the location of this point is not clear. It is comparatively clear in *Jiu Ying* and *Xun Jing*. Now, Dazhong (KI 4) is located on the medial side of the foot, posterior and inferior to the medial malleolus, and in the depression on the medial side of and anterior to the attachment of the Achilles tendon.

2. 8. 5 KI 5 Shuǐquán 水泉

Name: Seen in *Jia Yi*.

Location:

1) "1 *cun* inferior to Taixi (KI 3), below the medial malleolus." (*Jia Yi*, etc.)

2) "Directly below the medial malleolus, in the depression between two bones of the heel." (*Xun Jing*)

3) "Directly below Taixi (KI 3), inferior and a little posterior to the medial malleolus." (*Ji Cheng*)

Note: Most of the medical records follow *Jia Yi*. Now, Shuiquan (KI 5) is located on the medial side of the foot, posterior and inferior to the medial malleolus, 1 *cun* directly below Taixi (KI 3), and in the depression of the medial side of the tuberosity of the calcaneum. The location illustrated by *Xun Jing* is too anterior, and is not accepted.

2. 8. 6 KI 6 Zhàohǎi 照海

Name: Seen in *Jia Yi*.

Location:

1) "1 *cun* below the medial malleolus." (*Jia Yi*, etc.)

2) "One finger-breadth below the medial malleolus" or "0.4 *cun* below the medial malleolus." (*Qian Jin*)

3) "0.4 *cun* below the medial malleolus, tendons found anteriorly and posteriorly, malleolus bone superiorly and cartilage inferiorly." (*Da Cheng*, etc.)

Note: Medical literature through the ages holds similar views on the location of the point, i.e. inferior to the medial malleolus. But the distance between them varies from 0.4 *cun* to 1 *cun*. The description in *Da Cheng* is clearer, according to which Zhaohai (KI 6) is located on the medial side of the foot, in the depression below the tip of the medial malleolus.

2. 8. 7 KI 7 Fùliū 複溜

Name: Seen in *Ling Shu* and *Su Wen*.

Location:

1) "2 *cun* above the medial malleolus." (*Ling Shu*)

2) "In the depression 2 *cun* above the medial malleolus." (*Jia Yi*, etc.)

3) "2 *cun* superior to the medial malleolus, 0.5 *cun* posterior to the malleolus, directly above Taixi (KI 3)." (*Shen Ying*, etc.)

4) "In the depression of the tendons 2 *cun* superior to the medial malleolus; anteriorly Fuliu (KI 7) beside the bone, and posteriorly Jiaoxin (KI 8) beside the tendon, which is the border of these two points." (*Ju Ying*, etc.)

5) "0.5 *cun* posterior to Jiaoxin (KI 8), on the level of Jiaoxin (KI 8)." (*Ji Cheng*)

Note: Many of the medical literature through the ages follow *Jia Yi*. *Shen Ying* and others located the point "directly above Taixi (KI 3)," which is comparatively definite. But "below the malleolus" and "below the tip of the malleolus" are somewhat different. The location of Fuliu (KI 7) and Jiaoxin (KI 8) described in *Ju Ying* is contrary to the location adopted today. According to *Jia Yi*, "Jiaoxin (KI 8) is anterior to Shaoyin and posterior to Taiyin"; Jiaoxin (KI 8) should be beside the bone while Fuliu (KI 7) beside the tendon. In *Ji Cheng* the point is located accordingly, and this definition is followed now. So Fuliu (KI 7) is located on the medial side of the leg, directly above Taixi (KI 3) and anterior to the Achilles tendon.

2. 8. 8 KI 8 Jiāoxìn 交信

Name: Seen in *Jia Yi*.

Location:

1) "2 *cun* above the medial malleolus, anterior to Shaoyin, posterior to Taiyin, between the bone and the tendon." (*Jia Yi*, etc.)

2) "Posterior to and on the level of Fuliu (KI 7), Fuliu (KI 7) anteriorly beside the bone and Jiaoxin (KI 8) posteriorly beside the tendon, which is the border of these two points." (*Liu Ji*)

3) "A little posterior to Sanyinjiao (SP 6)." (*Xun Jing*)

Note: Most of the medical literature through the ages follow *Jia Yi*. The point is 2 *cun* above the medial malleolus. Its pertaining meridian curves forward from Fuliu (KI 7) to this point and crosses the Foot-Taiyin Meridian at Sanyinjiao (SP 6). So it is said that this point is anterior to Shaoyin and posterior to Taiyin. It is situated between the Achilles tendon and the medial border of the tibia. Now this view is accepted, and Jiaoxin (KI 8) is located on the medial side of the leg, 2 *cun* above Taixi (KI 3) and 0.5 *cun* anterior to Fuliu (KI 7), posterior to the medial border of the tibia. But the description in *Liu Ji* is wrong. See the note on Fuliu (KI 7).

2. 8. 9 KI 9 Zhùbīn 築賓

Name: Seen in *Jia Yi*.

Location:

1) "Above the medial malleolus, on the calf muscles." (*Jia Yi*, etc.)

2) "0.5 *cun* above the medial malleolus, on the calf muscles." (*Ju Ying*)

3) "Above the medial malleolus, on the calf muscles, on the big muscle behind the bone and inferior to the small muscle. To be located with the patient's knee flexed." (*Ru Men*)

4) "2 *cun* superior to and 1.5 *cun* posterior to Sanyinjiao (SP 6)." (*Ji Cheng*)

Note: Most of the medical literature follow *Jia Yi*, but its exact location is not clear. The "calf muscles" corresponds to the transitional part of the muscular and tendonous tissues of the triceps muscle of the leg. The location illustrated in *Ju Ying* is approximately 2 *cun* above Sanyinjiao (SP 6) and directly above Taixi (KI 3). *Ru Men* says it is "superior to the big muscle and inferior to the small muscle," but it is not clear. Now Zhubin (KI 9) is located on the medial side of the leg, on the line connecting Taixi (KI 3) and Yingu (KI 10), 5 *cun* above Taixi (KI 3), medial and inferior to the gastrocnemius muscle belly.

2. 8. 10 KI 10 Yīngǔ 陰谷

Name: Seen in *Ling Shu*.

Location:

1) "Posterior to the medial condyle of the tibia, inferior to the big muscle and superior to the small muscle. To be located by pressing and with the patient's knee flexed." (*Ling Shu*)

2) "Below the knee, posterior to the medial condyle of the tibia, inferior to the big muscle and superior to the small muscle. To be located by pressing and with the patient's knee flexed." (*Jia Yi*, etc.)

3) "0.5 *cun* posterior and a little inferior to Ququan (LR 8)." (*Ji Cheng*)

Note: Medical literature through the ages holds similar views on the location of the point. The "big and small muscles" refer to the semimembranous muscle and the semitendinous muscle respectively. When the knee is flexed, the point is located at the medial end of the popliteal crease, between the semimembranous and semitendinous muscles. Ququan (LR 8) is superior and anterior to Yingu (KI 10), as *Ji Cheng* says. Now, the point is located on the medial side of the popliteal fossa, between the tendons of semitendinous and semimembranous muscles when the knee is flexed.

2. 8. 11 KI 11 Hénggŭ 横骨

Name: Seen in *Mai Jing*.

Location:

1) "0.5 *cun* below Dahe (KI 12) (0.5 *cun* lateral to the midline)." (*Jia Yi*, etc.)

2) "1 *cun* below Dahe (KI 12) (1.5 *cun* lateral to the midline)." (*Zi Sheng*, etc.)

3) "1 *cun* below Dahe (KI 12) (1 *cun* lateral to the midline, like a crescent moon over the middle of the pubis)." (*Da Cheng*, etc.)

Note: The distance between the points of the Kidney Meridian from Henggu (KI 11) to Huangshu (KI 16) except Zhongzhu (SJ 3) is 1 *cun* apart from each other, which is recorded in *Jia Yi* and followed by other classics. The description in *Da Cheng* is not correct because it cites wrongly the description of Qugu (RN 2) in *Qian Jin*. The distance between the point and the midline of the abdomen varies in different books, such as 0.5 *cun* (*Jia Yi*), 1 *cun* (*Da Cheng*), 1.5 *cun* (*Zi Sheng*), etc. The opinion in *Jia Yi* is accepted nowadays, so Henggu (KI 11) is located on the lower abdomen, 5 *cun* below the centre of the umbilicus and 0.5 *cun* lateral to the anterior midline.

2. 8. 12 KI 12 Dàhè 大赫

Name: Seen in *Jia Yi*.

Location:

1) "1 *cun* below Qixue (KI 13) (0.5 *cun* lateral to the midline)." (*Jia Yi*, etc.)

2) "1 *cun* below Qixue (KI 13) (1.5 *cun* lateral to the midline)." (*Zi Sheng*, etc.)

3) "1 *cun* below Qixue (KI 13) (1 *cun* lateral to the midline)." (*Da Cheng*, etc.)

Note: Medical literature through the ages locates the point 1 *cun* below Qixue (KI 13), but the distance between the point and the anterior midline is different. The opinion in *Jia Yi* is adopted nowadays, so Dahe (KI 12) is located on the lower abdomen, 4 *cun* below the centre of the umbilicus and 0.5 *cun* lateral to the anterior midline.

2. 8. 13 KI 13 Qìxué 氣穴

Name: Seen in *Jia Yi*.

Location:

1) "1 *cun* below Siman (KI 14) (0.5 *cun* lateral to the midline)." (*Jia Yi*, etc.)

2) "1 *cun* below Siman (KI 14) (1.5 *cun* lateral to the midline)."(*Zi Sheng*, etc.)

3) "1 *cun* below Siman (KI 14) (1 *cun* lateral to the midline)." (*Da Cheng*, etc.)

Note: Medical literature locates it 1 *cun* below Siman (KI 14), but the distance between the point and the anterior midline is different. The opinion in *Jia Yi* is adopted nowadays, so Qixue (KI 13) is located on the lower abdomen, 3 *cun* below the centre of the umbilicus, and 0.5 *cun* lateral to the anterior midline.

2. 8. 14 KI 14 Sìmăn 四滿

Name: Seen in *Jia Yi*.

Location:

1) "1 *cun* below Zhongzhu (KI 15) (0.5 *cun* lateral to the midline)." (*Jia Yi*, etc.)

2) "1 *cun* below Zhongzhu (KI 15) (1.5 *cun* lateral to the midline)." (*Zi Sheng*, etc.)

3) "1 *cun* below Zhongzhu (KI 15) (1 *cun* lateral to the midline)." (*Da Cheng*, etc.)

Note: Medical literature through the ages locates the point 1 *cun* below Zhongzhu (KI 15), but the distance between the point and the anterior midline is different. The opinion in *Jia Yi* is adopted nowadays, so Siman (KI 14) is located on the lower abdomen, 2 *cun* below the centre of the umbilicus and 0.5 *cun* lateral to the anterior midline.

2. 8. 15 KI 15 Zhōngzhù 中注

Name: Seen in *Jia Yi*.

Location:

1) "0.5 *cun* below Huangshu (KI 16) (0.5 *cun* lateral to the midline)." (*Jia Yi*, etc.)

2) "1 *cun* below Huangshu (KI 16) (0.5 *cun* lateral to the midline)." (*Tong Ren*, etc.)

3) "1 *cun* below Huangshu (KI 16) (1.5 *cun* lateral to the midline)." (*Zi Sheng*, etc.)

4) "1 *cun* below Huangshu (KI 16) (1 *cun* lateral to the midline)." (*Da Cheng*, etc.)

Note: Most of the medical literature after the Song Dynasty locate the point 1 *cun* below Huangshu (KI 16), while *Jia Yi*, *Qian Jin* and others locate it 0.5 *cun* below Huangshu (KI 16). The opinion in *Tong Ren* is adopted nowadays, so Zhongzhu (KI 15) is located on the lower abdomen, 1 *cun* below the centre of the umbilicus and 0.5 *cun* lateral to the anterior midline.

2. 8. 16 KI 16 Huāngshū 肓俞

Name: Seen in *Jia Yi*.

Location:

1) "1 *cun* below Shangqu (KI 17) (0.5 *cun* lateral to the umbilicus)." (*Jia Yi*, etc.)

2) "1 *cun* below Shangqu (KI 17) (0.5 *cun* lateral to the umbilicus)." (*Zi Sheng*, etc.)

3) "1 *cun* below Shangqu (KI 17) (1 *cun* lateral to the umbilicus)." (*Da Cheng*, etc.)

4) "2 *cun* below Shangqu (KI 17) (1 *cun* wrongly defined in the old edition), 0.5 *cun* lateral to the umbilicus." (*Feng Yuan*)

Note: *Jia Yi* says "it is 0.5 *cun* lateral to the umbilicus," which is quite definite for this point, but the distance between the point and Shangqu (KI 17) is different. Now, Huangshu (KI 16) is located on the middle abdomen and 0.5 *cun* lateral to the centre of the umbilicus.

2. 8. 17 KI 17 Shāngqū 商曲

Name: Seen in *Jia Yi*.

Location:

1) "1 *cun* below Shiguan (KI 18) (0.5 *cun* lateral to the midline)." (*Jia Yi*, etc.)

2) "1 *cun* below Shiguan (KI 18) (0.5 *cun* lateral to the midline)." (*Zi Sheng*, etc.)

3) "2 *cun* from Huangshu (KI 16) (0.5 *cun* lateral to the midline)." (*Jin Jian*, etc.)

Note: Medical literature through the ages follows *Jia Yi*'s view about the location of the six points from Shangqu (KI 17) to Youmen (KI 21), namely Youmen (KI 21) is located in the depression 0.5 *cun* lateral to Juque (RN 14); Tonggu (KI 20) in the depression 1 *cun* below Youmen (KI 21); Yindu (KI 19) 1 *cun* below Tonggu (KL 20); Shiguan (KI 18) 1 *cun* below Yindu (KI 19); Shangqu (KI 17) 1 *cun* below Shiguan (KI 18); Huangshu (KI 16) 1 *cun* below Shangqu (KI 17) and 0.5 *cun* lateral to the umbilicus. Juque (RN 14) is 6 *cun* above the umbilicus, and from the umbilicus to Juque (RN 14) each *cun* apart lodges one point, and there should be seven points altogether, instead of six points. That is why *Jin Jian* says that the distance between Huangshu (KI 16) and Shangqu (KI 17) is 2 *cun*, which is accepted now. So Shangqu (KI 17) is located on the upper abdomen, 2 *cun* above the centre of the umbilicus and 0.5 *cun* lateral to the anterior midline.

2. 8. 18 KI 18 Shíguān 石關

Name: Seen in *Jia Yi*.

Location:

1) "1 *cun* below Yindu (KI 19) (0.5 *cun* lateral to the midline)." (*Jia Yi*, etc.)

2) "1 *cun* below Yindu (KI 19) (1.5 *cun* lateral to the midline)." (*Zi Sheng*, etc.)

Note: Most of the medical literature through the ages follow *Jia Yi*. Now, Shiguan (KI 18) is located on the upper abdomen, 3 *cun* above the centre of the umbilicus and 0.5 *cun* lateral to the anterior midline.

2. 8. 19 KI 19 Yīndū 陰都

Name: Seen in *Jia Yi*.

Location:

1) "1 *cun* below Tonggu (KI 20) (0.5 *cun* lateral to the midline)." (*Jia Yi*, etc.)

2) "1 *cun* below Tonggu (KI 20) (1.5 *cun* lateral to the midline)." (*Zi Sheng*, etc.)

Note: Most of the medical literature follow *Jia Yi*. Now, Yindu (KI 19) is located on the upper abdomen, 4 *cun* above the centre of the umbilicus and 0.5 *cun* lateral to the anterior midline.

2. 8. 20 KI 20 Fùtōnggŭ 腹通谷

Name: Seen in *Jia Yi* as "Tonggu," "fu" (abdomen) being added nowadays.

Location:

1) "In the depression 1 *cun* below Youmen (KI 21) (0.5 *cun* lateral to the midline)." (*Jia Yi*, etc.)

2) "On both sides of Shangwan (RN 13) (3 *cun* apart from each other and 1.5 *cun* lateral to the midline)." (*Sheng Hui*)

3) "1 *cun* below Youmen (KI 21) (taken as 1.5 *cun*) (0.5 *cun* lateral to Shangwan RN 13)." (*Feng Yuan*)

Note: Most of the medical literature through the ages follow *Jia Yi*. Now, Futonggu (KI 20) is located on the upper abdomen, 5 *cun* above the centre of the umbilicus and 0.5 *cun* lateral to the anterior midline. *Feng Yuan* wrongly says it is "1.5 *cun* below Youmen (KI 21) and lateral to Shangwan (RN 13)."

2. 8. 21 KI 21 Yōumén 幽門

Name: Seen in *Jia Yi*.

Location:

1) "In the depression 0.5 *cun* lateral to Juque (RN 14)." (*Jia Yi*, etc.)

2) "In the depression 1.5 *cun* lateral to Juque (RN 14)." (*Sheng Hui*, etc.)

Note: Medical literature through the ages locates the point on both sides of Juque (RN 14) as 6 *cun* above the umbilicus. As for the distance from the midline there is a difference of 0.5 *cun* and 1.5 *cun*. The opinion in *Jia Yi* is adopted nowadays, so Youmen (KI 21) is located on the upper abdomen, 6 *cun* above the centre of the umbilicus and 0.5 *cun* lateral to the anterior midline.

2. 8. 22 KI 22 Bùláng 步廊

Name: Seen in *Jia Yi*.

Location: "In the depression 1.6 *cun* below Shenfeng (KI 23), 2 *cun* lateral to the Ren Meridian on both sides. There are 12 points from Shufu (KI 27) to Bulang (KI 22)." (*Jia Yi*, etc.)

Note: All the points of this meridian on the chest are 2 *cun* lateral to the Ren Meridian. This point is in the depression 1.6 *cun* below Shenfeng (KI 23). Medical literature through the ages holds the same view on the location of the point. "1.6 *cun*" refers to the distance between the two ribs. Shenfeng (KI 23) is in the 4th intercostal space, so Bulang (KI 22) is located on the chest, in the 5th intercostal space and 2 *cun* lateral to the anterior midline.

2. 8. 23 KI 23 Shénfēng 神封

Name: Seen in *Jia Yi*.

Location: "In the depression 1.6 *cun* below Linxu (KI 24), 2 *cun* lateral to the Ren Meridian." (*Jia Yi*, etc.)

Note: Medical literature through the ages holds the same view on the location of the point. Now, Shenfeng (KI 23) is located on the chest, in the 4th intercostal space and 2 *cun* lateral to the anterior midline.

2. 8. 24 KI 24 Língxū 靈墟

Name: Seen in *Jia Yi*.

Location: "1.6 *cun* below Shencang (KI 25), 2 *cun* lateral to the Ren Meridian." (*Jia Yi*, etc.)

Note: Medical literature through the ages holds the same view on the location of the point. Now, Lingxu (KI 24) is located on the chest, in the 3rd intercostal space and 2 *cun* lateral to the anterior midline.

2. 8. 25 KI 25 Shéncáng 神藏

Name: Seen in *Jia Yi*.

Location: "In the depression 1.6 *cun* below Yuzhong (KI 26), 2 *cun* lateral to the Ren Meridian." (*Jia Yi*, etc.)

Note: Medical literature through the ages holds the same view on the location of the point. Now, Shencang (KI 25) is located on the chest, in the 2nd intercostal space and 2 *cun* lateral to the anterior midline.

2. 8. 26 KI 26 Yùzhōng 彧中

Name: Seen in *Jia Yi*.

Location:

1) "In the depression 1.6 *cun* below Shufu (KI 27), 2 *cun* lateral to the Ren Meridian." (*Jia Yi*, etc.)

2) "In the depression 1 *cun* to Shufu (KI 27)." (*Sheng Hui*)

Note: Medical literature through the ages holds similar views on the location of the point. "1.6 *cun* below Shufu (KI 27)" means that the point is one intercostal space inferior to Shufu (KI 27). Because the upper intercostal spaces are narrower than the lower ones, *Sheng Hui* locates the point "1 *cun* below Shufu (KI 27)." Now, Yuzhong (KI 26) is located on the chest, in the 1st intercostal space and 2 *cun* lateral to the anterior midline.

2. 8. 27 KI 27 Shūfǔ 俞府

Name: Seen in *Jia Yi*.

Location:

1) "Below the clavicle, in the depression 2 *cun* lateral to Xuanji (RN 21)." (*Jia Yi*, etc.)

2) "Below Qishe (ST 11), 2 *cun* lateral to Xuanji (RN 21). To be located with the patient's chin up." (*Da Cheng*)

3) "In the depression 1.6 *cun* below the clavicle. To be located with the patient's chin up, 2 *cun* lateral to Xuanji (RN 21)." (*Xun Jing*)

Note: Most of the medical literature through the ages follow *Jia Yi*, locating the point between the clavicle and the 1st rib, 2 *cun* lateral to Xuanji (RN 21) of the Ren Meridian. Now, Shufu (KI 27) is located on the chest, below the lower border of the clavicle and 2 *cun* lateral to the anterior midline.

2. 9 Points of the Pericardium Meridian of Hand-Jueyin, PC

手厥陰心包經穴

Shǒujuéyīn Xīnbáojīng Xué

2. 9. 1 PC 1 Tiānchí 天池

Name: Seen in *Ling Shu*.

Location:

1) "3 *cun* below the axilla." (*Ling Shu*)

2) "1 *cun* lateral to the breast, 3 *cun* below the axilla, near the hypochondriac region, in the intercostal space." (*Jia Yi*, etc.)

3) "2 *cun* lateral to the breast." (*Su Wen*, annotated by Wang)"

4) "1 or 2 *cun* lateral to the breast, approximately 3 *cun* below the axilla, in the intercostal space of the hypochondriac region." (*Jin Jian*)

5) "1 *cun* lateral and 0.5 *cun* inferior to the breast." (*Ji Cheng*)

Note: The nipples are situated in the 4th intercostal space, 3 *cun* from the axilla. Tianchi (PC 1) is located on the chest, 1 *cun* lateral to the nipple in the 4th intercostal space, and 5 *cun* lateral to the anterior midline. *Su Wen* (annotated by Wang Bing) says it is "2 *cun* lateral to the breast," which overlaps with the location of Tianxi (SP 18), and is undoubtedly a mistake. The location illustrated in *Jin Jian* is unclear and cannot be taken as a reference.

2. 9. 2 PC 2 Tiānquán 天泉

Name: Seen in *Jia Yi*.

Location:

1) "2 *cun* inferior to the axillary fold, on the medial side of the arm. Locate it with the patient's arm raised." (*Jia Yi*, etc.)

2) "2 *cun* below the axilla. Locate it with the patient's axilla exposed." (*Qian Jin*, etc.)

3) "3 *cun* below the axilla." (*Da Quan*)

4) "2 *cun* inferior to the anterior end of the axillary fold." (*Xun Jing*)

5) "Obliquely upward passing the axilla, 2 *cun* downward along the medial side of the arm. Locate it with the patient's arm raised." (*Jin Jian*)

6) "On the medial side of the arm, 1 *cun* or more directly below Jiquan (HT 1)."

Note: The distance between the point and the axillary fold is not unanimous in medical literature through the ages, i.e. 2 *cun*, 3 *cun*, and 1 *cun*, and 2 *cun* proposed by *Jia Yi* is commonly accepted. Since this meridian runs between the meridians Taiyin and Shaoyin, the point is located on the medial side of the arm, 2 *cun* below the anterior end of the axillary fold, between the long and short heads of the biceps muscle of the arm.

2. 9. 3 PC 3 Qūzé 曲澤

Name: Seen in *Ling Shu*.

Location:

1) "In the depression of the medial side of the elbow. Locate it with the patient's elbow flexed." (*Ling Shu*, etc.)

2) "In the depression of the medial side of the elbow, medial to the artery crossing the crease. Locate it with the patient's elbow flexed." (*Shen Ying*, etc.)

3) "In the depression of the medial side of the elbow, on the crease between the two tendons. Locate it with the patient's elbow flexed." (*Liu Ji*)

4) "On the medial side of the elbow, between the two tendons where the crease ends, on the level of Chize (LU 5), 1 *cun* apart from each other." (*Xun Jing*)

Note: Most of the medical literature through the ages follow *Ling Shu*, locating the point on the crease of the elbow and on the ulnar side of the biceps muscle of the arm, or on "the medial side of the big tendon when the elbow is flexed." The brachial artery is adjacent to this point, Chize (LU 5) is at the same level and lateral to it. Now, the point is located at the midpoint of the cubital crease and on the ulnar side of the tendon of the biceps muscle of the arm.

2. 9. 4 PC 4 Xìmén 郄門

Name: Seen in *Jia Yi*.

Location:

1) "5 *cun* from the wrist." (*Jia Yi*, etc.)

2) "Proximal to the hand, 5 *cun* from the wrist." (*Qian Jin*, etc.)

3) "5 *cun* proximal to the crease of the wrist between the two tendons." (*Xun Jing*)

Note: Medical literature through the ages holds similar views on the location of the point, i.e. on the palmar side of the forearm, on the line connecting Quze (PC 3) and Daling (PC 7), and 5 *cun* above the crease of the wrist.

2. 9. 5 PC 5 Jiānshǐ 間使

Name: Seen in *Ling Shu*.

Location:

1) "Between the two tendons, in the depression 3 *cun* proximally." (*Ling Shu*)

2) "In the depression 3 *cun* proximal to the hand, between the two tendons." (*Jia Yi*, etc.)

3) "1 *cun* from Neiguan (PC 6), 3 *cun* proximal to the hand." (*Da Quan*)

Note: Medical literature through the ages holds similar views on the location of the point. Now, Jianshi (PC 5) is located on the palmar side of the forearm, on the line connecting Quze (PC 3) and Daling (PC 7), 3 *cun* above the crease of the wrist, between the tendons of the long palmar muscle and radial flexor muscle of the wrist.

2. 9. 6 PC 6 Nèiguān 内關

Name: Seen in *Ling Shu*.

Location:

1) "2 *cun* from the wrist, between the two tendons." (*Ling Shu*, etc.)

2) "Proximal to the hand, 2 *cun* from the wrist." (*Jia Yi*)

3) "2 *cun* proximal to Daling (PC 7) opposite to Waiguan (SJ 5)." (*Xun Jing*)

Note: Medical literature through the ages holds similar views on the location of the point. Now, Neiguan (PC 6) is located on the palmar side of the forearm, on the line connecting Quze (PC 3) and Daling (PC 7), 2 *cun* above the crease of the wrist, between the tendons of the long palmar muscle and radial flexor muscle of the wrist.

2. 9. 7. PC 7 Dàlíng 大陵

Name: Seen in *Ling Shu*.

Location:

1) "In the depression proximal to the hand, between the two bones." (*Ling Shu*)

2) "In the depression proximal to the hand, between the two tendons." (*Jia Yi*, etc.)

3) "Proximal to the bone of the hand, between the two tendons." (*Ju Ying*)

Note: Medical literature through the ages holds similar views on the location of the point. The "two bones" refer to the ulna and the radius, and the "two tendons" to the tendons of the radial flexor muscle of the wrist and the long palmar muscle. Now, Daling (PC 7) is located at the midpoint of the crease of the wrist, between the tendons of the long palmar muscle and radial flexor muscle of the wrist.

2. 9. 8. PC 8 Láogōng 劳宫

Name: Seen in *Ling Shu*.

Location:

1) "On the palm, on the radial side of the 3rd metacarpal bone." (*Ling Shu*)

2) "In the centre of the palm, beside the artery." (*Jia Yi*, etc.)

3) "In the crease of the palm, beside the artery, at the place where the tip of the 4th finger lands when it is flexed." (*Sheng Hui*, etc.)

4) "At the place where the tip of the middle finger, not the 4th finger, lands when it is flexed." (*Zi Sheng*)

5) "In the centre of the palm, at the place where the 4th finger lands where it is flexed." (*Yu Long Jing*)

6) "At the place in between the tips of the middle and 4th fingers when they are flexed." (*Fa Hui*)

Note: Medical literature through the ages holds similar views. It is on the radial side of the 3rd metacarpal bone, indicating that the point is located in the central part of the palm, between the 2nd and the 3rd metacarpal bones and comparatively near the 3rd metacarpal bone. But, for the definite location, *Sheng Hui* locates it at the place where the tip of the 4th finger lands when it is flexed, i.e. between the 3rd and 4th metacarpal bones. *Zi Sheng* locates it between the 2nd and the 3rd metacarpal bones. *Fa Hui* makes a compromise, locating it on the palmar side of the 3rd metacarpal bone. Now, the point is located at the centre of the palm, between the 2nd and 3rd metacarpal bones, but close to the latter, and in the part where the tip of the middle finger lands when a fist is made.

2. 9. 9 PC 9 Zhōngchōng 中衝

Name: Seen in *Ling Shu*.

Location:

1) "On the tip of the middle finger." (*Ling Shu*)

2) "On the tip of the middle finger, in the depression about the width of a chive leaf from the nail." (*Jia Yi*, etc.)

3) "On the tip of the medial side of the middle finger, the width of a chive leaf from the nail." (*Da Quan*)

4) "Down from Laogong (PC 8) to the tip of the middle finger, in the depression about the width of a chive leaf from the corner of the nail." (*Jin Jian*, etc.)

Note: There are two locations of this point illustrated in the medical literature through the ages, i.e. "on the tip of the middle finger" (*Ling Shu*, *Jia Yi*, etc.) and "on the medial side of the tip of the middle finger." (*Da Quan*, *Jin Jian*, etc.) The former is accepted nowadays, and according to the ancient bronze statue Zhongchong (PC 9) is located at the centre of the tip of the middle finger.

2. 10 Points of the Sanjiao (Triple Energizer) Meridian of Hand-Shaoyang, SJ

手少陽三焦經穴

Shŏushàoyáng Sānjiāojīng Xué

2. 10. 1 SJ 1 Guānchōng 關衝

Name: Seen in *Ling Shu*.

Location:

1) "On the tip of the 4th finger." (*Ling Shu*)

2) "On the tip of the 4th finger, the width of a chive leaf from the corner of the nail." (*Jia Yi*, etc.)

3) "On the lateral side of the 4th finger, the width of a chive leaf from the corner of the nail." (*Ru Men*)

Note: According to the running course of the meridian, the point should be located on the ulnar side, identical to other Jing-Well points. So Guanchong (SJ 1) is located on the ulnar side of the distal segment of the 4th finger and 0.1 *cun* from the corner of the nail.

2. 10. 2 SJ 2 Yèmén 液門

Name: Seen in *Ling Shu*.

Location:

1) "Between the little finger and the 4th finger." (*Ling Shu*, etc.)

2) "In the depression between the little and 4th fingers." (*Jia Yi*)

3) "In the depression anterior to the junction of the 4th and little fingers." (*Xun Jing*)

Note: Medical literature through the ages holds similar views on the location of the point, i.e. on the dorsum of the hand, between the 4th and 5th fingers, at the junction of the red and white skin, proximal to the margin of the web.

2. 10. 3 SJ 3 Zhōngzhŭ 中渚

Name: Seen in *Ling Shu*.

Location:

1) "In the depression posterior (proximal) to the metacarpophalangeal joint." (*Ling Shu*)

2) "In the depression between the 4th and 5th metacarpal bones." (*Jia Yi*, etc.)

3) "In the depression between the 4th and 5th metacarpal bones." (*Ju Ying*, etc.)

4) "In the depression 0.5 *cun* proximal to the 4th and 5th metacarpophalangeal joints." (*Liu Ji*)

5) "In the depression 1 *cun* above Yemen (SJ 2)." (*Jin Jian*, etc.)

Note: "Posterior to the metacarpophalangeal joint" or "1 *cun* proximal to the web or Yemen (SJ 2)" refers to "in the depression between the distal ends of the 4th and 5th metacarpal bones on the dorsum of the hand." *Liu Ji* says, "0.5 *cun* proximal to the metacarpophalangeal joint." This distance between the two points should be settled according to the metacarpophalangeal joint. If 0.5 *cun* is added, the distance becomes too far. Now, the point is located on the dorsum of the hand, proximal to the 4th metacarpophalangeal joint, and in the depression between the 4th and 5th metacarpal bones.

2. 10. 4 SJ 4 Yángchí 陽池

Name: Seen in *Ling Shu*.

Location:

1) "In the depression of the wrist." (*Ling Shu*)

2) "In the depression of the dorsum of the wrist." (*Jia Yi*, etc.)

3) "In the depression of the dorsum of the wrist, on the line along the 4th metacarpal bone." (*Ju Ying*, etc.)

4) "From the 4th metacarpal bone towards the centre of the dorsum of the wrist, between the two tendons." (*Xun Jing*)

5) "In the depression of the wrist, on the line starting from Zhongzhu (SJ 3) along the 4th metacarpal bone." (*Jin Jian*)

Note: The description in *Jia Yi* is not clear. Most of the medical literature in the Ming Dynasty say: "It is at the centre of the wrist, on the line along the 4th metacarpal bone." *Jin Jian* gives a more definite location. According to the running course of the meridian, the above two opinions refer to a location going proximally along the 4th metacarpal bone to the wrist joint. Now, Yangchi (SJ 4) is located at the midpoint of the dorsal crease of the wrist, and in the depression on the ulnar side of the tendon of the extensor muscle of the finger. But the location illustrated in *Xun Jing* refers to the radial side of the tendon of the extensor muscle of the finger, where an extra point Zhongquan (EX-UE3) lodges.

2. 10. 5 SJ 5 Wàiguān 外關

Name: Seen in *Ling Shu*.

Location:

1) "2 *cun* above the wrist." (*Ling Shu*)

2) "In the depression 2 *cun* above the wrist." (*Jia Yi*, etc.)

3) "2 *cun* above the wrist, between the two tendons, 2 *cun* above Yangchi (SJ 4)." (*Ju Ying*)

4) "2 *cun* above the wrist, between the two bones, opposite to Neiguan (PC 6)." (*Da Cheng*)

Note: Medical literature through the ages holds similar views on the location of the point, i.e. 2 *cun* above the wrist. For "between the two tendons," read "between the two bones." Now, Waiguan (SJ 5) is located on the dorsal side of the forearm, on the line connecting Yangchi (SJ 4) and the tip of the olecranon, and 2 *cun* proximal to the dorsal crease of the wrist, between the radius and the ulna. The description in *Ju Ying* is self-contradictory.

2. 10. 6 SJ 6 Zhīgōu 支溝

Name: Seen in *Ling Shu*.

Location:

1) "3 *cun* above the wrist, in the depression between the two bones." (*Ling Shu*, etc.)

2) "3 *cun* above the wrist, in the depression between the two bones." (*Jia Yi*)

3) "3 *cun* above the wrist, on the lateral side of the arm, in the depression between the two bones." (*Ju Ying*, etc.)

4) "1 *cun* upward from Waiguan (SJ 5), between the two bones." (*Jin Jian*)

Note: Medical literature through the ages holds similar views on the location of the point, i.e. on the dorsal side of the forearm, on the line connecting Yangchi (SJ 4) and the tip of the olecranon, and 3 *cun* proximal to the dorsal crease of the wrist, between the radius and the ulna.

2. 10. 7 SJ 7 Huìzōng 會宗

Name: Seen in *Jia Yi*.

Location:

1) "In the depression 3 *cun* above the wrist." (*Jia Yi*)

2) "3 *cun* above the wrist, in the depression 1 *cun* apart." (*Tong Ren*, etc.)

3) "In the depression 1 *cun* lateral to Zhigou (SJ 6)." (*Ru Men*, etc.)

4) "3 *cun* above and 0.5 *cun* lateral to the wrist." (*Liu Ji*)

5) "3 *cun* above Yangchi (SJ 4), on the level of Zhigou (SJ 6), and 0.5 *cun* inferior." (*Ji Cheng*)

Note: Medical literature through the ages locates the point "3 *cun* above the wrist," but the distance between the point and Zhigou (SJ 6) is viewed differently. *Jia Yi* says it is "in the depression." *Tong Ren*, etc. say it is "1 *cun* apart," and *Liu Ji* says it is "0.5 *cun* lateral to." The opinion in *Jia Yi* is adopted nowadays, and Huizong (SJ 7) is located on the dorsal side of the forearm, 3 *cun* proximal to the dorsal crease of the wrist, on the ulnar side of Zhigou (SJ 6) and on the radial border of the ulna.

2. 10. 8 SJ 8 Sānyángluò 三陽絡

Name: Seen in *Jia Yi*.

Location:

1) "On the big crossing vessel of the arm, 1 *cun* above Zhigou (SJ 6)." (*Jia Yi*, etc.)

2) "In the depression 3 *cun* anterior (distal) to the lateral side of the elbow, 1 *cun* above Zhigou (SJ 6)." (*Sheng Hui*)

3) "2 *cun* above Zhigou (SJ 6)." (*Xun Jing*)

4) "1 *cun* obliquely upward and medially from Huizong (SJ 7), on the big crossing vessel of the arm." (*Jin Jian*)

Note: Most of the medical literature through the ages follow *Jia Yi*, locating the point on the dorsal side of the forearm, 4 *cun* proximal to the dorsal crease of the wrist, between the radius and the ulna. The "big crossing vessel of the arm" has no obvious connection with the artery and vein of the forearm, and is not important to the location of the point. The description in *Sheng Hui* is contradictory and *Xun Jing*'s location is also confusing and not accepted today.

2. 10. 9 SJ 9 Sìdú 四瀆

Name: Seen in *Jia Yi*.

Location:

1) "5 *cun* distal to the elbow, on the lateral side of the forearm." (*Jia Yi*, etc.)

2) "5 *cun* distal to the tip of the elbow, in the depression between the bone and the tendon." (*Xun Jing*)

Note: Medical literature through the ages holds similar views on the location of the point. Now, Sidu (SJ 9) is located on the dorsal side of the forearm, on the line connecting Yangchi (SJ 4) and the tip of the olecranon, and 5 *cun* distal to the tip of the olecranon, between the radius and the ulna.

2. 10. 10 SJ 10 Tiānjǐng 天井

Name: Seen in *Ling Shu*.

Location:

1) "In the depression of the big bone, on the lateral side of the elbow." (*Ling Shu*)

2) "Proximal to the big bone, on the lateral side of the elbow, in the depression between the two tendons." (*Jia Yi*)

3) "1 *cun* proximal to the big bone, on the lateral side of the elbow, in the depression between the two tendons." (*Qian Jin*, etc.)

4) "Proximal to the big bone, on the lateral side of the elbow, 1 *cun* above the elbow, in the depression between the two tendons of the radius." (*Ju Ying*, etc.)

Note: The big bone on the lateral side of the elbow refers to the olecranon of the ulna, and the "depression" refers to the notch of the olecranon. "1 *cun* proximal to the big bone" is taken when the elbow is flexed, and is accepted by the later practitioners. It corresponds to the depression posterior and superior to the olecranon of the ulna when the elbow is flexed. Now, Tianjing (SJ 10) is located on the lateral side of the upper arm, and in the depression 1 *cun* proximal to the tip of the olecranon when the elbow is flexed.

2. 10. 11 SJ 11 Qīnglěngyuān 清冷渊

Name: Seen in *Jia Yi*.

Location:

1) "1 *cun* (2 *cun* in another edition) above the elbow, with the arm raised and the elbow extended." (*Jia Yi*)

2) "3 *cun* above the elbow, with the arm raised and the elbow extended." (*Qian Jin*)

3) "2 *cun* above the elbow, with the arm raised and the elbow extended." (*Wai Tai*, etc.)

4) "1 *cun* upward from Tianjing (SJ 10), with the arm raised and the elbow extended." (*Jin Jian*)

5) "1.5 *cun* above the elbow, 1 *cun* from Tianjing (SJ 10)." (*Ji Cheng*)

Note: About the location of the point, *Jia Yi* has two ideas, i.e. "1 *cun*" and "2 *cun*" above the elbow. The latter is adopted by *Wai Tai* and followed by the later medical literature. Now, Qinglengyuan (SJ 11) is located on the lateral side of the upper arm 2 *cun* above the tip of the olecranon and 1 *cun* above Tianjing (SJ 10) with the elbow flexed. *Ji Cheng* locates the point 1.5 *cun* above the elbow and 1 *cun* from Tianjing (SJ 10), because Tianjing (SJ 10) is located in the depression "a little posterior to the elbow" in that book, which is comparatively low.

2. 10. 12 SJ 12 Xiāoluò 消濼

Name: Seen in *Jia Yi*.

Location:

1) "Inferior to the shoulder, on the lateral side of the arm." (*Jia Yi*, etc.)

2) "3 *cun* inferior to the shoulder, 6 *cun* superior to the tip of the elbow." (*Xun Jing*)

3) "Upward from Qinglengyuan (SJ 11), inferior to the shoulder, on the lateral side of the arm, between the muscles above the cubitus." (*Jin Jian*, etc.)

4) "2 *cun* inferior and less than 1 *cun* posterior to Naohui (SJ 13)." (*Ji Cheng*)

Note: Medical literature through the ages holds similar views on the location of the point, i.e. inferior to, and on the lateral side of the shoulder. When the shoulder is abducted, there appears an oblique groove on the deltoid muscle, which is described as "between the muscles." The location of "3 *cun* inferior to the shoulder" recorded in *Xun Jing* overlaps with Naohui (SJ 13), and is an apparent mistake. *Ji Cheng* says: "2 *cun* inferior (formerly superior) to Naohui (SJ 13)." If the arm is abducted horizontally, the distance between the shoulder and the elbow is 9 *cun*; 3 *cun* distal to the shoulder is Naohui (SJ 13), 5 *cun* is Xiaoluo (SJ 12), and 2 *cun* above the elbow is Qinglengyuan (SJ 11)." Thus the distance between Xiaoluo (SJ 12) and Qinglengyuan (SJ 11) is 2 *cun*. Now Xiaoluo (SJ 12) is located on the lateral side of the upper arm, at the midpoint of the line connecting Qinglengyuan (SJ 11) and Naohui (SJ 13).

2. 10. 13 SJ 13 Nàohuì 臑會

Name: Seen in *Jia Yi*.

Location:

1) "On the anterior side of the arm, 3 *cun* from the shoulder." (*Jia Yi*, etc.)

2) "Under the bone on the anterior side of the arm, 3 *cun* from the shoulder." (*Xun Jing*)

3) "A little anterior to and 2 *cun* above Xiaoluo (SJ 12)." (*Ji Cheng*)

Note: About the location of the point, medical literature through the ages follow *Jia Yi*, i.e. on the anterior aspect of the arm, 3 *cun* from the shoulder. Now, Naohui (SJ 13) is located on the lateral side of the upper arm, on the line connecting the tip of the olecranon and Jianliao (SJ 14), 3 *cun* below Jianliao (SJ 14), and on the posterior-inferior border of the deltoid muscle.

2. 10. 14 SJ 14 Jiānliáo 肩髎

Name: Seen in *Jia Yi*.

Location:

1) "On the acromion. To be located with the patient's arm raised obliquely." (*Jia Yi*, etc.)

2) "In the depression of the acromion." (*Wai Tai*, etc.)

3) "Superior to Naohui (SJ 13), in the depression formed when the arm is raised." (*Xun Jing*)

4) "1.3 *cun* posterior and a little inferior to Jianyu (LI 15)." (*Ji Cheng*)

Note: Medical literature through the ages holds similar views on the location of the point, i.e. "on the acromion," which refers to the upper part of the deltoid muscle, and the depression is posterior and inferior to the acromion when the arm is raised. The opinion in *Jia Yi* is accepted nowadays, and Jianliao (SJ 14) is located on the shoulder, posterior to Jianyu (LI 15) in the depression posterior and inferior to the acromion when the arm is abducted.

2. 10. 15 SJ 15 Tiānliáo 天髎

Name: Seen in *Jia Yi*.

Location:

1) "In the supraclavicular fossa, in the depression of the superior angle of the scapula." (*Jia Yi*, etc.)

2) "In the supraclavicular fossa, in the depression at the centre of the superior angle of the scapula." (*Ju Jing*, etc.)

3) "In the supraclavicular fossa, about 1 *cun* from Dazhu (BL 11) and Fufen (BL 41)." (*Xun Jing*)

4) "1 *cun* directly posterior to Jianjing (GB 21)."

5) "1 *cun* medial to and 0.8 *cun* posterior to Jianjing (GB 21), 1 *cun* above Jianwaishu (SI 14)." (*Ji Cheng*)

Note: *Su Wen*, annotated by Wang Bing, locates the point "in the supraclavicular fossa, in the depression of the corner of the scapula." So Tianliao (SJ 15) is located on the scapular, at the midpoint between Jianjing (GB 21) and Quyuan (SI 13), on the superior angle of the scapula.

2. 10. 16 SJ 16 Tiānyǒu 天牖

Name: Seen in *Ling Shu* and *Su Wen*.

Location:

1) "Between the muscles of the neck, above the supraclavicular fossa, behind Tianrong (SI

17), anterior to Tianzhu (BL 10), posterior to Wangu (GB 12), above the hairline." (*Jia Yi*, etc.)

2) "Above the supraclavicular fossa and the muscles of the neck, posterior to Tianrong (SI 17), anterior to Tianzhu (BL 10), behind Wangu (GB 12), in the depression 1 *cun* above the hairline." (*Sheng Hui*)

3) "Lateral to the big muscle of the neck, above the supraclavicular fossa, posterior to Tianchuang (SI 16), anterior to Tianzhu (BL 10), below Wangu (GB 12), above the hairline." (*Fa Hui*)

4) "About 1 *cun* above the hairline, below Yifeng (SJ 17), on the muscle at the end of the mandibular bone, or about 7.5 *cun* lateral to the Adam's apple." (*Xun Jing*)

5) "Upward from Tianliao (SJ 15), above the supraclavicular fossa and lateral to the big muscle of the neck, posterior to Tianrong (SI 17) of the Hand-Taiyang Meridian, anterior to Tianzhu (BL 10) of the Foot-Taiyang Meridian, below Wangu (GB 12) of the Gallbladder Meridian of Foot-Shaoyang, obliquely across the hairline, 1 *cun* behind the ear." (*Jin Jian*)

6) "1 *cun* below and a little lateral to Fengchi (GB 20)." (*Ji Cheng*)

Note: "Between the muscles of the neck" refers to the part between the sternocleidomastoid muscle and the trapezius muscle. "Posterior to Wangu" (GB 12) (or "below Wangu, GB 12," in *Qing Jin*) denotes that the point is directly below Wangu (GB 12), which is posterior and inferior to the mastoid process. It is posterior to Tianrong (SI 17) and anterior to Tianzhu (BL 10). Now, this view is accepted, and Tianyou (SJ 16) is located on the lateral side of the neck, directly below the posterior border of the mastoid process, on the level of the mandibular angle, on the posterior border of the sternocleidomastoid muscle. "1 *cun* above the hairline" or "about 1 *cun* above the hairline" described in *Sheng Hui*, *Xun Jing*, etc. are not correct because this position is already above Wangu (GB 12). The location described in *Jin Jian* and *Ji Cheng* is identical to that in *Jia Yi*.

2. 10. 17 SJ 17 Yìfēng 翳風

Name: Seen in *Jia Yi*.

Location:

1) "In the depression behind the ear." (*Jia Yi*, etc.)

2) "In the angular depression behind the ear." (*Sheng Hui*)

3) "Below the ear, in the depression behind the eardrop, in a hollow seen when the mouth is open." (*Xun Jing*)

Note: Medical literature through the ages holds similar views on the location of the point, i.e. posterior to the ear lobe and in the depression between the mastoid process and the mandibular angle.

2. 10. 18 SJ 18 Chìmài 瘈脈

Name: Seen in *Jia Yi*.

Location:

1) "Behind the ear root, where small vessels are visible." (*Jia Yi*, etc.)

2) "Behind the ear, superior to Yifeng (SJ 17), on the level of Tinghui (GB 2)." (*Xun Jing*)

3) "1 *cun* superior to Yifeng (SJ 17), adjacent to the ear root." (*Ji Cheng*)

Note: Now, Chimai (SJ 18) is located on the head, at the centre of the mastoid process, at the junction of the middle third and lower third of the line connecting Jiaosun (SJ 20) and Yifeng (SJ 17) along the curve of the ear helix.

2. 10. 19 SJ 19 Lúxī 盧息

Name: Seen in *Jia Yi*.

Location:

1) "Behind the ear where small vessels are visible." (*Jia Yi*, etc.)

2) "From Chimai (SJ 18) upward behind the ear, where small vessels are visible." (*Jin Jian*, etc.)

3) "A little more than 1 *cun* above Chimai (SJ 18)." (*Ji Cheng*)

Note: According to the above descriptions and with reference to the location of Chimai (SJ 18), Luxi (SJ 19) is located on the head, at the junction of the upper third and middle third of the line connecting Jiaosun (SJ 20) and Yifeng (SJ 17) along the curve of the ear helix.

2. 10. 20 SJ 20 Jiǎosūn 角孫

Name: Seen in *Ling Shu*.

Location:

1) "In the middle of the auricle, in a hollow seen with the mouth open." (*Jia Yi*, etc.)

2) "In the middle of the upper part of the auricle, below the upper hairline, in a hollow seen with the mouth open." (*Su Wen*, annotated by Wang)

Note: The description in *Jia Yi* is too simple and that in *Su Wen* annotated by Wang Bing is clearer. "In the middle of the upper part of the auricle" refers to the place above the auricle. Now, Jiaosun (SJ 20) is located on the head, above the ear apex above the hairline.

2. 10. 21 SJ 21 Ěrmén 耳門

Name: Seen in *Jia Yi*.

Location:

1) "On the the notch of the tragus." (*Jia Yi*, etc.)

2) "From Jiaosun (SJ 20) to the front of the ear, in the depression of the notch of the tragus." (*Jin Jian*)

3) "Lateral and inferior to the notch of the tragus." (*Ji Cheng*)

Note: Now, Ermen (SJ 21) is located on the face, anterior to the supratragic notch, in the depression behind the posterior border of the condyloid process of the mandible. *Ji Cheng* says it is "lateral and inferior (should read superior) to the notch of the tragus," because Tinghui (GB 2) is inferiorly located and the two points should not be confused.

2. 10. 22 SJ 22 Ěrhéliáo 耳和髎

Name: Seen in *Jia Yi*. Originally named Heliao.

Location: "Inferior to the hair of the temples where the superficial temporal artery is palpable." (*Jia Yi*, etc.)

Note: According to its description, now Erheliao (SJ 22) is located on the lateral side of the head, on the posterior margin of the temples, anterior to the anterior border of the root of the ear auricle and posterior to the superficial temporal artery.

2. 10. 23 SJ 23 Sīzhúkōng 絲竹空

Name: Seen in *Jia Yi*.

Location:

1) "In the depression posterior to the eyebrow." (*Jia Yi*, etc.)

2) "In the depression lateral to the eyebrow, in the hairline." (*Liu Ji*)

3) "Behind the lateral end of the eyebrow, in the depression 0.2 *cun* from the eyebrow." (*Xun Jing*)

Note: *Jia Yi* originally says it is in the depression lateral to the eyebrow. *Liu Ji* says it is "in the depression lateral to the eyebrow, in the hairline," which is confused with the points above the hairline. *Xun Jing*'s location is more or less similar to that adopted today. Now, the point is located on the face, in the depression of the lateral end of the eyebrow.

2. 11 Points of the Gallbladder Meridian of Foot-Shaoyang, GB

足少陽膽經穴

Zúshàoyáng Dǎnjīng Xué

2. 11. 1 GB 1 Tóngzǐliáo 瞳子髎

Name: Seen in *Jia Yi*.

Location: "0.5 *cun* lateral to the outer canthus." (*Jia Yi*, etc.)

Note: Medical literature through the ages holds similar views on the location of the point. Now, Tongziliao (GB 1) is located on the face, lateral to the outer canthus, and on the lateral border of the orbit.

2. 11. 2 GB 2 Tīnghuì 聽會

Name: Seen in *Jia Yi*.

Location:

1) "In the depression in front of the ear where the pulsation is palpable. To be located with the mouth open." (*Jia Yi*, etc.)

2) "1 *cun* posterior to the bone in front of the ear, in the depression inferior to the intertragic notch near an artery, in a hollow found with the patient's mouth open. To be located with the patient lying on his side and the mouth open." (*Jin Jian*)

Note: When the mouth is open, the mandible moves forward and a hollow is seen. Now, Tinghui (GB 2) is located on the face, anterior to the intertragic notch, and in the depression posterior to the condyloid process of the mandible when the patient's mouth is open.

2. 11. 3 GB 3 Shàngguān 上關

Name: Seen in *Su Wen*. Named Kezhuren in *Ling Shu*.

Location:

1) "In front of the ear, on the upper border of the zygomatic arch, in a hollow seen with the patient's mouth open." (*Jia Yi*, etc.)

2) "1 *cun* directly above Tinghui (GB 2), in a hollow seen with the patient's mouth open. To be located with the patient lying on his side and the mouth open." (*Jin Jian*)

Note: Medical literature through the ages holds similar views on the location of the point. In the middle of the lower border of the zygomatic arch is Xiaguan (ST 7), while on its upper border is Shangguan (GB 3). Now, Shangguan (GB 3) is located anterior to the ear, directly above Xiaguan (ST 7) and in the depression above the upper border of the zygomatic arch.

2. 11. 4 GB 4 Hányàn 頷厭

Name: Seen in *Jia Yi*.

Location:

1) "Superior to the anterior corner of the ear." (*Su Wen*)

2) "On the upper portion of the temples, above the hairline of the temporal region." (*Jia Yi*, etc.)

3) "On the upper portion of the temples, below the corner of the hairline of the temporal region." (*Su Wen*, annotated by Wang)

4) "Superior to Naokong (GB 19), above the hairline of the temporal region." (*Zi Sheng*)

5) "Above the temples, above the corner of the hairline of the temporal region." (*Jin Jian*)

Note: Now, Hanyan (GB 4) is located on the head, in the hair above the temples, and at the junction of the fourth and the lower three fourths of the curved line connecting Touwei (ST 8) and Qubin (GB 7). See details in Xuanli (GB 6).

2. 11. 5 GB 5 Xuánlú 懸盧

Name: Seen in *Ling Shu*.

Location:

1) "In the temples, above the hairline of the temporal region." (*Jia Yi*, etc.)

2) "In the temples, at the corner of the hairline of the temporal region." (*Su Wen*, annotated by Wang)

3) "Above the hairline of the temporal region, adjacent to Naokong (GB 19)." (*Zi Sheng*)

4) "Anterior to the ear, above the corner of the hairline of the temporal region, in the temples." (*Jin Jian*)

Note: Now, Xuanlu (GB 5) is located on the head, in the hair above the temples, and at the midpoint of the curved line connecting Touwei (ST 8) and Qubin (GB 7). See details in Xuanli (GB 6).

2. 11. 6 GB 6 Xuánlí 懸釐

Name: Seen in *Jia Yi*.

Location:

1) "Below the anterior corner of the ear." (*Su Wen*)

2) "On the lower border of the temples, above the hairline of the temporal region." (*Jia Yi*, etc.)

3) "In the corner of the hairline, on the lower border of the temples." (*Su Wen*, annotated by Wang)

4) "Above the hairline of the temporal region, below Naokong (GB 19)." (*Zi Sheng*)

5) "At the corner of the hairline of the temporal region, in front of the ear, in the lower portion of the temples." (*Jin Jian*)

Note: According to medical literature through the ages, it is known that Hanyan (GB 4), Xuanlu (GB 5) and Xuanli (GB 6) are three points in the temple area anterior to the ear." *Jia Yi* divides the corner of the hairline into upper, middle and lower parts, where the three points lodge accordingly. Now, the points are located in the line connecting Touwei (ST 8) (0.5 *cun* above the hairline of the corner of the forehead) and Qubin (GB 7) (on the hairline in front of the ear). Midway of the line is Xuanlu (GB 5), at the junction of the upper fourth and lower three fourths is Hanyan (GB 4), and at the junction of the upper three fourths and lower fourth is Xuanli (GB 6).

2. 11. 7 GB 7 Qūbìn 曲鬢

Name: Seen in *Jia Yi*.

Location:

1) "Above the ear and the hairline, in the depression above the curved hairline in front of the ear, in a hollow seen with the patient's cheeks blown." (*Jia Yi*, etc.)

2) "Superior to the ear, in the depression above the curved hairline in front of the ear, in

a hollow seen with the patient's cheeks blown." (*Jin Jian*)

Note: Medical literature through the ages holds similar views on the location of the point. Now, Qubin (GB 7) is located on the head, at a crossing point of the vertical posterior border of the temples and the horizontal line through the apex of the ear.

2. 11. 8 GB 8 Shuàigǔ 率谷

Name: Seen in *Jia Yi*.

Location:

1) "1.5 *cun* above the hairline anterior to the ear; locate it with the patient's jaw clenched." (*Jia Yi*, etc.)

2) "In the depression 0.3 *cun* anterior and superior to the ear, 1.5 *cun* above the hairline." (*Fa Hui*, etc.)

Note: Medical literature through the ages holds similar views on the location of the point. The opinion in *Jia Yi* is adopted nowadays, and Shuaigu (GB 8) is located on the head, directly above the ear apex and 1.5 *cun* above the hairline, directly above Jiaosun (SJ 20).

2. 11. 9 GB 9 Tiānchōng 天衝

Name: Seen in *Jia Yi*.

Location:

1) "Above and 0.3 *cun* posterior to the ear." (*Jia Yi*, etc.)

2) "Above and 3 *cun* posterior to the ear." (*Qian Jin*, etc.)

3) "2 *cun* above the hairline posterior to the ear, 0.3 *cun* posterior to the apex of the ear." (*Fa Hui*, etc.)

Note: The location recorded in *Jia Yi* is not clear. The description "3 *cun* superior to the ear" in *Qian Jin* should read "0.3 *cun* superior to the ear." *Fa Hui*'s description is comparatively clearer. Now, Tianchong (GB 9) is located on the head, directly above the posterior border of the ear root, 2 *cun* above the hairline, and 0.5 *cun* posterior to Shuaigu (GB 8). As for the distance to Shuaigu (GB 8), the measurement is directly above the apex of the ear, or directly above the hairline posterior to the ear, both of which are in accordance with the order of points in the running course of the meridian.

2. 11. 10 GB 10 Fúbái 浮白

Name: Seen in *Su Wen*.

Location:

1) "Posterior to the ear, 1 *cun* within (above) the hairline." (*Jia Yi*, etc.)

2) "Downward from Tianchong (GB 9) behind the ear, 1 *cun* within the hairline." (*Jin Jian*)

Note: Medical literature through the ages holds similar views on the location of the point. Now, Fubai (GB 10) is located on the head, posterior and superior to the mastoid process, and at the junction of the middle third and upper third of the curved line connecting Tianchong (GB 9) and Wangu (GB 12).

2. 11. 11 GB 11 Tóuqiàoyīn 頭竅陰

Name: Seen in *Zi Sheng*. Originally named Qiaoyin in *Jia Yi*.

Location:

1) "Superior to the mastoid process of the temporal bone, inferior to the occipital bone." (*Jia Yi*, etc.)

2) "Downward from Fubai (GB 10) behind the ear, inferior to the occipital bone." (*Jin*

Jian)

Note: Medical literature through the ages holds similar views on the location of the point, i.e. posterior to the mastoid process, inferior to the horizontal level of the tuberosity of the occipital bone. Now, Touqiaoyin (GB 11) is located on the head, posterior and superior to the mastoid process, and at the junction of the middle third and lower third of the curved line connecting Tianchong (GB 9) and Wangu (GB 12).

2. 11. 12 GB 12 Wángŭ 完骨

Name: Seen in *Ling Shu* and *Su Wen*.

Location: "0.4 *cun* within (above) the hairline behind the ear." (*Jia Yi*, etc.)

Note: Medical literature through the ages holds similar views on the location of the point. "Wangu" is named after the mastoid process of the occipital bone. The point is located on the head, in the depression posterior and inferior to the mastoid process.

2. 11. 13 GB 13 Běnshén 本神

Name: Seen in *Jia Yi*.

Location:

1) "1.5 *cun* lateral to Qucha (BL 4), on the hairline, or directly above the ear, 0.4 *cun* within (above) the hairline." (*Jia Yi*, etc.)

2) "3 *cun* lateral to Shenting (DU 24), directly above the ear, 0.4 *cun* within the hairline." (*Jia Yi*, etc.)

Note: Qucha (BL 4) is 1.5 *cun* lateral to Shenting (DU 24), which is 1.5 *cun* to Qucha (BL 4) and 3 *cun* to Shenting (DU 24). The point is said to be "on the hairline" or "0.4 *cun* above the hairline." Starting from *Sheng Hui*, Shenting (DU 24) is located 0.5 *cun* above the hairline, and so are the adjacent points. Now, Benshen (GB 13) is located on the head, 0.5 *cun* above the anterior hairline, 3 *cun* lateral to Shenting (DU 24), at the junction of the medial two thirds and lateral third of the line connecting Shenting (DU 24) and Touwei (ST 8).

2. 11. 14 GB 14 Yángbái 陽白

Name: Seen in *Jia Yi*.

Location: "1 *cun* above the eyebrow, directly above the pupil." (*Jia Yi*, etc.)

Note: Medical literature through the ages holds similar views on the location of the point. When one looks straight forward, the pupil is at the centre of the eye. Yangbai (GB 14) is located on the forehead, directly above the pupil, and 1 *cun* above the eyebrow.

2. 11. 15 GB 15 Tóulínqì 頭臨泣

Name: Seen in *Zi Sheng*. Originally named Linqi in *Jia Yi*.

Location:

1) "In the depression above the eye, 0.5 *cun* within (above) the hairline." (*Jia Yi*, etc.)

2) "Above the eye, 0.5 *cun* within the hairline." (*Tong Ren*, etc.)

3) "Directly above Yangbai (GB 14), in the depression 0.5 *cun* within the hairline. To be located with the patient's eyes looking straight forward." (*Jin Jian*)

Note: Medical literature through the ages holds similar views on the location of the point. Toulinqi (GB 15) is located on the head, directly above the pupil, 0.5 *cun* above the anterior hairline, and at the midpoint of the line connecting Shenting (DU 24) and Touwei (ST 8).

2. 11. 16 GB 16 Mùchuāng 目窗

Name: Seen in *Jia Yi*.

Location:

1) "1 *cun* posterior to Linqi (GB 15)." (*Jia Yi*, etc.)

2) "0.5 *cun* posterior to Linqi (GB 15)." (*Da Cheng*)

Note: Medical literature through the ages holds similar views on the location of the point, with the exception of only a few books, such as *Da Cheng* and *Xun Jing*, which locate the point 0.5 *cun* posterior to Linqi (GB 15). The opinion in *Jia Yi* is adopted. Now, Muchuang (GB 16) is located on the head 1.5 *cun* above the anterior hairline, and 2.25 *cun* lateral to the midline of the head.

2. 11. 17 GB 17 Zhèngyíng 正營

Name: Seen in *Jia Yi*.

Location:

1) "1 *cun* posterior to Muchuang (GB 16)." (*Jia Yi*, etc.)

2) "0.5 *cun* posterior to Muchuang (GB 16)." (*Da Cheng*)

Note: Medical literature through the ages holds similar views on the location of the point, with the exception of *Da Cheng* and a few other books, which locate the point 0.5 *cun* posterior to Muchuang (GB 16), 2.25 *cun* lateral to the midline. Now, this point is located on the head, 2.5 *cun* above the anterior hairline, 2.25 *cun* lateral to the midline of the head.

2. 11. 18 GB 18 Chénglíng 承靈

Name: Seen in *Jia Yi*.

Location: "1.5 *cun* posterior to Zhengying (GB 17)." (*Jia Yi*, etc.)

Note: Medical literature through the ages holds the same view on the location of the point. Accordingly, Chengling (GB 18) is located on the head, 4 *cun* above the anterior hairline, and 2.25 *cun* lateral to the midline of the head.

2. 11. 19 GB 19 Nǎokōng 腦空

Name: Seen in *Jia Yi*.

Location: "1.5 *cun* posterior to Chengling (GB 18)." (*Jia Yi*, etc.)

Note: Medical literature through the ages holds the same view on the location of the point. The occipital bone is the landmark for locating it. Naokong (GB 19) is located on the head, on the level of the upper border of the external occipital protuberance or Naohu (DU 17), and 2.25 *cun* lateral to the midline of the head.

2. 11. 20 GB 20 Fēngchí 風池

Name: Seen in *Ling Shu*.

Location:

1) "Behind Naokong (GB 19), in the depression above the posterior hairline." (*Jia Yi*, etc.)

2) "In the depression above the hairline, lateral to the trapezius muscle on the nape." (*Qian Jin*)

3) "In the depression behind the ear. On pressing, a sensation can be felt in the ear." (*Su Wen*, annotated by Wang)

4) "In the depression above the posterior hairline on the nape." (*Sheng Hui*)

5) "In the depression above the posterior hairline, posterior to Naokong (GB 19)." (*Zi Sheng*, etc.)

6) "Downward from Naokong (GB 19) to the area behind the ear, in the depression above the hairline, lateral to the big muscle. On pressing, a sensation can be felt in the ear." (*Jin Jian*, etc.)

Note: What is mentioned in *Su Wen*, annotated by Wang, is the location of Yifeng (SJ 17), which should not be confused with Fengchi (GB 20). Other books all locate the point inferior to the occipital bone, in the hairline area, in the depression lateral to the big muscle on the nape. Accordingly, Fengchi (GB 20) is located on the nape below the occipital bone, on the level of Fengfu (DU 16), and in the depression between the upper ends of the sternocleidomastoid and trapezius muscles.

2. 11. 21 GB 21 Jiānjǐng 肩井

Name: Seen in *Jia Yi*.

Location:

1) "In the depression on the shoulder, above the supraclavicular fossa, superior to the spine of the scapula." (*Jia Yi*, etc.)

2) "In the depression on the shoulder, above the supraclavicular fossa, 1.5 *cun* superior to the spine of the scapula." (*Sheng Hui*, etc.)

Note: Medical literature through the ages holds similar views on the location of the point. Now, Jianjing (GB 21) is located on the shoulder, directly above the nipple, at the midpoint of the line connecting Dazhui (DU 14) and the acromion.

2. 11. 22 GB 22 Yuānyè 淵腋

Name: Seen in *Ling Shu*.

Location: "In the depression 3 *cun* below the axilla. Locate it with the patient's arm raised." (*Jia Yi*, etc.)

Note: Medical literature through the ages holds the same view on the location of the point. Now, Yuanye (GB 22) is located on the lateral side of the chest, on the midaxillary line when the patient's arm is raised, 3 *cun* below the axilla, in the 4th intercostal space.

2. 11. 23 GB 23 Zhéjīn 輒筋

Name: Seen in *Jia Yi*.

Location:

1) "3 *cun* below and 1 *cun* anterior to the axilla, on the rib." (*Jia Yi*)

2) "3 *cun* below and 1 *cun* anterior to the axilla, at the end of the 3rd rib, 7.5 *cun* lateral to the xiphoid process, on the level of the nipple. Locate it with the patient lying on his side, his hip flexed." (*Da Cheng*)

Note: Most of the medical literature follow *Jia Yi*. *Ju Ying* wrongly defines the location of Riyue (GB 24) for Zhejin (GB 23). *Da Cheng*, affected by *Ju Ying*, makes a wrong location too. The opinion in *Jia Yi* is adopted now. Zhejin (GB 23) is located on the lateral side of the chest, 1 *cun* anterior to Yuanye (GB 22), on the level of the nipple and in the 4th intercostal space.

2. 11. 24 GB 24 Rìyuè 日月

Name: Seen in *Mai Jing*.

Location:

1) "1.5 *cun* below Qimen (LR 14)." (*Jia Yi*)

2) "0.5 *cun* below Qimen (LR 14)." (*Qian Jin*)

3) "On the 3rd rib, 2.5 *cun* lateral to the xiphoid process, directly below the nipple." (*Su Wen*, annotated by Wang)

4) "0.5 *cun* below Qimen (LR 14), two ribs directly below the nipple." (*Tong Ren*)

5) "0.5 *cun* below Qimen (LR 14), 4 *cun* lateral to the Ren Meridian, on the level of the xiphoid process." (*Liu Ji*)

6) "1.5 *cun* lateral to and 0.5 *cun* directly below Qimen (LR 14)." (*Xun Jing*)

7) "0.5 *cun* below Qimen (LR 14), three ribs inferior, on the level of the xiphoid process." (*Feng Yuan*)

Note: In most of the medical literature, Qimen (LR 14) is taken as the chief landmark for locating the point. *Jia Yi* says: "Qimen (LR 14) is at the end of the 2nd rib, 1.5 *cun* lateral to Burong (ST 19). The nipples are directly above it. Riyue (GB 24) is located three ribs below the nipple." Now, Riyue (GB 24) is located on the upper abdomen, directly below the nipple, in the 7th intercostal space and 4 *cun* lateral to the anterior midline. The descriptions in *Liu Ji* and *Xun Jing* are contradictory to that in *Jia Yi*, and are not acceptable.

2. 11. 25 GB 25 Jīngmén 京門

Name: Seen in *Mai Jing*.

Location:

1) "Below the iliac bone, on the waist, lateral to the spinal column, 1.8 *cun* below the hypochondrium." (*Jia Yi*)

2) "On the iliac bone, the waist and the hypochondrium, lateral to the spinal column." (*Qian Jin*)

3) "On the iliac bone, the waist and the hypochondrium, lateral to the spinal column." (*Su Wen*, annotated by Wang)

4) "From Riyue (GB 24) to the iliac bone and the hypochondrium, lateral to the spinal column, 0.5 *cun* above and 9.5 *cun* lateral to the umbilicus. Locate it with the patient lying on his side, his upper leg flexed, his lower leg straight, and his arm raised." (*Jin Jian*)

Note: The location of Jingmen (GB 25) recorded in the popular edition of *Jia Yi* is confused with Daimai (GB 26). But its hand-written copy of the Ming Dynasty described it as on the iliac bone and hypochondrium, lateral to the spinal column, which is the same as that in *Qing Jin*. Now, Jingmen (GB 25) is located on the lateral side of the waist, 1.8 *cun* posterior to Zhangmen (LR 13), below the free end of the 12th rib.

2. 11. 26 GB 26 Dàimài 帶脈

Name: Seen in *Ling Shu*.

Location:

1) "1.8 *cun* below the hypochondrium." (*Jia Yi*)

2) "Below Jingmen (GB 25), in the depression 1.8 *cun* below the hypochondrium, 0.2 *cun* above and 8.5 *cun* lateral to the umbilicus." (*Jin Jian*)

3) "In the depression 1.8 *cun* below the hypochondrium, 0.2 *cun* above and 7.5 *cun* lateral to the umbilicus." (*Feng Yuan*)

Note: "Below the hypochondrium" refers to the location of Zhangmen (LR 13). Daimai (GB 26) is on the lateral side of the abdomen, 1.8 *cun* below Zhangmen (LR 13) and at the crossing point of a vertical line through the free end of the 11th rib and a horizontal line through the umbilicus. The saying "0.2 *cun* above the umbilicus" comes from the location of Zhangmen (LR 13), which is "2 *cun* above the umbilicus." According to *Tu Yi*, the distance between Zhangmen (LR 13) and the umbilicus should be 1.8 *cun*.

2. 11. 27 GB 27 Wǔshū 五樞

Name: Seen in *Jia Yi*.

Location:

1) "3 *cun* below Daimai (GB 26), or 1.5 *cun* lateral to Shuidao (ST 28)." (*Jia Yi*)

2) "3 *cun* below Daimai (GB 26), 5.5 *cun* lateral to Shuidao (ST 28)." (*Da Cheng*)

3) "3 *cun* below Daimai (GB 26), or 1.5 *cun* below Shuidao (ST 28)." (*Qian Jin*)

Note: Medical literature through the ages holds similar views on the location of the point, i.e. 3 *cun* below Daimai (GB 26), lateral to Shuidao (ST 28), but the distance between Shuidao (ST 28) and Wushu (GB 27) is different. According to the running course of meridians, if it is 1.5 *cun* lateral to Shuidao (ST 28), it is on the meridian of Foot-Taiyin; if it is 5.5 *cun* lateral to Shuidao (ST 28), it seems too posterior; if it is 1.5 *cun* below Shuidao (ST 28), it is on the meridian of Foot-Yangming. Now, taking the medial border of the iliac crest as the landmark, Wushu (GB 27) is located on the lateral side of the abdomen, anterior to the anterior superior iliac spine and 3 *cun* below the level of the umbilicus.

2. 11. 28 GB 28 Wéidào 維道

Name: Seen in *Jia Yi*.

Location: "5.3 *cun* below Zhangmen (LR 13)." (*Jia Yi*)

Note: Medical literature through the ages holds similar views on the location of the point. 1.8 *cun* below Zhangmen (LR 13) is Daimai (GB 26), again 3 *cun* below is Wushu (GB 27), again 0.5 *cun* below is Weidao (GB 28), so the total distance is 5.3 *cun*. Now, Weidao (GB 28) is located on the lateral side of the abdomen, anterior and inferior to the anterior superior iliac spine, and 0.5 *cun* anterior and inferior to Wushu (GB 27).

2. 11. 29 GB 29 Jūliáo 居髎

Name: Seen in *Jia Yi*.

Location:

1) "8.3 *cun* below Zhangmen (LR 13), in the depression on the iliac bone." (*Jia Yi*)

2) "4.3 *cun* below Zhangmen (LR 13), in the depression on the iliac bone." (*Su Wen*, annotated by Wang)

3) "1 *cun* above Huantiao (GB 30)." (*Yu Long Jing*)

4) "8.3 *cun* below Zhangmen (LR 13), in the depression on the iliac bone. It is 1 *cun* from and level with Huantiao (GB 30) when the patient bends the back." (*Liu Ji*)

5) "2.5 *cun* above Huantiao (GB 30)." (*Xun Jing*)

6) "2 *cun* below and 0.5 *cun* posterior to Weidao (GB 28), anterior and slightly superior to and 3 *cun* from Huantiao (GB 30)." (*Ji Cheng*)

Note: Juliao (GB 29) is lateral to the iliac bone, in the depression between the anterior superior iliac spine and the prominence of the great trochanter. "8.3 *cun* below Zhangmen (LR 13)" refers to the fact that the distance between Zhangmen (LR 13) and Weidao (GB 28) is 5.3 *cun*, and the point is located further posteriorly. The location described in *Su Wen*, annotated by Wang Bing, is obviously wrong. The distance between Zhangmen (LR 13) and Huantiao (GB 30) is 3 *cun*, and another statement of 1 *cun* only denotes their vertical distance. Since either transverse or vertical distance is not definitely mentioned, it is rather confusing, and all the descriptions are only for reference. Now, Juliao (GB 29) is located on the hip, at the midpoint of the line connecting the anterior superior iliac spine and the prominence of the great trochanter.

2. 11. 30 GB 30 Huántiào 環跳

Name: Seen in *Jia Yi*.

Location:

1) "On the hip joint, to be located when the patient lies on his side with the upper leg flexed and the lower leg extended." (*Jia Yi*, etc.)

2) "Posterior to the hip joint." (*Su Wen*, annotated by Wang)

3) "In the depression near the great trochanter." (*Sheng Hui*)

4) "Locate the point when the patient lies on his side with the upper leg flexed and the lower leg extended. One finger-breath posterior to the great trochanter, where a deep depression can be felt." (*Xun Jing*)

5) "Below Juliao (GB 29) and on the hip joint. Locate it when the patient lies on his side with the upper leg flexed and the lower leg extended." (*Jin Jian*)

Note: Huantiao (GB 30) is located in the depression posterior and superior to the great trochanter. When the patient lies on his side with the hip flexed, Huantiao (GB 30) is located on the lateral side of the thigh, at the middle third and lateral third of the line connecting the prominence of the great trochanter and the sacral hiatus when the patient lies on his side with the thigh flexed.

2. 11. 31 GB 31 Fēngshì 風市

Name: Seen in *Zhou Hou*.

Location:

1) "On the lateral side of the thigh, at the spot touched by the middle finger when the hands of the patient are hanging down and close to the thigh."(*Zhou Hou*)

2) "Between two muscles lateral to the knee, in the depression which can be touched by the middle finger when the patient stands erect with his arms close to the thigh." (*Sheng Hui*, etc.)

3) "7 *cun* above the lateral side of the knee, at the spot touched by the tip of the middle finger." (*Yu Long Jing*, etc.)

Note: The statements in *Zhou Hou* and *Sheng Hui* only illustrate a general location of the point. *Yu Long Jing* denotes a more detailed measurement. Now, Fengshi (GB 31) is located on the lateral midline of the thigh, 7 *cun* above the popliteal crease, or at the place touched by the tip of the middle finger when the patient stands erect with arms hanging down freely.

2. 11. 32 GB 32 Zhōngdú 中瀆

Name: Seen in *Jia Yi*.

Location: "Lateral to the femur, 5 *cun* above the knee, in the depression between muscles." (*Jia Yi*, etc.)

Note: Medical literature through the ages holds similar views on the location of the point. Zhongdu (GB 32) is located on the lateral side of the thigh, 5 *cun* above the popliteal crease, between the lateral vastus muscle and the biceps muscle of the thigh.

2. 11. 33 GB 33 Xīyángguān 膝陽關

Name: Seen in *Jia Yi*. Originally named Yangguan.

Location:

1) "3 *cun* above Yanglingquan (GB 34), in the depression lateral to Dubi (ST 35)." (*Jia Yi*, etc.)

2) "2 *cun* above Yanglingquan (GB 34), in the depression lateral to Dubi (ST 35)." (*Zi Sheng*)

3) "Below Zhongdu (GB 32), 2 *cun* above the knee, in the depression lateral to Dubi (ST 35)." (*Jin Jian*)

Note: Different medical schools take Yanglingquan (GB 34) as the basis to locate Xiyangguan (GB 33), which is located on the lateral side of the knee, 3 *cun* above Yanglingquan

(GB 34), and in the depression above the external epicondyle of the femur.

2. 11. 34 GB 34 Yánglíngquán 陽陵泉

Name: Seen in *Ling Shu*.

Location:

1) "In the depression lateral to the knee joint." (*Ling Shu*)

2) "1 *cun* below the knee, in the depression on the lateral side." (*Jia Yi*, etc.)

3) "Below the knee joint, about 1 *cun* below the bone tuberosity, in the depression slightly anterior to the big muscle. Locate it when the patient is in a squatting posture." (*Xun Jing*)

4) "1 *cun* below Xiyangguan (GB 33), in the depression on the lateral side of the knee joint, anterior to the sharp bone, between the muscle and the bone. Locate it when the patient is in a squatting posture." (*Jin Jian*, etc.)

Note: The point is located with the head of the fibula as the landmark, and is anterior and inferior to it. Now, Yanglingquan (GB 34) is located on the lateral side of the leg, in the depression anterior and inferior to the head of the fibula.

2. 11. 35 GB 35 Yángjiāo 陽交

Name: Seen in *Jia Yi*.

Location:

1) "7 *cun* above the external malleolus." (*Jia Yi*, etc.)

2) "Below Yanglingquan (GB 34), 7 *cun* above the external malleolus." (*Jin Jian*)

Note: Now, Yangjiao (GB 35) is located on the lateral side of the leg, 7 *cun* above the tip of the external malleolus, and on the posterior border of the fibula.

2. 11. 36 GB 36 Wàiqiū 外丘

Name: Seen in *Jia Yi*.

Location:

1) "7 *cun* above the internal malleolus." (*Jia Yi*)

2) "7 *cun* above the external malleolus." (*Qian Jin*)

3) "7 *cun* above the external malleolus, on the level of Yangjiao (GB 35), 1 *cun* posterior to it." (*Liu Ji*)

4) "6 *cun* above the external malleolus, on the oblique line when the patient's heel is turned outward." (*Xun Jing*)

5) "7 *cun* laterally and obliquely above the external malleolus." (*Xun Jing*, etc.)

Note: The "internal malleolus" in the current edition of *Jia Yi* should be a slip of the pen in its original edition and should obviously read "external malleolus." Yangjiao (GB 35) and Waiqiu (GB 36) are 7 *cun* above the external malleolus. Yangjiao (GB 35) posteriorly crosses the Foot-Taiyang Meridian, while Waiqiu (GB 36) lies on the same vertical line of Yanglingquan (GB 34). "6 *cun* above the external malleolus" is inconsistent with the record in *Jia Yi*. Now the latter is adopted, so Waiqiu (GB 36) is located on the lateral side of the leg, 7 *cun* above the tip of the external malleolus, on the anterior border of the fibula, on the level of Yangjiao (GB 35).

2. 11. 37 GB 37 Guāngmíng 光明

Name: Seen in *Ling Shu*.

Location:

1) "5 *cun* above the external malleolus." (*Ling Shu*)

2) "5 *cun* above the external malleolus." (*Jia Yi*, etc.)

Note: Medical literature through the ages holds the same view on the location of the point. So Guangming (GB 37) is located on the lateral side of the leg, 5 *cun* above the tip of the external malleolus, and on the anterior border of the fibula.

2. 11. 38 GB 38 Yángfǔ 陽輔

Name: Seen in *Ling Shu*.

Location:

1) "Above the external malleolus, at the end of the fibula." (*Su Wen*)

2) "4 *cun* above the external malleolus, anterior to the fibula, 0.3 *cun* anterior to the end of the fibula, 7 *cun* from Qiuxu (GB 40)." (*Jia Yi*, etc.)

3) "Above the external malleolus, anterior to the fibula, 0.3 *cun* anterior to the end of the fibula, 7 *cun* from Qiuxu (GB 40)." (*Qian Jin*)

4) "4 *cun* above the external malleolus, 0.3 *cun* anterior to the end of the fibula, 7 *cun* from Qiuxu (GB 40)." (*Ju Ying*, etc.)

5) "1 *cun* below Guangming (GB 37), 0.3 *cun* obliquely medial to the end of the fibula." (*Jin Jian*)

Note: Medical literature through the ages holds similar views on the location of the point. Now "4 *cun* above and 0.3 *cun* anterior to the external malleolus" are taken as the standard, and Yangfu (GB 38) is located on the lateral side of the leg, 4 *cun* above the tip of the external malleolus, slightly anterior to the anterior border of the fibula. "7 *cun* from Qiuxu (GB 40)" is not adopted, since the length of measurement is too long.

2. 11. 39 GB 39 Xuánzhōng 懸鍾

Name: Seen in *Jia Yi*.

Location:

1) "3 *cun* above the external malleolus, where the pulsation is palpable." (*Jia Yi*, etc.)

2) "3 *cun* above the external malleolus, on the artery where a sharp bone can be felt." (*Da Cheng*, etc.)

Note: Medical literature through the ages holds similar views on the location of the point. Now, according to the record of "the pulsation is palpable," Xuanzhong (GB 39) is located on the lateral side of the leg, 3 *cun* above the tip of the external malleolus, in the depression on the anterior border of the fibula.

2. 11. 40 GB 40 Qiūxū 丘墟

Name: Seen in *Ling Shu*.

Location:

1) "In the depression anterior to the external malleolus." (*Ling Shu*, etc.)

2) "Below Xuanzhong (GB 39), distal and obliquely anterior to the external malleolus." (*Jin Jian*)

Note: Medical literature through the ages holds similar views on the location of the point. Qiuxu (GB 40) is located anterior and interior to the external malleolus, and in the depression lateral to the tendon of the long extensor muscle of the toes.

2. 11. 41 GB 41 Zúlínqì 足臨泣

Name: Seen in *Da Quan*. Originally named Linqi in *Ling Shu*.

1) "In the depression between the 4th and 5th metatarsal bones, 1.5 *cun* from Xiaxi (GB 43)." (*Jia Yi*, etc.)

2) "3 *cun* below Qiuxu (GB 40), in the depression between the 4th and 5th metatarsal bones." (*Jin Jian*)

Note: Medical literature through the ages holds similar views on the location of the point. Now, Zulinqi (GB 41) is located on the lateral side of the instep of the foot, posterior to the 4th metatarsophalangeal joint, and in the depression lateral to the tendon of the extensor muscle of the little toe.

2. 11. 42 GB 42 Dìwǔhuì 地五會

Name: Seen in *Jia Yi*.

Location:

1) "In the depression posterior to the proximal end of the 4th and 5th metatarsal bones." (*Jia Yi*, etc.)

2) "Posterior to the proximal end of the 4th and 5th metatarsal bones." (*Qian Jin*, etc.)

3) "In the depression posterior to the proximal ends of the 4th and 5th metatarsal bones, 1 *cun* from Xiaxi (GB 43)."

Note: Medical literature through the ages holds similar views on the location of the point. Now Diwuhui (GB 42) is located on the lateral side of the instep of the foot, posterior to the 4th metatarsophalangeal joint, between the 4th and 5th metatarsal bones, medial to the tendon of the extensor muscle of the little toe.

2. 11. 43 GB 43 Xiáxī 俠谿

Name: Seen in *Ling Shu*.

Location:

1) "Between the little and the 4th toes." (*Ling Shu*)

2) "In the depression between the 4th and 5th metatarsal bones, anterior (distal) to the metatarsophalangeal joint." (*Su Wen*, etc.)

3) "1 *cun* below Diwuhui (GB 42), in the depression anterior to the metatarsophalangeal joint. (*Jin Jian*)

Note: Medical literature through the ages holds similar views on the location of the point. Now, Xiaxi (GB 43) is located on the lateral side of the instep of the foot, between the 4th and 5th toes, and at the junction of the red and white skin proximal to the margin of the web.

2. 11. 44 GB 44 Zúqiàoyīn 足竅陰

Name: Seen in *Da Quan*. Originally named Qiaoyin in *Ling Shu*.

Location:

1) "At the tip of the 4th toe." (*Ling Shu*)

2) "At the tip of the 4th toe, about the width of a chive leaf from the corner of the nail." (*Jia Yi*, etc.)

3) "At the tip of the 4th toe, about the width of a chive leaf from the corner of the nail." (*Qian Jin Yi*)

4) "On the lateral side of the 4th toe, about the width of a chive leaf from the corner of the nail." (*Da Cheng*, etc.)

Note: Medical literature through the ages holds the same view on the location of the point. Zuqiaoyin (GB 44) is located on the lateral side of the distal segment of the 4th toe, about 0.1 *cun* from the corner of the toenail.

2. 12 Points of the Liver Meridian of Foot-Jueyin, LR

足厥陰肝經穴

Zújuéyīn Gānjīng Xué

2. 12. 1 LR 1 Dàdūn 大敦

Name: Seen in *Ling Shu* and *Su Wen*.

Location:

1) "At the tip of the great toe, the width of a chive leaf from the corner of the toenail, surrounded by the hair." (*Jia Yi*, etc.)

2) "Inside the hair of the great toe." (*Qian Jin*)

3) "At the tip of the great toe, the width of a chive leaf from the corner of the toenail." (Annotated *Su Wen*)

4) "At the tip of the great toe, about the width of a chive leaf from the corner of the nail, inside the hair on the lateral side of the great toe." (*Jin Jian*)

5) "0.4 *cun* posterior to the corner of the nail of the great toe, anterior (distal) to its joint." (*Ji Cheng*)

Note: Medical literature through the ages holds similar views on the location of the point. According to the annotations to *Su Wen*, Dadun (LR 1) is located on the lateral side of the distal phalanx of the great toe, 0.1 *cun* from the corner of the toenail. *Ji Cheng* refers it to the place between the lateral corner of the toenail of the great toe and the interphalangeal joint, which corresponds to the location illustrated in *Ling Shu*. The location is a little posterior to other Jing-Well points, so "0.4 *cun* posterior to the corner of the nail" may be taken as a reference.

2. 12. 2 LR 2 Xíngjiān 行間

Name: Seen in *Ling Shu*.

Location:

1) "In the depression on the pulsating artery of the great toe." (*Jia Yi*, etc.)

2) "Proximal to the 1st metatarsal bone, between the two tendons below and above and the two small bones anteriorly and posteriorly, exactly in the depression where the pulsation is palpable." (*Shen Ying*)

3) "Between the 1st and 2nd toes." (*Xun Jing*)

4) "Above Dadun (LR 1), between the 1st and 2nd toes, in the depression where the pulsation is palpable." (*Jin Jian*)

Note: Medical literature through the ages holds similar views on the location of the point. Xingjian (LR 2) is located on the instep of the foot, between the 1st and 2nd toes, and at the junction of the red and white skin, proximal to the margin of the web.

2. 12. 3 LR 3 Tàichōng 太衝

Name: Seen in *Ling Shu*.

Location:

1) "In the depression 2 *cun* above Xingjian (LR 2)." (*Ling Shu*)

2) "2 *cun* posterior to the distal end of the 1st metatarsal bone, or in the depression 1.5 *cun* posterior to it." (*Jia Yi*)

3) "2.5 *cun* posterior to the distal end of the 1st metatarsal bone, or in the depression, 1.5 *cun* posterior to it." (*Wai Tai*)

Note: Medical literature through the ages holds similar views on the location of the point. Taichong (LR 3) is located posterior to the distal end of the 1st metatarsal bone. Only the distance is quite different, i.e. 1.5 *cun*, 2 *cun*, 2.5 *cun*, etc. The depression between the 1st and 2nd metatarsal bones should be taken as the landmark. "2.5 *cun*" in *Wai Tai* should read "2 *cun*," which has been corrected in the illustration of the five Shu points. Now, Taichong (LR 3) is located on the instep of the foot, in the depression at the posterior end of the 1st interosseous space.

2. 12. 4 LR 4 Zhōngfēng 中封

Name: Seen in *Ling Shu*.

Location:

1) "In the depression 1.5 *cun* anterior to the medial malleolus." (*Ling Shu*, etc.)

2) "1 *cun* anterior to the medial malleolus, in the depression when the ankle is flexed. To be located with the patient's ankle stretched." (*Jia Yi*, etc.)

3) "On the level of and 1.5 *cun* anterior to the tip of the medial malleolus between the two tendons. To be located with the patient's ankle extended." (*Xun Jing*)

Note: Medical literature through the ages holds similar views on the location of the point. Now, Zhongfeng (LR 4) is located on the instep of the foot, anterior to the medial malleolus, on the line connecting Shangqiu (SP 5) and Jiexi (ST 41), and in the depression medial to the tendon of the anterior tibial muscle.

2. 12. 5 LR 5 Lígōu 蠡溝

Name: Seen in *Ling Shu*.

Location:

1) "0.5 *cun* from the medial malleolus." (*Ling Shu*)

2) "Lateral to the calf muscle." (*Su Wen*)

3) "5 *cun* above the medial malleolus." (*Jia Yi*)

Note: Medical literature through the ages holds similar views on the location of the point. The statement of a location on the medial side of the shank is not clear or definite. According to the running course of the Liver Meridian and the position of Zhongdu (LR 6), Ligou (LR 5) is located on the medial side of the leg, 5 *cun* above the tip of the medial malleolus and on the midline of the medial surface of the tibia.

2. 12. 6 LR 6 Zhōngdū 中都

Name: Seen in *Jia Yi*.

Location:

1) "7 *cun* above the medial malleolus, in the middle of the tibia." (*Jia Yi*, etc.)

2) "7 *cun* above the medial malleolus, in the middle of the tibia." (*Wai Tai*)

3) "2 *cun* above Ligou (LR 5), in the middle of the tibia." (*Jin Jian*)

Note: Medical literature through the ages holds similar views on the location of the point. Zhongdu (LR 6) is located 7 *cun* above the tip of the medial malleolus and on the medial side of the leg, on the midline of the medial surface of the tibia.

2. 12. 7 LR 7 Xīguān 膝關

Name: Seen in *Jia Yi*.

Location:

1) "In the depression 2 *cun* below Dubi (ST 35)." (*Jia Yi*)

2) "In the depression 3 *cun* below Dubi (ST 35)." (*Qian Jin*)

3) "In the depression lateral to and 2 *cun* below Dubi (ST 35)." (*Ju Ying*, etc.)

4) "In the depression on the medial side of and inferior to the patella, on the same level of Dubi (ST 35) and 2 *cun* from it." (*Liu Ji*)

Note: "2 *cun* below Dubi (ST 35)" refers to the location being 2 *cun* below the knee. According to the running course of the Liver Meridian, it runs posteriorly along the medial border of the patella. So Xiguan (LR 7) is posterior to Yinlingquan (SP 9). Now, Xiguan (LR 7) is located on the medial side of the leg, posterior and inferior to the medial epicondyle of the tibia, 1 *cun* posterior to Yinlingquan (SP 9), at the upper end of the medial head of the gastrocnemius muscle.

2. 12. 8 LR 8 Qūquán 曲泉

Name: Seen in *Ling Shu*.

Location:

1) "Below the medial epicondyle of the femur and above the big tendon. To be located with the patient's knee flexed." (*Ling Shu*)

2) "In the depression below the medial epicondyle of the femur, above the big tendon and below the small tendon. To be located with the patient's knee flexed." (*Jia Yi*, etc.)

3) "At the medial end of the popliteal crease." (*Qian Jin*, etc.)

4) "In the depression between the medial and lateral tendons when the patient's knee is flexed, or at the end of the crease when the knee is flexed." (*Zi Sheng*)

5) "On the knee, in the depression below the medial epicondyle of the femur, above the big tendon and below the small tendon, at the end of the popliteal crease when the patient's knee is flexed." (*Ju Ying*)

6) "1 *cun* posterior to Yingu (KI 10)." (*Xun Jing*)

Note: What is recorded in *Ling Shu* should be considered as the standard. The "big tendon" refers to the tendon of the semimembranous muscle, and the point is located above it. The "small tendon" mentioned in *Jia Yi* is not so important. The description in *Qian Jin* may be taken as a reference. Yingu (KI 10) should be posterior to Ququan (LR 8).

2. 12. 9 LR 9 Yīnbāo 陰包

Name: Seen in *Jia Yi*.

Location: "4 *cun* above the knee, on the medial side of the thigh between the two tendons." (*Jia Yi*, etc.)

Note: The records in various ancient literature are unanimous. Yinbao (LR 9) is located on the medial side of the thigh, 4 *cun* above the medial epicondyle of the femur, in the depression between the medial vastus muscle and the sartorius muscle.

2. 12. 10 LR 10 Zúwǔlǐ 足五裏

Name: Seen in *Zi Sheng*. Originally named Wuli in *Jia Yi*.

Location:

1) "Below Yinlian (LR 11), 3 *cun* from Qichong (ST 30), beside the artery on the medial side of the thigh." (*Jia Yi*, etc.)

2) "2 *cun* below Yinlian (LR 11)." (*Qian Jin*, etc.)

3) "3 *cun* below Qichong (ST 30), beside the artery on the medial side of the thigh." (*Tong Ren*, etc.)

4) "1 *cun* below Yinlian (LR 11), 3 *cun* from Qichong (ST 30), beside the artery on the medial aspect of the thigh." (*Liu Ji*)

Note: Yinlian (LR 11) is 2 *cun* below Qichong (ST 30), and Zuwuli (LR 10) is 3 *cun* below Qichong (ST 30), i.e. 1 *cun* below Yinlian (LR 11). *Qian Jin* wrongly says it is 2 *cun* below Yinlian (LR 11). Accordingly, Zuwuli (LR 10) is located on the medial side of the thigh, 3 *cun* directly below Qichong (ST 30), at the proximal end of the thigh, below the pubic tubercle, and on the lateral border of the long abductor muscle of the thigh.

2. 12. 11 LR 11 Yīnlián 陰廉

Name: Seen in *Jia Yi*.

Location:

1) "Below the 'goat feces,' 0.3 *cun* from Qichong (ST 30), on the artery." (*Jia Yi*, etc.)

2) "Above Wuli (LR 10), below the 'goat feces,' 0.3 *cun* medial to and 2 *cun* above Qichong (ST 30), in the depression on the artery." (*Jin Jian*, etc.)

Note: Medical literature through the ages holds similar views on the location of the point. The "goat feces" is a metaphor for the lymph nodes in the inguinal region. Accordingly, Yinlian (LR 11) is located on the medial side of the thigh, 2 *cun* directly below Qichong (ST 30), at the proximal end of the thigh, below the pubic tubercle, and on the lateral border of the long abductor muscle of the thigh.

2. 12. 12 LR 12 Jímài 急脈

Name: Seen in *Su Wen*.

Location:

1) "Inside the pubic hair." (*Sun Wen*)

2) "Inside the pubic hair. 2.5 *cun* lateral to the pubic symphysis." (*Su Wen*, annotated by Wang, etc.)

Note: Medical literature through the ages holds similar views on the location of the point. Accordingly, Jimai (LR 12) is located lateral to the pubic tubercle lateral and inferior to Qichong (ST 30), in the inguinal groove where the pulsation of the femoral artery is palpable, and 2.5 *cun* lateral to the anterior midline.

2. 12. 13 LR 13 Zhāngmén 章門

Name: Seen in *Mai Jing*.

Location:

1) "Lateral to Daheng (SP 15), on the level of the umbilicus, at the end of the 11th rib. To be located when the patient lies on his side with the upper leg flexed, the lower leg extended and the arm raised." (*Jia Yi*, etc.)

2) "2 *cun* above and 6 *cun* lateral to the umbilicus." (*Shen Ying*, etc.)

3) "Lateral to Daheng (SP 15), at the end of the 11th rib, 3 *cun* above and 9 *cun* lateral to the umbilicus." (*Ju Ying*, etc.)

4) "At the spot on the lateral side of the chest touched by the tip of the elbow." (*Ju Ying*, etc.)

5) "On the spot touched by the tip of the elbow when the patient lies on his side with the upper leg flexed and the lower leg extended, and the finger touching the earlobe, or 2 *cun* above and 6 *cun* (8 *cun* in the obese person) lateral to the umbilicus." (*Xun Jing*)

6) "1.8 *cun* above and 8.5 *cun* lateral to the umbilicus, at the end of the 11th rib." (*Tu Yi*)

Note: "At the end of the 11th rib" does not mean it is directly lateral to the umbilicus, so "on the level of the umbilicus" cannot be accepted. "1.8 *cun*" above the umbilicus is more reasonable. In locating Zhangmen (LR 13), Jingmen (GB 25) and Daimai (GB 26) should be taken as a reference. The distance lateral to the anterior midline cannot be taken as the standard. Now, Zhangmen (LR 13) is located on the lateral side of the abdomen, below the free end of the 11th rib.

2. 12. 14 LR 14 Qīmén 期門

Name: Seen in *Shang Han Lun*.

Location:

1) "At the end of the 2nd rib, 1.5 *cun* lateral to Burong (ST 19), directly below the nipples." (*Jia Yi*, etc.)

2) "In the 2nd intercostal space below the nipple." (*Qian Jin*)

3) "1.5 *cun* lateral to and 1.5 *cun* directly below the nipple." (*Da Cheng*)

Note: Most of the medical literature through the ages follow *Jia Yi*. Burong (ST 19) is 2 *cun* lateral to the Ren Meridian, and Qimen is 3.5 *cun* lateral to the Ren Meridian. Since "the nipple is directly above the point," it should be 4 *cun* lateral to the Ren Meridian. Now, Qimen (LR 14) is located according to the description in *Jia Yi* and *Qian Jin*, i.e. directly below the nipple, in the 6th intercostal space, 4 *cun* lateral to the anterior midline. The description in *Da Cheng* is not adopted.

2. 13 Points of the Du Meridian, DU

督脈穴

Dūmài Xué

2. 13. 1 DU 1 Chángqiáng 長强

Name: Seen in *Ling Shu*.

Location:

1) "At the end of the coccyx." (*Jia Yi*, etc.)

2) "In the depression inferior to the coccyx." (*Sheng Hui*)

3) "0.3 *cun* inferior to the end of the coccyx." (*Ju Ying*)

Note: *Ju Ying* says that there is a certain distance between the location of Changqiang (DU 1) and the tip of the coccyx. For convenience of locating and puncturing this point, Changqiang (DU 1) is located below the tip of the coccyx, at the midpoint of the line connecting the tip of the coccyx and anus.

2. 13. 2 DU 2 Yāoshū 腰俞

Name: Seen in *Su Wen*.

Location: "In the depression below the 21st vertebra." (*Jia Yi*)

Note: Medical literature through the ages holds similar views on the location of the point. The "21st vertebra" corresponds to the 4th sacral vertebra. Yaoshu (DU 2) is located on the sacrum, on the posterior midline, just at the sacral hiatus.

2. 13. 3 DU 3 Yāoyángguān 腰陽關

Name: Seen in *Da Quan*. Originally named Yangguan in *Su Wen*, annotated by Wang.

Location: "Below the 16th vertebra." (*Su Wen*, annotated by Wang)

Note: Medical literature through the ages holds similar views on the location of the point.

The "16th vertebra" corresponds to the 4th lumbar vertebra. Yaoyangguan (DU 3) is located on the low back, on the posterior midline and in the depression below the spinous process of the 4th lumbar vertebra.

2. 13. 4 DU 4 Mìngmén 命門

Name: Seen in *Jia Yi*.

Location: "Below the 14th vertebra." (*Jia Yi*, etc.)

Note: Medical literature through the ages holds the same view on the location of the point. Mingmen (DU 4) is located on the low back, on the posterior midline and in the depression below the spinous process of the 2nd lumbar vertebra.

2. 13. 5 DU 5 Xuánshū 懸樞

Name: Seen in *Jia Yi*.

Location: "Below the 13th vertebra." (*Jia Yi*, etc.)

Note: Medical literature through the ages holds the same view on the location of the point. Xuanshu (DU 5) is located on the low back, on the posterior midline and in the depression below the spinous process of the 1st lumbar vertebra.

2. 13. 6 DU 6 Jǐzhōng 脊中

Name: Seen in *Jia Yi*.

Location: "Below the 11th vertebra." (*Jia Yi*, etc.)

Note: Medical literature through the ages holds the same view on the location of the point. Jizhong (DU 6) is located on the back, on the posterior midline and in the depression below the spinous process of the 11th thoracic vertebra.

2. 13. 7 DU 7 Zhōngshū 中樞

Name: Seen in *Su Wen*, annotated by Wang.

Location: "Below the 10th vertebra." (*Su Wen*, annotated by Wang)

Note: There is no record of this point in *Jia Yi*. In the Qing Dynasty, *Jin Jian*, *Feng Yuan* and other books began to introduce Wang's annotations to *Su Wen*, which included Zhongshu (DU 7) in the Du Meridian. Accordingly, Zhongshu (DU 7) is located on the back, on the posterior midline and in the depression below the spinous process of the 10th thoracic vertebra.

2. 13. 8 DU 8 Jīnsuō 筋縮

Name: Seen in *Jia Yi*.

Location: "Below the 9th vertebra." (*Jia Yi*)

Note: Medical literature through the ages holds the same view on the location of the point. Jinsuo (DU 8) is located on the back, on the posterior midline and in the depression below the spinous process of the 9th thoracic vertebra.

2. 13. 9 DU 9 Zhìyáng 至陽

Name: Seen in *Jia Yi*.

Location: "Below the 7th vertebra." (*Jia Yi*)

Note: Medical literature through the ages holds the same view on the location of the point. Zhiyang (DU 9) is located on the back, on the posterior midline and in the depression below the spinous process of the 7th thoracic vertebra.

2. 13. 10 DU 10 Língtái 靈台

Name: Seen in *Su Wen*, annotated by Wang.

Location: "Below the 6th vertebra." (*Su Wen*, annotated by Wang, etc.)

Note: Medical literature through the ages holds the same view on the location of the point.

Lingtai (DU 10) is located on the back, on the posterior midline and in the depression below the spinous process of the 6th thoracic vertebra.

2. 13. 11 DU 11 Shéndào 神道

Name: Seen in *Jia Yi*.

Location: "Below the 5th vertebra." (*Jia Yi*)

Note: Medical literature through the ages holds the same view on the location of the point. Shendao (DU 11) is located on the back, on the posterior midline and in the depression below the spinous process of the 5th thoracic vertebra.

2. 13. 12 DU 12 Shēnzhù 身柱

Name: Seen in *Jia Yi*.

Location: "Below the 3rd vertebra." (*Jia Yi*, etc.)

Note: Medical literature through the ages holds the same view on the location of the point. Shenzhu (DU 12) is located on the back, on the posterior midline, and in the depression below the spinous process of the 3rd thoracic vertebra.

2. 13. 13 DU 13 Táodào 陶道

Name: Seen in *Jia Yi*.

Location:

1) "Below the big vertebra." (*Jia Yi*, etc.)

2) "Below the 1st vertebra." (*Da Cheng*, etc.)

3) "Below the 2nd vertebra." (*Liu Ji*)

Note: Most of the medical literature through the ages follow *Jia Yi*. "Below the big vertebra" corresponds to "below the spinous process of the 1st thoracic vertebra," which is in conformity with the description in *Da Cheng*. The statement in *Liu Ji* is wrong and not accepted. Now, the point is located on the back, on the posterior midline and in the depression below the spinous process of the 1st thoracic vertebra.

2. 13. 14 DU 14 Dàzhuī 大椎

Name: Seen in *Su Wen*.

Location:

1) "In the depression of the 1st vertebra." (*Jia Yi*)

2) "In the depression above the 1st vertebra." (*Qian Jin*, etc.)

3) "In the depression below the 1st vertebra, on the nape." (*Sheng Hui*, etc.)

Note: *Jia Yi* always shows the exact locations of the points of this meridian, as either "above" or "below" the vertebra, but there is no such description for Dazhui (DU 14), maybe because of missing words. The statement in *Qian Jin* is simple and clear, and accepted by others thereafter. The "1st vertebra" in *Sheng Hui* should be considered as the most prominent spinous process on the nape, i.e. the spinous process of the 7th cervical vertebra, and not as that of the 1st thoracic vertebra. "Dazhui" (the big vertebra) is named after the big prominence of the spinous process of the 7th cervical vertebra.

2. 13. 15 DU 15 Yǎmén 啞門

Name: Seen in *Su Wen*.

Location:

1) "Inferior to the occiput on the nape." (*Su Wen*)

2) "In the depression on the posterior hairline." (*Jia Yi*, etc.)

3) "In the depression on the hairline of the nape, 1 *cun* from Fengfu (DU 16). (*Su Wen*,

annotated by Wang)

4) "In the middle of the nape, in the depression 0.5 *cun* above the hairline." (*Tong Ren*, etc.)

Note: Medical literature before the Song Dynasty believed that Yamen (DU 15) was above the posterior hairline, on the midline of the head and neck, 1 *cun* from Fengfu (DU 16). *Tong Ren* located it as in the middle of the nape, in the depression 0.5 *cun* above the hairline, and this location has been followed ever since.

2. 13. 16 DU 16 Fēngfǔ 風府

Name: Seen in *Ling Shu* and *Su Wen*.

Location:

1) "1 *cun* above the hairline on the nape, in the depression between the big tendons." (*Jia Yi*, etc.)

2) "1 *cun* above Yamen (DU 15)." (*Qian Jin*)

Note: For the location of this point, *Jia Yi* has been followed by the later generations. Now, Fengfu (DU 16) is located on the nape, 1 *cun* directly above the midpoint of the posterior hairline, directly below the external occipital protuberance and in the depression between the trapezius muscle of both sides.

2. 13. 17 DU 17 Nǎohù 腦户

Name: Seen in *Jia Yi*.

Location:

1) "On the occipital bone, 1.5 *cun* posterior to Qiangjian (DU 18)." (*Jia Yi*)

2) "1.5 *cun* above Fengfu (DU 16), on the occipital bone." (*Jin Jian*)

Note: The above-mentioned locations are more or less the same. So Naohu (DU 17) is located on the head, 2.5 *cun* directly above the midpoint of the posterior hairline, 1.5 *cun* above Fengfu (DU 16), in the depression on the upper border of the external occipital protuberance.

2. 13. 18 DU 18 Qiángjiān 强間

Name: Seen in *Jia Yi*.

Location: "1.5 *cun* posterior to Houding (DU 19)." (*Jia Yi*)

Note: Medical literature through the ages holds similar views on the location of the point. Qiangjian (DU 18) is located on the head, 4 *cun* directly above the midpoint of the posterior hairline, and 1.5 *cun* above Naohu (DU 17).

2. 13. 19 DU 19 Hòudǐng 後頂

Name: Seen in *Jia Yi*.

Location: "1.5 *cun* posterior to Baihui (DU 20), on the occipital bone." (*Jia Yi*)

Note: Medical literature through the ages holds the same view on the location of the point. Houding (DU 19) is located on the head, 5.5 *cun* directly above the midpoint of the posterior hairline and 3 *cun* above Naohu (DU 17).

2. 13. 20 DU 20 Bǎihuì 百會

Name: Seen in *Jia Yi*.

Location:

1) "1.5 *cun* posterior to Qianding (DU 21), inside the whirl of the hair on the top of the head, in the depression about the size of the finger tip." (*Jia Yi*, etc.)

2) "At the midpoint between Yintang (EX-HN3) and the posterior hairline." (*Yu Long Jing*)

Note: For the location of Baihui (DU 20), many medical schools accept "1.5 *cun* posterior to Qianding (DU 21)" or "1.5 *cun* above Houding (DU 19)," which represents the same location, i.e. 5 *cun* directly above the midpoint of the anterior hairline. The location of the whirl of the hair on the top of the head varies among individuals, and should not be adopted. According to the bone proportional measurement, the location of Baihui (DU 20) illustrated in *Yu Long Jing* should be 4.5 *cun* from the anterior hairline, with a difference of 0.5 *cun*.

2. 13. 21 DU 21 Qiándǐng 前頂

Name: Seen in *Jia Yi*.

Location:

1) "1.5 *cun* posterior to Xinhui (DU 22), in the depression of the bone." (*Jia Yi*, etc.)

2) "1 *cun* anterior to Baihui (DU 20)." (*Sheng Hui*)

Note: Medical literature through the ages follows *Jia Yi*. But *Sheng Hui* says it is "1.5 *cun* posterior to Xinhui (DU 22)," corresponding to 3.5 *cun* above the anterior hairline, or 1.5 *cun* anterior to Baihui, and again "1 *cun* anterior to Baihui (DU 20)," which is self-contradictory. The location of Qianding (DU 21) recorded in *Jia Yi* is adopted nowadays.

2. 13. 22 DU 22 Xìnhuì 顖會

Name: Seen in *Ling Shu*.

Location:

1) "1 *cun* posterior to Shangxing (DU 23), in the depression of the bone." (*Jia Yi*, etc.)

2) "1.5 *cun* anterior to Qianding (DU 21)." (*Jin Jian*, etc.)

Note: Medical literature through the ages holds the same view on the location of the point. Xinhui (DU 22) is located on the head, 2 *cun* directly above the midpoint of the anterior hairline and 3 *cun* anterior to Baihui (DU 20).

2. 13. 23 DU 23 Shàngxīng 上星

Name: Seen in *Jia Yi*.

Location: "On the head, directly above the nose, in the depression 1 *cun* above the anterior hairline." (*Jia Yi*, etc.)

Note: Medical literature through the ages holds the same view on the location of the point. Shangxing (DU 23) is located on the head, 1 *cun* directly above the midpoint of the anterior hairline.

2. 13. 24 DU 24 Shéntíng 神庭

Name: Seen in *Jia Yi*.

Location:

1) "On the hairline, directly above the nose." (*Jia Yi*, etc.)

2) "Directly above the nose, 0.5 *cun* above the hairline." (*Sheng Hui*)

Note: *Jia Yi* locates the point on the hairline, which is followed by *Qian Jin* and *Su Wen*. *Sheng Hui* first located it "0.5 *cun* above the hairline." Later Wang Weiyi adopted this view, which is followed nowadays.

2. 13. 25 DU 25 Sùliáo 素髎

Name: Seen in *Jia Yi*.

Location: "At the upper end of the nasal pillar." (*Jia Yi*, etc.)

Note: Medical literature through the ages holds the same view on the location of the point. Suliao (DU 25) is located on the face, at the centre of the nose apex.

2. 13. 26 DU 26 Shuǐgōu 水溝

Name: Seen in *Jia Yi*.

Location:

1) "In the philtrum below the nasal pillar." (*Jia Yi*, etc.)

2) "Below the nasal pillar." (*Tong Ren*, etc.)

3) "0.3 *cun* below the nose, on the prominence when water is held in the mouth." (*Yu Long Jing*, etc.)

4) "In the philtrum below the nasal pillar, in the depression near the nostrils." (*Ju Ying*, etc.)

5) "In the philtrum below the nasal pillar." (*Ru Men*)

6) "0.3 *cun* below the nasal pillar, on the prominence when water is held in the mouth." (*Liu Ji*)

Note: Below the nasal pillar is the philtrum, in which this point lodges. *Yu Long Jing* and *Liu Ji* propose it should be "0.3 *cun* below the nose" or "0.3 *cun* below the nasal pillar." *Ju Ying*, *Da Cheng* and *Jin Jian* all say it is "near the nostrils." Both views are of the same meaning. So Shuigou (DU 26) is located on the face, at the junction of the upper third and middle third of the philtrum.

2. 13. 27 DU 27 Duìduān 兑端

Name: Seen in *Jia Yi*.

Location: "On the upper portion of the lip." (*Jia Yi*, etc.)

Note: Medical literature through the ages holds the same view on the location of the point. Duiduan (DU 27) is located on the face on the labial tubercle of the upper lip, and on the vermilion border between the philtrum and upper lip.

2. 13. 28 DU 28 Yínjiāo 齦交

Name: Seen in *Su Wen*.

Location: "Inside of the lip, on the upper gum." (*Jia Yi*, etc.)

Note: Medical literature through the ages holds the same view on the location of the point. Yinjiao (DU 28) is inside the upper lip, at the junction of the labial frenum and upper gum.

2. 14 Points of the Ren Meridian, RN
任脈穴
Rènmài Xué

2. 14. 1 RN 1 Huìyīn 會陰

Name: Seen in *Jia Yi*.

Location:

1) "Between the urinal orifice and the anus." (*Jia Yi*, etc.)

2) "From Qugu (RN 2) downward, below the genitals between the urinal orifice and the anus." (*Su Wen*, annotated by Wang)

3) "Between the urinal orifice and the anus, at the midpoint behind the scrotum in male." (*Liu Ji*)

Note: This point is located on the perineum, at the midpoint between the posterior border of the scrotum and anus in male, and between the posterior commissure of the labium majus and anus in female.

2. 14. 2 RN 2 Qūgǔ 曲骨

Name: Seen in *Jia Yi*.

Location:

1) "On the pubic bone, 1 *cun* below Zhongji (RN 3), in the depression on the hairline, where the pulsation is palpable." (*Jia Yi*, etc.)

2) "In the middle of the bilateral pubic bones above the genitals." (*Qian Jin*)

Note: This point is located 1 *cun* below Zhongji (RN 3), or 5 *cun* below the umbilicus, so it is "on the pubic bone." Now Qugu (RN 2) is located on the lower abdomen, on the anterior midline, and at the midpoint of the upper border of the pubic symphysis.

2. 14. 3 RN 3 Zhōngjí 中極

Name: Seen in *Su Wen*.

Location: "4 *cun* below the centre of the umbilicus." (*Jia Yi*, etc.)

Note: Medical literature through the ages holds the same view on the location of the point.

2. 14. 4 RN 4 Guānyuán 關元

Name: Seen in *Ling Shu* and *Su Wen*.

Location: "3 *cun* below the centre of the umbilicus." (*Ling Shu*, etc.)

Note: Medical literature through the ages holds the same view on the location of the point.

2. 14. 5 RN 5 Shímén 石門

Name: Seen in *Jia Yi*.

Location: "2 *cun* below the centre of the umbilicus." (*Jia Yi*)

Note: Medical literature through the ages holds the same view on the location of the point.

2. 14. 6 RN 6 Qìhǎi 氣海

Name: Seen in *Mai Jing*. Also named "Boyang" in *Ling Shu*.

Location: "1.5 *cun* below the centre of the umbilicus." (*Jia Yi*, etc.)

Note: Medical literature through the ages holds the same view on the location of the point.

2. 14. 7 RN 7 Yīnjiāo 陰交

Name: Seen in *Jia Yi*.

Location: "1 *cun* below the centre of the umbilicus." (*Jia Yi*, etc.)

Note: Medical literature through the ages holds the same view on the location of the point.

2. 14. 8 RN 8 Shénquè 神闕

Name: Seen in *Tong Ren*.

Location: "At the centre of the umbilicus." (*Jia Yi*, etc.)

Note: Medical literature through the ages holds the same view on the location of the point.

2. 14. 9 RN 9 Shuǐfēn 水分

Name: Seen in *Jia Yi*.

Location: "1 *cun* below Xiawan (RN 10), 1 *cun* above the centre of the umbilicus." (*Jia Yi*, etc.)

Note: Medical literature through the ages holds the same view on the location of the point.

2. 14. 10 RN 10 Xiàwǎn 下脘

Name: Seen in *Ling Shu*.

Location: "1 *cun* below Jianli (RN 11)." (*Jia Yi*, etc.)

Note: Medical literature through the ages holds the same view on the location of the point, i.e. 2 *cun* directly above the centre of the umbilicus.

2. 14. 11 RN 11 Jiànlǐ 建裏

Name: Seen in *Jia Yi*.

Location: "1 *cun* below Zhongwan (RN 12)." (*Jia Yi*, etc.)

Note: Medical literature through the ages holds the same view on the location of the point, i.e. 3 *cun* directly above the centre of the umbilicus.

2. 14. 12 RN 12 Zhōngwǎn 中脘

Name: Seen in *Mai Jing*.

Location:

1) "4 *cun* or 3 *cun* below the xiphoid process."

2) "1 *cun* below Shangwan (RN 13), at the midpoint between the xiphoid process and the umbilicus." (*Jia Yi* , etc.)

3) "4 *cun* below the xiphoid process, four finger-breaths above the umbilicus." (*Qian Jin*)

Note: Since the length of the xiphoid process varies among individuals it is difficult to feel it in short persons and in tall persons it amounts to 1 *cun*. So *Mai Jing* locates the point 4 *cun* or 3 *cun* below the xiphoid process. In *Qian Jin* four finger-breaths represent 3 *cun* or 4 *cun*. *Jia Yi* locates the point 1 *cun* below Shangwan (RN 13), corresponding to 4 *cun* above the centre of the umbilicus. The above locations are more or less the same.

2. 14. 13 RN 13 Shàngwǎn 上脘

Name: Seen in *Ling Shu*.

Location:

1) "1.5 *cun* below Juque (RN 14) and 3 *cun* from the xiphoid process." (*Jia Yi*, etc.)

2) "1 *cun* below Juque (RN 14), 3 *cun* from the xiphoid process or 2 *cun* below the heart." (*Qian Jin*)

3) "1 *cun* below Juque (RN 14) and 5 *cun* above the umbilicus." (*Da Cheng*)

Note: Most of the medical literature say "3 *cun* from the xiphoid process." The distance between the xiphoid process and the umbilicus is 8 *cun*, so Shangwan (RN 13) should be located "5 *cun* above the umbilicus." If the bone proportional measurement is applied to the upper abdomen, the distance between the sternocostal angle and the umbilicus is 8 *cun*, so Shangwan (RN 13) is located at the point 5 *cun* directly above the centre of the umbilicus.

2. 14. 14 RN 14 Jùquè 巨闕

Name: Seen in *Mai Jing*.

Location:

1) "1 *cun* below Jiuwei (RN 15)." (*Jia Yi*, etc.)

2) "5.5 *cun* above the umbilicus." (*Xun Shu*)

3) "1 *cun* below Jiuwei (RN 15) and 2.5 *cun* above Zhongwan (RN 12)." (*Xun Jing*)

4) "Above Shangwan (RN 13), 2 *cun* below the xiphoid process." (*Jin Jian*)

Note: *Jia Yi* and other books locate Juque (RN 14) "1 *cun* below Jiuwei (RN 15)." Since Jiuwei (RN 15) is 1 *cun* from the xiphoid process, Juque (RN 14) is located 2 *cun* below the xiphoid process, or 6 *cun* above the centre of the umbilicus. However, the distance between Juque (RN 14) and Shangwan (RN 13) is 1.5 *cun*, so Juque (RN 14) is "2.5 *cun* above Zhongwan (RN 12)." "5.5 *cun* above the umbilicus" in *Xin Shu* may be a mistake of "6.5 *cun* above the umbilicus." Now Juque (RN 14) is located 1 *cun* above Shangwan (RN 13), or 6 *cun* above the centre of the umbilicus.

2. 14. 15 RN 15 Jiūwěi 鳩尾

Name: Seen in *Ling Shu* and *Su Wen*.

Location:

1) "0.5 *cun* below the xiphoid process." (*Jia Yi*, etc.)

2) "For those who have no xiphoid process, the point is located 1 *cun* below the sternocostal angle." (*Zi Sheng*, etc.)

3) "1 *cun* above Juque (RN 14)." (*Jin Jian*)

Note: Since the length of the xiphoid process varies, Jiuwei (RN 15) can be located 1 *cun* below the xiphosternal synchondrosis, 1 *cun* from Juque (RN 14), or 7 *cun* above the centre of the umbilicus.

2. 14. 16 RN 16 Zhōngtíng 中庭

Name: Seen in *Jia Yi*.

Location:

1) "In the depression 1.6 *cun* below Danzhong (RN 17)." (*Jia Yi*, etc.)

2) "In the depression 1 *cun* below Jiuwei (RN 15)." (*Jing Jian*)

Note: "1.6 *cun*" in *Jia Yi* refers to the distance between the two intercostal spaces. Danzhong (RN 17) is located on the level of the 5th intercostal space. So Zhongting (RN 16) is located on the level of the 5th intercostal space. The location in *Jin Jian* corresponds to the sternocostal angle.

2. 14. 17 RN 17 Dánzhōng 膻中

Name: Seen in *Ling Shu*.

Location: "1.6 *cun* below Yutang (RN 18), in the depression midway between the two nipples." (*Nan Jing*)

Note: Medical literature through the ages holds the same view on the location of the point. Danzhong (RN 17) is located on the anterior midline, on the level of the 4th intercostal space and at the midpoint of a line connecting both nipples.

2. 14. 18 RN 18 Yùtáng 玉堂

Name: Seen in *Nan Jing*.

Location: "In the depression 1.6 *cun* below Zigong (RN 19)." (*Jia Yi*, etc.)

Note: Medical literature through the ages holds the same view on the location of the point. That is to say, Yutang (RN 18) is located on the anterior midline, on the level of the 3rd intercostal space.

2. 14. 19 RN 19 Zǐgōng 紫宫

Name: Seen in *Jia Yi*.

Location: "In the depression 1.6 *cun* below Huagai (RN 20)." (*Jia Yi*, etc.)

Note: Medical literature through the ages holds the same view on the location of the point. Zigong (RN 19) is located on the anterior midline, on the level of the 2nd intercostal space.

2. 14. 20 RN 20 Huágài 華蓋

Name: Seen in *Jia Yi*.

Location:

1) "In the depression 1 *cun* below Xuanji (RN 21)." (*Jia Yi*, etc.)

2) "2 *cun* below Xuanji (RN 21)." (*Fa Hui*)

3) "In the depression 1.6 *cun* below Xuanji (RN 21)." (*Da Cheng*, etc.)

Note: The points on the midline of the chest are generally located with the intercostal spaces as landmarks. The distance between the two adjacent points on the lower chest are considered as 1.6 *cun*, and on the upper chest as 1 *cun*. According to the measurement illustrated in *Jia Yi*, the distance between Tiantu (RN 22) and Zhongting (RN 16) is only 8.4 *cun*, which is not in accord with 9 *cun* of the bone proportional measurement. *Fa Hui* says it is "2 *cun* below Xuanji (RN 21)," so the distance between Tiantu (RN 22) and Zhongting (RN 16) should be 9.4 *cun*, which is also not in accord with the bone proportional measurement. *Da Cheng* considers that the space between the two points from Tiantu (RN 22) to Zhongting (RN 16) is 1.6 *cun* and the total distance amounts to 9.6 *cun*. If there is a distance of 1 *cun* between Tiantu (RN 22) and Xuanji (RN 21), as illustrated in *Jia Yi*, the total distance is just 9 *cun*.

2. 14. 21 RN 21 Xuánjī 璇璣

Name: Seen in *Jia Yi*.

Location:

1) "In the depression 1 *cun* below Tiantu (RN 22)." (*Jia Yi*, etc.)

2) "In the depression 1.6 *cun* below Tiantu (RN 22)." (*Da Cheng*)

3) "In the depression 1 *cun* above Huagai (RN 20)." (*Jin Jian*)

Note: The distance between Tiantu (RN 22) and Xuanji (RN 21) is less than one intercostal space, so *Jia Yi* defines it as 1 *cun*, which is followed by others. *Da Cheng* defines it as 1.6 *cun*, thus the total length is more than 9 *cun* according to the bone proportional measurement. The description in *Jin Jian* says it is consistent with that in *Jia Yi*. See Huagai (RN 20).

2. 14. 22 RN 22 Tiāntū 天突

Name: Seen in *Ling Shu* and *Su Wen*.

Location:

1) "On the Ren Meridian, in the suprasternal fossa." (*Ling Shu*)

2) "In the depression 2 *cun* below the Adam's apple." (*Jia Yi*, etc.)

3) "In the depression 5 *cun* below the Adam's apple." (*Qian Jin*, etc.)

4) "In the depression 4 *cun* below the Adam's apple." (*Su Wen*, annotated by Wang)

5) "In the depression four finger-breadths below the Adam's apple." (*Sheng Hui*)

Note: The location illustrated in *Ling Shu* is clear and definite. When *Jia Yi* says "2 *cun* below the Adam's apple," it may be a mistake of "5 *cun*." In addition, other books say it is 2 *cun*, 3 *cun* or 4 *cun* below the Adam's apple, but what is described in *Su Wen*, annotated by Wang Bing, is correct. So Tiantu (RN 22) is located on the neck at the centre of the suprasternal fossa.

2. 14. 23 RN 23 Liánquán 廉泉

Name: Seen in *Ling Shu* and *Su Wen*.

Location: "Below the chin, above the Adam's apple. Below the root of the tongue." (*Jia Yi*, etc.)

Note: Medical literature through the ages holds similar views on the location of the point. Now, Lianquan (RN 23) is located on the neck, above the laryngeal protuberance, and in the depression above the upper border of the hyoid bone.

2. 14. 24 RN 24 Chéngjiāng 承漿

Name: Seen in *Jia Yi*.

Location:

1) "In front of the cheek, below the lip." (*Jia Yi*, etc.) (Or below the lower lip in *Qian Jin*.)

2) "In the depression inferior to the lip." (*Zhou Hou*)

Note: Medical literature through the ages holds similar views on the location of the point. Chengjiang (RN 24) is located on the face, in the depression at the midpoint of the mentolabial sulcus.

3. Extra Points, EX

經外穴

Jīngwài Xué

3. 1 Points of the Head and Neck, EX-HN

頭頸部穴

Tóujǐngbù Xué

3. 1. 1 EX-HN 1 Sìshéncōng 四神聰

Name: Seen in *Zhen Jiu Xue*. Originally named Shencong in *Sheng Hui*.

Location:

1) "Around Baihui (DU 20), 1 *cun* from Baihui (DU 20)." (*Sheng Hui*, etc.)

2) "Baihui (DU 20) as the centre, 2.5 *cun* to Baihui (DU 20) in four directions." (*Yin Jing*)

3) "1 *cun* respectively anterior, posterior and lateral to Baihui (DU 20), totally four points." (*Zhen Jiu Xue*)

Note: Most of the medical literature follow *Sheng Hui*. Now, they are located on the vertex of the head, 1 *cun* anterior, ppsterior and lateral to Baihui (DU 20), totally four points.

3. 1. 2 EX-HN 2 Dāngyáng 當陽

Name: Seen in *Qian Jin*.

Location:

1) "Above the pupil, 1 *cun* within (above) the hairline." (*Qian Jin*)

2) "Directly above the pupil, 1 *cun* within the hairline and 0.5 *cun* from Linqi (GB 15)." (*Tu Yi*)

Note: Medical literature through the ages holds similar views on the location of the point. Now, Dangyang (EX-HN 2) is located at the frontal part of the head, directly above the pupil and 1 *cun* above the anterior hairline.

3. 1. 3 EX-HN 3 Yìntáng 印堂

Name: Seen in *Yu Long Jing*. Named Qumei in *Qian Jin Yi*.

Location:

1) "For a patient with malaria, first ask him the cause of the disease, then treat the cause first... For cases with severe headache, first puncture the site between the two eyebrows to cause bleeding." (*Su Wen*)

2) "In treatment of hemiplegia to dispel wind, first give moxibustion, ... then puncture the point between the two eyebrows." (*Qian Jin Yi*)

3) "In the depression midway between the two eyebrows." (*Yu Long Jing*)

4) "Midway between the two eyebrows." (*Da Quan*)

5) "Midway between the two eyebrows." (*Zhen Jiu Xue*)

Note: Medical literature through the ages holds similar views on the location of the point. Now, Yintang (EX-HN 3) is located on the forehead, at the midpoint between the bilateral eyebrows.

3. 1. 4 EX-HN 4 Yúyāo 魚腰

Name: Seen in *Yu Long Jing*. Named Guangming in *Yin Jing*.

Location:

1) "In the middle of the eyebrow, above the pupil." (*Yin Jing*)

2) "In the middle of the eyebrow, for aching of eyes." (*Xiao Xue*)

3) "In the middle of the eyebrow." (*Qi Xiao*)

4) "In the middle of the eyebrow." (*Zhen Jiu Xue*)

Note: Medical literature through the ages holds similar views on the location of the point. Now, Yuyao (EX-HN 4) is located on the forehead, directly above the pupil, and in the eyebrow.

3. 1. 5 EX-HN 5 Tàiyáng 太陽

Name: Seen in *Sheng Hui*.

Location:

1) "Qianguan is another name for Taiyang (EX-HN 5) and is 0.5 *cun* lateral to the eye." (*Sheng Hui*)

2) "1 *cun* lateral to the small canthus of the eye." (*Sheng Ji*)

3) "0.5 *cun* from the outer canthus." (*Yin Jing*)

4) "On the vein of the temple." (*Yu Long Jing*)

5) "Superior and lateral to the two eyebrows on the temple." (*Xiao Xue*)

6) "In the depression lateral to the eyebrow, on the vein of the temple." (*Qi Xiao*)

7) "In the depression 1 *cun* lateral to the superciliary ridge." (*Zhen Jiu Xue*)

8) "In the depression 1 *cun* posterior to the midpoint between the lateral end of the eyebrow and the outer corner of the eyes." (*Gai Lun*)

Note: There are three locations of Taiyang (EX-HN 5); i.e., 0.5 *cun* and 1 *cun* posterior to the outer canthus, and on the vein of the forehead. Now the definitions in *Sheng Ji* and *Zhen Jiu Xue* are followed. Taiyang (EX-HN 5) is located at the temporal part of the head, in the depression one finger-breadth posterior to the midpoint between the lateral end of the eyebrow and the outer canthus.

3. 1. 6 EX-HN 6 Ěrjiān 耳尖

Name: Seen in *Qi Xiao*.

Location: "On the ear apex. To be located on the tip of the ear with the patient's auricle folded." (*Qi Xiao*, etc.)

Note: Medical literature through the ages holds similar views on the location of the point. Erjian (EX-HN 6) is located above the apex of the ear auricle, touched by the tip of the auricle when the ear is folded forward.

3. 1. 7 EX-HN 7 Qiúhòu 球後

Name: Seen in *Zhejiang Journal of Traditional Chinese Medicine* (8): 18, 1957.

Location:

1) "The lateral third of the infraorbital margin." (Any point from the junction of the medial and the lateral third of the infraorbital margin to the crossing point of the

infraorbital and supraorbital margin can be needled.) (*Zhejiang Journal of TCM*)

2) "Slightly superior to the infraorbital margin, at the junction of the lateral fourth and the medial three fourths of the infraorbital margin. To be located with the patient's eyes looking straight forward." (*Jian Bian*)

Note: Qiuhou (EX-HN 7) is a new point, which is located on the face, at the junction of the lateral fourth and medial three fourths of the infraorbital margin.

3. 1. 8 EX-HN 8 Shàngyíngxiāng 上迎香

Name: Seen in *Yin Jing*.

Location:

1) "On both sides of the nasal ridge." (*Ci Ding*)

2) "On the nose, at the junction of the cartilage of the nasal ala and the nasal bone." (*Jian Bian*)

3) "On the middle part of the nose, laterally close to the cheek." (*Gai Lun*)

Note: Medical literature through the ages holds similar views on the location of the point. It is located on the face, at the junction of the alar cartilage of the nose and the nasal concha, near the upper end of the nasolabial groove.

3. 1. 9 EX-HN 9 Nèiyíngxiāng 内迎香

Name: Seen in *Yu Long Jing*.

Location:

1) "Some serious patients due to noxious factors can be cured by puncturing the inner surface of the nose with onion to cause bleeding." (*Qian Jin*)

2) "Inside the nostril." (*Yu Long Jing*)

3) "Inside the nostril." (*Qi Xiao*, etc.)

4) "At the upper part of the nostril." (*Zhen Jiu Xue*)

Note: Medical literature through the ages holds similar views on the location of the point. Neiyingxiang (EX-HN 9) is located in the nostril, at the junction between the mucosa of the alar cartilage of the nose and the nasal concha.

3. 1. 10 EX-HN 10 Jùquán 聚泉

Name: Seen in *Da Quan*.

Location:

1) "In the centre of the tongue, in the depression on the groove appearing when the tongue protrudes." (*Qi Xiao*, etc.)

2) "In the centre of the upper tongue surface." (*Zhen Jiu Xue*)

Note: Medical literature through the ages holds similar views on the location of the point. Juquan (EX-HN 10) is located in the mouth, at the midpoint of the dorsal midline of the tongue.

3. 1. 11 EX-HN 11 Hăiquán 海泉

Name: Seen in *Da Quan*.

Location:

1) "If bleeding becomes persistent after the sublingual central vessel is punctured, the patient may turn dumb." (*Su Wen*)

2) "*Acupuncture Illustrations and Verses for Treating Mental Disorders* says puncturing the tongue 1 *cun* deep and penetrating from the sublingual median groove to the tongue surface is known as 'Guifeng'." (*Qian Jin*)

3) "On the muscle of the tongue." (*Da Quan*)

4) "On the sublingual medial blood vessel." (*Qi Xiao*)

5) "On the central sublingual frenulum, a little posterior to the midpoint between Jinjin (EX-HN 12) and Yuye (EX-HN 13)." (*Zhen Jiu Xue*)

Note: Medical literature through the ages holds similar views on the location of the point. Haiquan (EX-HN 11) is located in the mouth, at the midpoint of the frenulum of the tongue.

3. 1. 12 EX-HN 12 Jīnjīn 金津

Name: Seen in *Xiao Xue*.

Location:

1) "In treatment of malaria ... puncture two sublingual vessels to cause bleeding." (*Su Wen*)

2) "Puncture the lateral sublingual vessels (not the central) to cause bleeding." (*Qian Jin*)

3) "There are two points on the sublingual veins, i.e. Jinjin (EX-HN 12) on the left and Yuye (EX-HN 13) on the right." (*Xiao Xue*)

4) "On the sublingual veins on both sides. To be located with the patient's tongue curled up." (*Qi Xiao*)

Note: Medical literature through the ages holds similar views on the location of the point. Two points are located in the mouth, Jinjin (EX-HN 12) is on the vein on the left side of the frenulum of the tongue and Yuye (EX-HN 13), on the right.

3. 1. 13 EX-HN 13 Yùyè 玉液

See Jinjin (EX-HN 12).

3. 1. 14 EX-HN 14 Yìmíng 翳明

Name: Seen in *Chinese Medical Journal* (6): 535, 1956.

Location:

1) "Inferior to the high bone behind the ear lobe, on the level of the ear lobe, about 1 *cun* from Tianyou (SJ 16). On pressing, a sensation of soreness and pain is felt." (*Chinese Medical Journal*)

2) "1 *cun* posterior to Yifeng (SJ 17)." (*Jian Bian*)

Note: Yiming (EX-HN 14) is a new point, which is located on the nape, 1 *cun* posterior to Yifeng (SJ 17).

3. 1. 15 EX-HN 15 Jǐngbǎiláo 頸百勞

Name: Seen in *Fang An*. Named Bailao in *Ji Cheng*.

Location:

1) "From Dazhui (DU 14) to the hairline is 2 *cun*. Divide this distance into two portions and mark the midpoint with ink. Through the midpoint draw a line transversely, and its left and right ends are the point." (*Ji Cheng*)

2) "2 *cun* above and 1 *cun* lateral to Dazhui (DU 14)." (*Zhen Jiu Xue*)

Note: Dazhui (DU 14) is known in ancient medical books as Bailao. For the sake of avoiding confusion, this point is called Jingbailao (EX-HN 15). Medical literature through the ages holds similar views on the location of the point. Jingbailao (EX-HN 15) is located on the nape, 2 *cun* above Dazhui (DU 14) and 1 *cun* lateral to the posterior midline.

3. 2 Points of the Chest and Abdomen, EX-CA

胸腹部穴

Xiōngfùbù Xué

3. 2. 1 EX-CA 1 Zǐgōng 子宫

Name: Seen in *Da Quan.*

Location:

1) "In treating prolapse of the uterus, moxibustion is done to the point 3 *cun* lateral to Yuquan (another name of Zhongji, RN 3) three times, according to the age of the patient." (*Qian Jin*)

2) "2 *cun* lateral to Zhongji (RN 3)." (*Da Quan*)

3) "3 *cun* lateral to Zhongji (RN 3)." (*Da Cheng*, etc.)

There are two locations of Zigong (EX-CA 1), i.e. 2 *cun* and 3 *cun* on both sides of Zhongji (RN 3). The former is only seen in *Da Quan*, and later medical books follow *Da Cheng*. So Zigong (EX-CA 1) is located on the lower abdomen, 4 *cun* below the centre of the umbilicus and 3 *cun* lateral to Zhongji (RN 3).

3. 3 Points of the Back, EX-B

背部穴

Bèibù Xué

3. 3. 1 EX-B 1 Dìngchuǎn 定喘

Name: Seen in *Jian Bian.*

Location:

1) "0.3-0.5 *cun* or one finger-breadth lateral to Dazhui (DU 14)." (*Beijing Journal of Traditional Chinese Medicine*, 11: 29, 1954)

2) "In the upper portion of the back, 0.5-1 *cun* lateral to the spinous process of the 7th cervical vertebra." (*Jian Bian*)

Note: Dingchuan (EX-B 10) is a new point, which is located on the back, below the spinous process of the 7th cervical vertebra and 0.5 *cun* lateral to the posterior midline.

3. 3. 2 EX-B 2 Jiájǐ 夾脊

Name: Seen in *Su Wen.*

Location:

1) "Involvement of the Foot-Taiyang Meridian leads to spasm and pain of the back referring to the intercostal region. Puncture the tender points 0.3 *cun* lateral to the spinal column from the nape downwards. Pain can thus be relieved." (*Su Wen*)

2) "In the depression 1 *cun* lateral to the vertebra." (*Zhou Hou*)

3) "Many points on the back, 1 *cun* lateral to the spinal column." (*Biographical Records of Hua Tuo*)

4) "A group of 34 points on both sides of the spinal column, 0.5 *cun* lateral to the spinous process from the 1st thoracic vertebra to the 5th lumbar vertebra." (*Zhen Jiu Xue*)

Note: This group of points were first mentioned in *Su Wen*. Hua Tuo, a famous physician in the Three Kingdoms Period, applied them in his clinical practice and pointed out their definite locations. Later, *Yi Xin Fang* denoted that there are 19 points "1 *cun* lateral to the spine on each side, each of which is named." The Jiaji points are also known as Huatuojiaji points, in which those on the neck are not included. Now, Jiaji (EX-B 2) points are located on the back and low back, totally 34 points on both sides, below the spinous process from the 1st thoracic vertebra to the 5th lumbar vertebra, and 0.5 *cun* lateral to the posterior midline.

3. 3. 3 EX-B 3 Wèiwǎnxiàshū 胃脘下俞

Name: Seen in *Qian Jin*. ("Wan" is also called "Guan.")

Location:

1) "On the back, below and 3 *cun* lateral to the 8th vertebra." (*Qian Jin*)

2) "1.5 *cun* lateral to the midline, between the 8th and 9th thoracic vertebrae." (*Zhen Jiu Xue*)

Note: Weiwanxiashu (EX-B 3) is located on the back, below the spinous process of the 8th thoracic vertebra and 1.5 *cun* lateral to the posterior midline.

3. 3. 4 EX-B 4 Pǐgēn 痞根

Name: Seen in *Xiao Xue*.

Location:

1) "3.5 *cun* lateral to the lower border of the 13th vertebra." (*Ru Men*)

2) "On both sides below the 11th thoracic vertebra, in the depression 3.5 *cun* from the vertebra." (*Zhen Jiu Xue*)

3) "In the lumbar region, 3.5 *cun* lateral to the depression between the spinous process of the 1st and the 2nd lumbar vertebrae." (*Jian Bian*)

Note: The location recorded in medical literature through the ages is definite. But there are two locations in modern medical books, "below the 11th thoracic vertebra" and "below the 1st lumbar vertebra." According to ancient literature Pigen (EX-B 4) is located on the low back, below the spinous process of the 1st lumbar vertebra and 3.5 *cun* lateral to the posterior midline.

3. 3. 5 EX-B 5 Xiàjíshū 下極俞

Name: Seen in *Qian Jin*.

Location:

1) "The 15th vertebra is named Xiajishu." (*Qian Jin*)

2) "On the midline of the low back, in the depression of the third and fourth lumbar vertebrae." (*Tu Pu*)

Note: Medical literature through the ages holds smililar views on the location of the point. Xiajishu (EX-B 5) is located on the midline of the low back, below the third lumbar spinous process.

3. 3. 6 EX-B 6 Yāoyí 腰宜

Name: Seen in *Bian Lan*.

Location:

1) "Above the coccygosacral bone, four finger-breaths lateral to the lower border of the 16th vertebra." (*Bian Lan*)

2) "3 *cun* lateral to the midline of the lumbar region, on the level of the midpoint between the 4th and 5th lumbar vertebrae." (*Tu Pu*)

Note: Yaoyi (EX-B 6) is a new point, which is located on the low back, below the spinous process of the 4th lumbar vertebra and 3 *cun* lateral to the posterior midline.

3. 3. 7 EX-B 7 Yāoyǎn 腰眼

Name: Seen in *Zhou Hou*.

Location:

1) "3 *cun* below Shenshu (BL 23), 1.5 *cun* lateral to the spinal column." (*Qian Jin*)

2) "Locate the point in the two depressions between the 4th and 5th lumbar vertebrae when the patient is in a prone position, with the knee extended and the palms overlapped over the forehead." (*Zhen Jiu Xue*)

3) "In the depression 3 to 4 *cun* lateral to the spinous process of the 3rd lumbar vertebra, corresponding to the depression formed by the lateral border of the prominence of the sacrospinal muscle and the posterior superior iliac spine." (*Jian Bian*)

Note: There's a slight difference in ancient medical literature. Now according to the location in *Zhen Jiu Xue*, Yaoyan (EX-B 7) is located on the low back, below the spinous process of the 4th lumbar vertebra, and in the depression 3.5 *cun* lateral to the posterior midline.

3. 3. 8 EX-B 8 Shíqīzhūi 十七椎

Name: Seen in *Qian Jin Yi*.

Location: "On correcting the malposition of the fetus, ... give moxibustion to the 17th spinal vertebra with 50 moxa cones." (*Qian Jin Yi*)

Note: Medical literature through the ages holds similar views on the location of the point. Now, Shiqizhui (EX-B 8) is located on the low back, on the posterior midline, at the spinous process of the 5th lumbar vertebra.

3. 3. 9 EX-B 9 Yāoqí 腰奇

Name: Seen in *Journal of Traditional Chinese Medicine* (9): 46, 1955.

Location: "2 *cun* directly above the tip of the coccygosacral bone." (*Journal of TCM*, etc.)

Note: Yaoqi (EX-B 9) is a new point. Medical literature holds similar views on the location of the point. It is located on the low back, 2 *cun* directly above the tip of the coccyx, in the depression between the sacral horns.

3. 4 Points of the Upper Extremities, EX-UE

上肢穴

Shàngzhī Xué

3. 4. 1 EX-UE 1 Zhǒujiān 肘尖

Name: Seen in *Qian Jin Yi*.

Location:

1) "Give moxibustion to the styloid process of the ulna with the patient's elbow flexed." (*Qian Jin*)

2) "At the tip of the elbow when the patient's elbow is flexed." (*Qi Xiao*, etc.)

Note: Medical literature through the ages holds similar views on the location of the point. Zhoujian (EX-UE 1) is located on the posterior side of the elbow, at the tip of the olecranon when the patient's elbow is flexed.

3. 4. 2 EX-UE 2 Èrbái 二白

Name: Seen in *Yu Long Jing*.

Location:

1) "4 *cun* above the dorsal crease of the hand, one point between the tendons, and the

other on the lateral side of the big tendon." (*Yu Long Jing*)

2) "Four points of Erbai (EX-UE 2) are located when the patient's hand is pronated." (*Xiao Xue*)

3) "On the dorsum of the hand, 4 *cun* directly above Daling (PC 7) and 0.2 *cun* on both sides of Ximen (PC 4)." (*Zhen Jiu Xue*)

Note: Medical literature through the ages holds similar views on the location of the point. Erbai (EX-UE 2) is located on the palmar side of each forearm, 4 *cun* proximal to the crease of the wrist, and on each side of the tendon of the radial flexor muscle of the wrist.

3. 4. 3 EX-UE 3 Zhōngquán 中泉

Name: Seen in *Qi Xiao*.

Location:

1) "On the dorsum of the hand and wrist, in the depression between Yangxi (LI 5) and Yangchi (SJ 4)." (*Qi Xiao*, etc.)

2) "In the depression between Yangchi (SJ 4) and Yangxi (LI 5)." (*Zhen Jiu Xue*)

Note: Medical literature through the ages holds similar views on the location of the point. Zhongquan (EX-UE 3) is located on the dorsal crease of the wrist, in the depression on the radial side of the tendon of the common extensor muscle of the fingers.

3. 4. 4 EX-UE 4 Zhōngkuí 中魁

Name: Seen in *Yu Long Jing*.

Location:

1) "If a patient suffers from deviation of the mouth ... give moxibustion to the knuckle of the middle finger. If the mouth is deviated to the right, treat the left side, and vice versa." (*Zhou Hou*)

2) "At the distal end of the 2nd knuckle of the middle finger." (*Yu Long Jing*)

3) "At the distal end of the 2nd knuckle when the patient's middle finger is flexed." (*Tu Yi*)

Note: Medical literature through the ages holds similar views on the location of the point. Zhongkui (EX-UE 4) is located on the dorsal side of the middle finger, at the centre of the proximal interphalangeal joint.

3. 4. 5 EX-UE 5 Dàgǔkōng 大骨空

Name: Seen in *Yu Long Jing*.

Location:

1) "For a patient with cataract, give moxibustion with 3 moxa cones at the crease of the thumb. Moxibustion is applied on the right side for cataract of the left eye, and vice versa." (*Zhou Hou*)

2) "For cases with persistent nasal bleeding, ask the patient to hold his hands with the thumb flexed, then moxibustion of three cones is applied at the top of the bone. The size of each cone is as big as a millet." (*Bei Ji*)

3) "On the interphalangeal joint of the thumb, in the depression of the tip of the joint when the patient's thumb is flexed." (*Yu Long Jing*)

Note: Medical literature through the ages holds similar views on the location of the point. Dagukong (EX-UE 5) is located on the dorsal side of the thumb, at the centre of the interphalangeal joint.

3. 4. 6 EX-UE 6 Xiǎogǔkōng 小骨空

Name: Seen in *Yu Long Jing*.

Location:

1) "On the top of the 2nd interphalangeal joint of the little finger." (*Yu Long Jing*)

2) "On the top of the 2nd interphalangeal joint of the little finger." (*Xiao Xue*)

3) "In the middle of the 1st and 2nd interphalangeal joints, on the dorsal side of the little finger. Apply moxibustion with 3-5 cones." (*Zhen Jiu Xue*)

4) "On the dorsal side of the little finger, in the midpoint of the two interphalangeal joints, two points on each side." (*Tu Pu*)

Note: Medical literature through the ages holds similar views on the location of the point. In modern medical books, there are two locations: on the proximal or the distal interdigital joint. Now according to *Zhen Jiu Xue*, Xiaogukong (EX-UE 6) is located on the dorsal side of the little finger, at the centre of the proximal interphalangeal joint.

3. 4. 7 EX-UE 7 Yāotòngdiǎn 腰痛點

Name: Seen in *Jian Bian*.

Location: "On the dorsal side of the hand, on both sides of the tendon of the common extensor muscle of the fingers, 1 *cun* proximal to the dorsal wrist crease, directly posterior (proximal) to the interspace between the 2nd and the 3rd metacarpal bone." (*Jian Bian*)

Note: Yaotongdian (EX-UE 7) is a new point, which is also known as Yaotuidian in modern medical books. It is located on the dorsum of each hand, between the 1st and 2nd and between the 3rd and 4th metacarpal bones, and at the midpoint between the dorsal crease of the wrist and the metacarpophalangeal joint.

3. 4. 8 EX-UE 8 Wàiláogōng 外勞宮

Name: Seen in *Mi Zhi*. Named Xiangqiang or Luozhen now.

Location:

1) "In the centre of the palm touched by the finger when a fist is made." (*Mi Zhi*)

2) "In the depression proximal to the metacarpophalangeal joint of the middle and index fingers, about 1 *cun* posterior to Yishanmen point." (*Hui Bian*)

3) "On the dorsum of the hand, at the junction between the anterior and middle third of the interspace between the 2nd and 3rd metacarpal bones." (*Jian Bian*)

Note: This point was discovered later, and its name is inconsistent at present, but the location is identical. Now, Wailaogong (EX-UE 8) is located on the dorsum of the hand, between the 2nd and 3rd metacarpal bones and 0.5 *cun* proximal to the metacarpophalangeal joint.

3. 4. 9 EX-UE 9 Bāxié 八邪

Name: Seen in *Xiao Xue*.

Location:

1) "For cases of malaria with the pulse not palpable, puncture the interspace between the ten fingers to cause bleeding." (*Su Wen*)

2) "For spasms of the foot and hand, apply moxibustion to the tip of the fingers and toes, and also the proximal end of the proximal knuckles." (*Qian Jin*)

3) "In the interspaces between the ten fingers, for Bi-syndrome." (*Xiao Xue*)

4) "Four points on each hand, in the interspaces between the five fingers of each hand." (*Qi Xiao*, etc.)

Note: Medical literature through the ages holds similar views on the location of the point. Baxie (EX-UE 9) is located on the dorsum of each hand, at the junction of the red and white skin proximal to the margin of the webs between each two of the five fingers of a hand.

3. 4. 10 EX-UE 10 Sìfèng 四縫

Name: Seen in *Qi Xiao*.

Location:

1) "On the proximal interphalangeal joint of the four fingers." (*Qi Xiao*, etc.)

2) "On the palmar side of the four fingers (the thumb not included), at the two ends of the crease between the proximal and middle phalanges of the fingers, two points on each finger." (*Zhen Jiu Xue*)

3) "On the palmar surface, at the midpoint of the crease of the 1st interphalangeal joints of the index, middle, ring and little fingers." (*Jian Bian*)

Note: Medical literature through the ages holds similar views on the location of the point. Some of the modern medical books believe that there are two locations, i.e. at the two ends of the crease (two points on each finger) and at the midpoint of the crease (one point on each finger). Now, according to the definition in most medical books, Sifeng (EX-UE 10) is located on the palmar side of the 2nd to the 5th finger, and at the centre of the proximal interphalangeal joint.

3. 4. 11 EX-UE 11 Shíxuān 十宣

Name: Seen in *Da Quan*.

Location:

1) "For spleen-wind syndrome with dysphasia and twitching of the limbs, apply moxibustion to the tips of the ten fingers. For cases with severe cough due to exogenous pathogenic factors, apply moxibustion to the tips (0.1 *cun* from the nails) of the ten fingers." (*Qian Jin*)

2) "On the tips of the ten fingers, 0.1 *cun* from the corners of the nails, one point on each finger, and ten points on both hands." (*Qi Xiao*)

Note: Medical literature through the ages holds similar views on the location of the point. Shixuan (EX-UE 11) is located at the tips of the ten fingers and 0.1 *cun* from the free margin of the nails.

3. 5 Points of the Lower Extremities, LE
下肢穴
Xiàzhī Xué

3. 5. 1 EX-LE 1 Kuāngǔ 髋骨

Name: Seen in *Yu Long Jing*.

Location:

1) "1 *cun* above the patella, 5 *cun* from Liangqiu (ST 34) on both sides." (*Yu Long Jing*)

2) "1.5 *cun* from Liangqiu (ST 34) on both sides, totally four points on both legs." (*Qi Xiao*, etc.)

3) "Above the patella, 1 *cun* from Liangqiu (ST 34)." (*Tu Yi*)

Note: Medical literature through the ages holds different views on the location of the point. "5 *cun* from Liangqiu (ST 34)" is not true. Now, according to the location in *Qi Xiao* and others, Kuangu (EX-LE 1) is located in the lower part of the surface of the thigh and 1.5 *cun* lateral and medial to Liangqiu (ST 34).

3. 5. 2 EX-LE 2 **Hèdǐng** 鶴頂

Location:

1) "On the top of the patella." (*Gang Mu*)

2) "1 *cun* above the centre of the patella." (*Zhen Jiu Xue*)

Note: Medical literature through the ages holds similar views on the location of the point. Now, Heding (EX-LE 2) is located above the knee, in the depression at the midpoint of the upper border of the patella.

3. 5. 3 EX-LE 3 Baǐchóngwō 百蟲窩

Name: Seen in *Da Cheng*.

Location:

1) "3 *cun* above the medial side of the knee." (*Da Cheng*)

2) "In the depression 3 *cun* above the medial side of the knee." (*Ji Cheng*)

3) "On the tibial side of the thigh, above the medial epicondycle, and 3 *cun* superior to the transverse crease of the popliteal fossa." (*Tu Pu*)

Note: Medical literature through the ages holds similar views on the location of the point. Baichongwo (EX-LE 3) is located 3 *cun* above the medial superior corner of the patella of the thigh, i.e. 1 *cun* above Xuehai (SP 10). It is stated in *Da Cheng* that this point is Xuehai (SP 10) point. However, Xuehai (SP 10) is located 2 *cun* above the medial side of the knee, 1 *cun* away from Caichongwo (EX-LE 3). It is therefore not the same point.

3. 5. 4 EX-LE 4 Nèixīyǎn 内膝眼

Name: See Xiyan (EX-LE 5).

3. 5. 5 EX-LE 5 Xīyǎn 膝眼

Name: Seen in *Qian Jin*. Named Ximu in *Qian Jin Yi*.

Location:

1) "In the depression on both sides of and below the patella." (*Qian Jin*, etc.)

2) "At the junction inferior to the patella, in the depression lateral to the tendon." (*Wai Tai*)

3) "Below the knee." (*Yu Long Jing*)

4) "Below and on both sides of the patella." (*Zhen Jiu Xue*)

Note: Medical literature through the ages holds similar views on the location of the point. Now, Xiyan (EX-LE 5) is located in the depression on both sides of the patellar ligament when the patient's knee is flexed, the medial and lateral points being named "Neixiyan" and "Waixiyan" respectively.

3. 5. 6 EX-LE 6 Dǎnnáng 膽囊

Name: Seen in *Chinese Journal of Surgery* (8): 743, 1959.

Location:

1) "On the tender spot, about 1 *cun* below Yanglingquan (GB 34)." (*Chinese Journal of Surgery*)

2) "On the proximal part of the lateral aspect of the leg, 1 to 2 *cun* below Yanglingquan (GB 34)." (*Jian Bian*)

Note: Dannang (EX-LE 6) is a new point. Now it is located at the upper part of the lateral surface of the leg, 2 *cun* directly below the depression anterior and inferior to the head of the fibula.

3. 5. 7 EX-LE 7 Lánwěi 闌尾

Name: Seen in *Journal of New Traditional Chinese Medicine* 8 (2): 44, 1957.

Location: "On the anterior tibial muscle, on the lateral side of the right leg, slightly anterior to and 2 *cun* below Zusanli (ST 36)." (*Journal of New TCM*)

Note: The article in the *Journal of New TCM* is a translation by Xiao Lin from Deutsche Zeichrift Frer Akupunktuv, No. 3-4, 1956; 醫道の日本, No. 10, 1956. In this article, it is mentioned that this point was discovered by Nile Klak, a German medical doctor. According to this record, Lanwei (EX-LE 7) is located at the upper part of the anterior surface of the leg, 5 *cun* below Dubi (ST 35) and one finger-breadth lateral to the anterior crest of the tibia.

3. 5. 8 EX-LE 8 Nèihuáijiān 内踝尖

Name: Seen in *Bei Ji*.

Location: "At the tip of the medial malleolus." (*Qi Xiao*, etc.)

Note: Medical literature through the ages holds the same view on the location of the point. Neihuaijian (EX-LE 8) is located on the medial side of the foot, at the tip of the medial malleolus.

3. 5. 9 EX-LE 9 Wàihuáijiān 外踝尖

Name: Seen in *Qian Jin*.

Location:

1) "In treating acute urination disorders, apply moxibustion to the centre of the external malleolus on both sides." (*Qian Jin*)

2) "At the tip of the external malleolus." (*Qi Xiao*, etc.)

3) "3 *cun* above the tip of the external malleolus." (*Tu Yi*)

Note: In ancient medical literature, there are two locations, i.e. on the tip of the external malleolus and 3 *cun* above the tip of the external malleolus. The latter is easily confused with Xuanzhong (GB 39) of the Gallbladder Meridian of Foot-Shaoyang. So Waihuaijian (EX-LE 9) is located on the lateral side of the foot, at the tip of the lateral malleolus.

3. 5. 10 EX-LE 10 Bāfēng 八風

Name: Seen in *Qi Xiao*.

Location:

1) "In treating malaria, ... with aching in the leg, puncture the interspaces of the ten toes." (*Su Wen*)

2) "0.1 *cun* from the free margin of the webs between the ten toes, totally eight points on two feet, known as Bachong." (*Qian Jin*, etc.)

3) "Between the metatarsophalangeal joints of the five toes, totally eight points on two feet." (*Qi Xiao*, etc.)

Note: Medical literature through the ages holds similar views on the location of the point. Bafeng (EX-LE 10) is located on the instep of both feet, at the junction of the red and white skin, proximal to the margin of the webs between each two neighbouring toes.

3. 5. 11 EX-LE 11 Dúyīn 獨陰

Name: Seen in *Qi Xiao*.

Location:

1) "Zhang Wenzhong's moxibustion therapy for sudden intolerable cardiac pain ... Apply directly moxibustion to the crease of the great toe and the 2nd toe." (*Sheng Hui*)

2) "On the crease of the 2nd toe." (*Qi Xiao*, etc.)

Note: Medical literature through the ages holds similar views on the location of the point. Duyin (EX-LE 11) is located on the plantar side of the 2nd toe, at the centre of the distal interphalangeal joint.

3. 5. 12 EX-LE 12 Qìduān 氣端

Name: Seen in *Qian Jin*.

Location: "At the tips of the ten toes." (*Qian Jin*)

Note: Medical literature through the ages holds similar views on the location of the point. Qiduan (EX-LE 12) is located at the tips of the ten toes of both feet, 0.1 *cun* from the free margin of each toenail.

PART THREE

The Regional Anatomy of Points

1. Points of the Lung Meridian of Hand-Taiyin, LU
手太陰肺經穴
Shǒutàiyīn Fèijīng Xué

2. 1. 1 LU 1 Zhōngfǔ 中府

Skin---subcutaneous tissue---greater pectoral muscle---smaller pectoral muscle---axillary cavity.

In the superficial layer, there are the intermediate supraclavicular nerve, the lateral cutaneous branches of the first intercostal nerve and the cephalic vein and so on. In the deep layer, there are the thoracoacromial artery and vein, the medial and lateral pectoral nerves.

2. 1. 2 LU 2 Yúnmén 雲門

Skin---subcutaneous tissue---deltoid muscle--clavipectoral fascia---coracoclavicular ligament.

In the superficial layer, there are the cephalic vein and the intermediate supraclavicular nerve. In the deep layer, there are the branches of the thoracoacromial artery and vein, the branches of the medial and lateral pectoral nerves.

2. 1. 3 LU 3 Tiānfǔ 天府

Skin---subcutaneous tissue---brachial muscle.

In the superficial layer, there are the cephalic vein and the lateral cutaneous nerve of the arm. In the deep layer, there are the muscular branches of the brachial artery and vein and the branches of the musculocutaneous nerve.

2. 1. 4 LU 4 Xiábái 俠白

Skin---subcutaneous tissue---brachial muscle.

In the superficial layer, there are the cephalic vein and the lateral cutaneous nerve of the arm. In the deep layer, there are the muscular branches of the brachial artery and vein and the branches of the musculocutaneous nerve.

2. 1. 5 LU 5 Chǐzé 尺澤

Skin---subcutaneous tissue---brachioradial muscle---radial nerve---brachial muscle.

In the superficial layer, there are the cephalic vein and the lateral cutaneous nerve of the forearm and so on. In the deep layer, there are the radial nerve, the anterior branches of the raidal collateral artery and vein and the radial recurrent artery and vein.

2. 1. 6 LU 6 Kǒngzùi 孔最

Skin---subcutaneous tissue---brachioradial muscle---radial flexor muscle of wrist---between superficial flexor muscle of fingers and round pronator muscle---long flexor muscle of thumb.

In the superficial layer, there are the cephalic vein and the branches of the lateral cutaneous nerve of the forearm. In the deep layer, there are the radial artery and vein and the superficial branches of the radial nerve.

2. 1. 7 LU 7 Lièquē 列缺

Skin---subcutaneous tissue---long abductor muscle of the thumb---tendon of brachioradial muscle---quadrate pronator muscle.

In the superficial layer, there are the cephalic vein, the lateral cutaneous nerve of the forearm and the superficial branches of the radial nerve. In the deep layer, there are the branches of the radial artery and vein.

2. 1. 8 LU 8 Jīngqú 經渠

Skin---subcutaneous tissue---ulnar border of tendon of brachioradial muscle---quadrate pronator muscle.

In the superficial layer, there are the lateral cutaneous nerve of the forearm and the superficial branches of the radial nerve. In the deep layer, there are the radial artery and vein.

2. 1. 9 LU 9 Tàiyuān 太淵

Skin---subcutaneous tissue---between tendons of radial flexor muscle of wrist and long abductor muscle of thumb.

In the superficial layer, there are the lateral cutaneous nerve of the forearm, the superficial branches of the radial nerve and the superficial palmar branches of the radial artery. In the deep layer, there are the radial artery and vein.

2. 1. 10 LU 10 Yújì 魚際

Skin---subcutaneous tissue---short abductor muscle of thumb---opponens muscle of thumb ---short flexor muscle of thumb.

In the superficial layer, there are the cutaneous branches of the median nerve and the superficial branches of the radial nerve. In the deep layer, there are the muscular branches of the median and ulnar nerves.

2. 1. 11 LU 11 Shàoshāng 少商

Skin---subcutaneous tissue---root of nail

There are the dorsal digital branches of the proper palmar digital nerve of the median nerve, the arteriovenous network formed by the principal arteries and veins of the thumb and the 1st dorsal metacarpal arteries and veins in this area.

2. Points of the Large Intestine Meridian of Hand-Yangming, LI
手陽明大腸經穴
Shǒuyángmíng Dàchángjīng Xué

2. 2. 1 LI 1 Shāngyáng 商陽

Skin---subcutaneous tissue---root of nail.

There are the dorsal digital branches of the proper palmar digital nerve of the median nerve, the arteriovenous network formed by the arteries and veins in the radial side of the index finger and the branches of the first dorsal metacarpal artery and vein in this area.

2. 2. 2 LI 2 Èrjiān 二間

Skin---subcutaneous tissue---first lumbrical muscle tendon---base of proximal phalanx of index finger.

In the superficial layer, there are the dorsal digital nerve of the radial nerve, the proper palmar digital nerve of the median nerve, the branches of the first dorsal metacarpal artery and vein and the branches of the radial artery and vein of the index finger. In the deep layer, there are the muscular branches of the median nerve.

2. 2. 3 LI 3 Sānjiān 三間

Skin---subcutaneous tissue---first dorsal interosseous muscle---between first lumbrical muscle and second metacarpal bone---between tendons of superficial and deep flexor muscles of index finger and first palmar interosseous muscle.

In the superficial layer, there are the dorsal digital nerve of the radial nerve and the proper palmar digital nerve of the median nerve, the dorsal venous network of the hand, the branches of the first dorsal metacarpal artery and vein and the branches of the radial artery and vein of the index finger. In the deep layer, there are the deep branches of the ulnar nerve and the muscular branches of the median nerve.

2. 2. 4 LI 4 Hégǔ 合谷

Skin---subcutaneous tissue---first dorsal interosseous muscle---adductor muscle of thumb.

In the superficial layer, there are the superficial branches of the radial nerve, the radial part of the dorsal venous network of the hand and the branches or tributaries of the first dorsal metacarpal artery and vein. In the deep layer, there are the deep branches of the ulnar nerve.

2. 2. 5 LI 5 Yángxī 陽谿

Skin---subcutaneous tissue---between short extensor muscle tendon of thumb and long extensor muscle tendon of thumb---front part of long radial extensor muscle of wrist.

In the superficial layer, there are the branches of the cephalic vein and the superficial branches of the radial nerve. In the deep layer, there are the branches or tributaries of the radial artery and vein.

2. 2. 6 LI 6 Piānlì 偏歷

Skin---subcutaneous tissue---short extensor muscle of thumb---long radial extensor muscle tendon of wrist---long abductor muscle tendon of thumb.

In the superficial layer, there are the tributaries of the cephalic vein, the lateral cutaneous nerve of the forearm and the superficial branches of the radial nerve. In the deep layer, there are the branches of the posterior interosseous nerve of the radial nerve.

2. 2. 7 LI 7 Wēnliū 温溜

Skin---subcutaneous tissue---long radial extensor muscle tendon of wrist---short radial extensor muscle of wrist.

In the superficial layer, there are the cephalic vein, the lateral cutaneous nerve of the forearm and the posterior cutaneous nerve of the forearm. In the deep layer, there are the superficial branches of the radial nerve before the tendons of the long and short radial extensor muscles of the wrist.

2. 2. 8 LI 8 Xiàlián 下廉

Skin---subcutaneous tissue---brachioradial muscle---short radial extensor muscle of wrist ---supinator muscle.

In the superficial layer, there are the lateral and posterior cutaneous nerves of the forearm. In the deep layer, there are the deep branches of the radial nerve.

2. 2. 9 LI 9 Shànglián 上廉

Skin---subcutaneous tissue---posterior part of long radial extensor muscle of wrist---short radial extensor muscle of wrist---supinator muscle---long abductor muscle of thumb.

In the superficial layer, there are the lateral and posterior cutaneous nerves of the forearm and the superficial vein. In the deep layer, there is the supinator muscle perforated by the deep branches of the radial nerve.

2. 2. 10 LI 10 Shǒusānlǐ 手三裏

Skin---subcutaneous tissue---long radial extensor muscle of wrist---short radial extensor muscle of wrist---front part of extensor muscle of fingers---supinator muscle.

In the superficial layer, there are the lateral and posterior cutaneous nerves of the forearm. In the deep layer, there are the branches or tributaries of the radial recurrent artery and vein and the deep branches of the radial nerve.

2. 2. 11 LI 11 Qūchí 曲池

Skin---subcutaneous tissue---long radial extensor muscle of wrist and short radial extensor muscle of wrist----brachioradial muscle.

In the superficial layer, there are the tributaries of the cephalic vein and the posterior cutaneous nerve of the forearm. In the deep layer, there are the radial nerve and the anastomotic branches of the radial recurrent artery and vein and the radial collateral artery and vein.

2. 2. 12 LI 12 Zhǒuliáo 肘髎

Skin---subcutaneous tissue---brachioradial muscle---brachial muscle.

In the superficial layer, there is the posterior cutaneous nerve of the forearm. In the deep layer, there are the branches or tributaries of the radial collateral artery and vein.

2. 2. 13 LI 13 Shǒuwǔlǐ 手五裏

Skin---subcutaneous tissue---brachial muscle.

In the superficial layer, there are the lateral inferior cutaneous nerve of the arm and the posterior cutaneous nerve of the forearm. In the deep layer, there are the radial collateral artery and vein and the radial nerve.

2. 2. 14 LI 14 Bìnào 臂臑

Skin---subcutaneous tissue---deltoid muscle.

In the superficial layer, there are the inferior and superior lateral cutaneous nerves of the arm. In the deep layer, there are the muscular branches of the brachial artery.

2. 2. 15 LI 15 Jīanyú 肩髃

Skin---subcutaneous tissue---deltoid muscle---subdeltoid bursa---supraspinous muscle tendon.

In the superficial layer, there are the lateral supraclavicular nerve and the superior lateral cutaneous nerve of the arm. In the deep layer, there are the posterior humeral circumflex artery and vein and the branches of the axillary nerve.

2. 2. 16 LI 16 Jùgǔ 巨骨

Skin---subcutaneous tissue---acromioclavicular ligament---supraspinous muscle.

In the superficial layer, there is the lateral supraclavicular nerve. In the deep layer, there are the branches of the suprascapular nerve and the branches or tributaries of the suprascapular artery and vein.

2. 2. 17 LI 17 Tiāndǐng 天鼎

Skin---subcutaneous tissue---posterior border of sternocleidomastoid muscle---interspace of scalene muscle.

In the superficial layer, there are the transverse nerve of the neck, the external jugular vein and the platysma muscle. In the deep layer, there are the branches or tributaries of the ascending cervical artery and vein and the brachial plexus in the interspace of the scalene muscle.

2. 2. 18 LI 18 Fútū 扶突

Skin---subcutaneous tissue---between sternal head and clavicular head of sternocleidomastoid muscle---posterior border of carotid sheath.

In the superficial layer, there are the transverse nerve of the neck and the platysma muscle. In the deep layer, there is the carotid sheath.

2. 2. 19 LI 19 Kǒuhéliáo 口禾髎

Skin---subcutaneous tissue---orbicular muscle of mouth.

In the superficial layer, there are the branches of the infraorbital nerve of the maxillary nerve and so on. In the deep layer, there are the artery and vein of the upper lip and the buccal branches of the facial nerve.

2. 2. 20 LI 20 Yíngxiāng 迎香

Skin---subcutaneous tissue---levator muscle of upper lip.

In the superficial layer, there are the branches of the infraorbital nerve from the maxillary nerve. In the deep layer, there are the buccal branches of the facial nerve and the branches or tributaries of the facial artery and vein.

3. Points of the Stomach Meridian of Foot-Yangming, ST
足陽明胃經穴
Zúyángmíng Wèijīng Xué

2. 3. 1 ST 1 Chéngqì 承泣

Skin---subcutaneous tissue---orbicular muscle of eye---adipose body of orbit---inferior oblique muscle.

In the superficial layer, there are the branches of the infraorbital nerve and the zygomatic branches of the facial nerve. In the deep layer, there are the branches of the oculomotor nerve and the branches or tributaries of the ophthalmic artery and vein.

2. 3. 2 ST 2 Sìbái 四白

Skin---subcutaneous tissue---orbicular muscle of eye, levator muscle of upper lip---infraorbital foramen or maxilla.

In the superficial layer, there are the branches of the infraorbital nerve and the zygomatic branches of the facial nerve. In the deep layer, the infraorbital artery, vein and nerve pass through the infraorbital foramen.

2. 3. 3 ST 3 Jùliáo 巨髎

Skin---subcutaneous tissue---levator muscle of upper lip---levator muscle of angle of mouth.

There are the infraorbital nerve of the maxillary nerve, the buccal branches of the facial nerve, the anastomotic branches formed by the branches or tributaries of the facial artery and vein and the infraorbital artery and vein in this area.

2. 3. 4 ST 4 Dìcāng 地倉

Skin---subcutaneous tissue---orbicular muscle of mouth---depressor muscle of angle of mouth.

There are the buccal and infraorbital branches of the trigeminal nerve and the branches or tributaries of the facial artery and vein in this area.

2. 3. 5 ST 5 Dàyíng 大迎

Skin---subcutaneous tissue---depressor muscle of angle of mouth and platysma muscle ---anterior border of masseter muscle.

In the superficial layer, there are the buccal nerve of the mandibular branch of the trigeminal nerve and the marginal mandibular branch of the facial nerve. In the deep layer, there are the facial artery and vein.

2. 3. 6 ST 6 Jiáché 頰車

Skin---subcutaneous tissue---masseter muscle.

There are the branches of the great auricular nerve and the marginal mandibular branches of the facial nerve in this area.

2. 3. 7 ST 7 Xiàguān 下關

Skin---subcutaneous tissue---parotid gland---between masseter muscle and zygomatic process of temporal bone---lateral pterygoid muscle.

In the superficial layer, there are the branches of the auriculotemporal nerve, the zygomatic branches of the facial nerve and the transverse facial artery and vein. In the deep layer, there are the maxillary artery and vein, the lingual nerve, the inferior alveolar nerve, the middle meningeal artery and the pterygoid plexus.

2. 3. 8 ST 8 Tóuwéi 頭維

Skin---subcutaneous tissue---epicranial aponeurosis---subaponeurotic loose connective tissue ---pericranium.

There are the branches of the auriculotemporal nerve, the temporal branches of the facial nerve and the frontal branches of the superficial temporal artery and vein in this area.

2. 3. 9 ST 9 Rényíng 人迎

Skin---subcutaneous tissue and platysma muscle---superficial layer of cervical proper fascia and anterior border of sternocleidomastoid muscle---deep layer of cervical proper fascia and posterior border of omohyoid muscle---constrictor muscle of pharynx.

In the superficial layer, there are the transverse nerve of the neck and the cervical branches of the facial nerve. In the deep layer, there are the branches or tributaries of the superior thyroid artery and vein and the branches of the loop of the hypoglossal nerve.

2. 3. 10 ST 10 Shuǐtū 水突

Skin---subcutaneous tissue and platysma muscle---superficial layer of cervical proper fascia and sternocleidomastoid muscle-deep layer of cervical proper fascia, omohyoid muscle and sternothyroid muscle.

In the superficial layer, there is the transverse nerve of the neck. In the deep layer, there is the thyroid gland.

2. 3. 11 ST 11 Qìshè 氣舍

Skin---subcutaneous tissue and platysma muscle---between sternal head and clavicular head of sternocleidomastoid muscle.

In the superficial layer, there are the branches of the medial supraclavical nerve, the transverse nerve of the neck and the cervical branches of the facial nerve. In the deep layer, there are the arch connecting the bilateral anterior jugular veins and the brachiocephalic vein.

2. 3. 12 ST 12 Quēpén 缺盆

Skin---subcutaneous tissue and platysma muscle---between clavicle and trapezius muscle ---between inferior belly of omohyoid muscle and subclavicular muscle---brachial plexus.

In the superficial layer, there is the intermediate supraclavicular nerve. In the deep layer, there are the transverse cervical artery and vein and the supraclavicular portion of the brachial plexus.

2. 3. 13 ST 13 Qìhù 氣户

Skin---subcutaneous tissue---greater pectoral muscle.

In the superficial layer, there is the intermediate supraclavicular nerve. In the deep layer, there are the axillary artery and the thoracoacromial artery.

2. 3. 14 ST 14 Kùfáng 庫房

Skin---subcutaneous tissue---greater pectoral muscle---smaller pectoral muscle.

In the superficial layer, there are the supraclavicular nerve and the cutaneous branches of the intercostal nerve. In the deep layer, there are the branches or tributaries of the thoracoacromial artery and vein and the branches of the medial pectoral and lateral pectoral nerves.

2. 3. 15 ST 15 Wūyì 屋翳

Skin---subcutaneous tissue---greater pectoral muscle---smaller pectoral muscle.

In the superficial layer, there are the lateral cutaneous branches of the second intercostal nerve. In the deep layer, there are the branches or tributaries of the thoracoacromial artery and vein and the branches of the medial pectoral and lateral pectoral nerves.

2. 3. 16 ST 16 Yīngchuāng 膺窗

Skin---subcutaneous tissue---greater pectoral muscle---intercostal muscle.

In the superficial layer, there are the lateral cutaneous branches of the intercostal nerve and the tributaries of the thoracoepigastric vein. In the deep layer, there are the medial and lateral pectoral nerves, the branches or tributaries of the thoracoacromial artery and vein, the third intercostal nerve and the third posterior intercostal artery and vein.

2. 3. 17 ST 17 Rǔzhōng 乳中

Skin of mammary nipple---subcutaneous tissue---greater pectoral muscle.

In the superficial layer, there are the lateral cutaneous branches of the fourth intercostal nerve. In males, the subcutaneous tissue is mainly composed of the connective tissue and trace, but not parenchyma, of the mammary gland. In the deep layer, there are the branches of the medial and lateral pectoral nerves and the branches or tributaries of the lateral pectoral artery and vein.

2. 3. 18 ST 18 Rǔgēn 乳根

Skin---subcutaneous tissue---greater pectoral muscle.

In the superficial layer, there are the lateral cutaneous branches of the 5th intercostal nerve and the tributaries of the thoracoepigastric vein. In the deep layer, there are the branches or tributaries of the lateral pectoral artery and vein, the branches of the medial and lateral pectoral nerves, the 5th intercostal nerve and the 5th posterior intercostal artery and vein.

2. 3. 19 ST 19 Bùróng 不容

Skin---subcutaneous tissue---anterior sheath of rectus muscle of abdomen---rectus muscle of abdomen.

In the superficial layer, there are the lateral and anterior cutaneous branches of the anterior branches of the 6th to 8th thoracic nerves and the superficial epigastric vein. In the deep layer, there are the branches or tributaries of the superior epigastric artery and vein and the muscular branches of the anterior branches of the 6th and 7th thoracic nerves.

2. 3. 20 ST 20 Chéngmǎn 承滿

Skin---subcutaneous tissue---anterior sheath of rectus muscle of abdomen---rectus muscle of abdomen.

In the superficial layer, there are the lateral and anterior cutaneous branches of the anterior branches of the 6th to 8th thoracic nerves and the superficial epigastric vein. In the deep layer, there are the branches or tributaries of the superior epigastric artery and vein and the muscular branches of the anterior branches of the 6th to 8th thoracic nerves.

2. 3. 21 ST 21 Liángmén 梁門

Skin---subcutaneous tissue---anterior sheath of rectus muscle of abdomen---rectus muscle of abdomen.

In the superficial layer, there are the lateral and anterior cutaneous branches of the anterior branches of the 7th to 9th thoracic nerves and the superficial epigastric vein. In the deep layer, there are the branches or tributaries of the superior epigastric artery and vein and the muscular branches of the anterior branches of the 7th to 9th thoracic nerves.

2. 3. 22 ST 22 Guānmén 關門

Skin---subcutaneous tissue---anterior sheath of rectus muscle of abdomen---rectus muscle of abdomen.

In the superficial layer, there are the lateral and anterior cutaneous branches of the anterior branches of the 7th to 9th thoracic nerves and the superficial epigastric vein. In the deep layer, there are the branches or tributaries of the superior epigastric artery and vein and the muscular branches of the anterior branches of the 7th to 9th thoracic nerves.

2. 3. 23 ST 23 Tàiyǐ 太乙

Skin---subcutaneous tissue---anterior sheath of rectus muscle of abdomen---rectus muscle of abdomen.

In the superficial layer, there are the lateral and anterior cutaneous branches of the anterior branches of the 8th to 10th thoracic nerves and the superficial epigastric vein. In the deep layer, there are the branches or tributaries of the superior epigastric artery and vein and the muscular branches of the anterior branches of the 8th to 10th thoracic nerves.

2. 3. 24 ST 24 Huáròumén 滑肉門

Skin---subcutaneous tissue---anterior sheath of rectus muscle of abdomen---rectus muscle of abdomen.

In the superficial layer, there are the lateral and anterior cutaneous branches of the anterior branches of the 8th to 10th thoracic nerves and the periumbilical venous network. In the deep layer, there are the branches of tributaries of the superior epigastric artery and vein and the muscular branches of the anterior branches of the 8th to 10th thoracic nerves.

2. 3. 25 ST 25 Tiānshū 天樞

Skin---subcutaneous tissue---anterior sheath of rectus muscle of abdomen---rectus muscle of abdomen.

In the superficial layer, there are the lateral and anterior cutaneous branches of the anterior branches of the 9th to 11th thoracic nerves and the periumbilical venous network. In the deep layer, there are the anastomotic branches of the superior and inferior epigastric arteries and veins and the muscular branches of the anterior branches of the 9th to 11th thoracic nerves.

2. 3. 26 ST 26 Wàilíng 外陵

Skin---subcutaneous tissue---anterior sheath of rectus muscle of abdomen---rectus muscle of abdomen.

In the superficial layer, there are the lateral and anterior cutaneous branches of the anterior branches of the 10th to 12th thoracic nerves and the superficial epigastric vein. In the deep layer, there are the branches or tributaries of the inferior epigastric artery and vein and the muscular branches of the anterior branches of the 10th to 12th thoracic nerves.

2. 3. 27 ST 27 Dàjù 大巨

Skin---subcutaneous tissue---anterior sheath of rectus muscle of abdomen---rectus muscle of abdomen.

In the superficial layer, there are the lateral and anterior cutaneous branches of the anterior branches of the 10th to 12th thoracic nerves and the superficial epigastric artery and vein. In the deep layer, there are the branches or tributaries of the inferior epigastric artery and vein and the muscular branches of the anterior branches of the 10th to 12th thoracic nerves.

2. 3. 28 ST 28 Shuǐdào 水道

Skin---subcutaneous tissue---lateral border of anterior sheath of rectus muscle of abdomen ---lateral border of rectus muscle of abdomen.

In the superficial layer, there are the anterior and lateral cutaneous branches of the anterior branches of the 11th and 12th thoracic nerves and the 1st lumbar nerve, and the superficial epigastric artery and vein. In the deep layer, there are the muscular branches of the anterior branches of the 11th and 12th thoracic nerves.

2. 3. 29 ST 29 Guīlái 歸來

Skin---subcutaneous tissue---lateral border of anterior sheath of rectus muscle of abdomen ---lateral border of rectus muscle of abdomen.

In the superficial layer, there are the lateral and anterior cutaneous branches of the anterior branches of the 11th and 12th thoracic nerves and the 1st lumbar nerve, and the branches or tributaries of the superficial epigastric artery and vein. In the deep layer, there are the branches or tributaries of the inferior epigastric artery and vein, and the muscular branches of the anterior branches of the 11th and 12th thoracic nerves.

2. 3. 30 ST 30 Qìchōng 氣衝

Skin---subcutaneous tissue---aponeurosis of external oblique muscle of abdomen---internal oblique muscle of abdomen---transverse muscle of abdomen.

In the superficial layer, there are the superficial epigastric artery and vein, the lateral and anterior cutaneous branches of the anterior branches of the 12th thoracic nerve and the 1st lumbar nerve. In the deep layer, there are the spermatic cord (or round ligament of the uterus), the ilioinguinal nerve, and the genital branch of the genitofemoral nerve in the inguinal canal at the inferior lateral side of this point.

2. 3. 31 ST 31 Bìguān 髀關

Skin---subcutaneous tissue---between tensor muscle of fascia lata and sartorius muscle ---rectus muscle of thigh---lateral vastus muscle of thigh.

In the superficial layer, there is the lateral cutaneous nerve of the thigh. In the deep layer, there are the ascending branches of the lateral circumflex femoral artery and vein and the muscular branches of the femoral nerve.

2. 3. 32 ST 32 Fútù 伏兔

Skin---subcutaneous tissue---rectus muscle of thigh---intermediate vastus muscle of thigh.

In the superficial layer, there are the lateral femoral vein, the anterior cutaneous branches of the femoral nerve and the lateral cutaneous nerve of the thigh. In the deep layer, there are the descending branches of the lateral circumflex artery and vein and the muscular branches of the femoral nerve.

2. 3. 33 ST 33 Yīnshì 陰市

Skin---subcutaneous tissue---between tendons of rectus muscle and lateral vastus muscle of thigh---intermediate vastus muscle of thigh.

In the superficial layer, there are the anterior cutaneous branches of the femoral nerve and the lateral cutaneous nerve of the thigh. In the deep layer, there are the descending branches of the lateral circumflex femoral arterv and vein and the muscular branches of the femoral nerve.

2. 3. 34 ST 34 Liángqiū 梁丘

Skin---subcutaneous tissue---between tendons of rectus muscle of thigh and lateral vastus muscle of thigh---lateral side of the tendon of intermediate vastus muscle of thigh.

In the superficial layer, there are the anterior cutaneous branches of the femoral nerve and the lateral cutaneous nerve of the thigh. In the deep layer, there are the descending branches of the lateral circumflex femoral artery and vein and the muscular branches of the femoral nerve.

2. 3. 35 ST 35 Dúbí 犢鼻

Skin---subcutaneous tissue---between ligament of patella and lateral patellar retinaculum ---capsule of knee joint and alar folds.

In the superficial layer, there are the lateral cutaneous nerve of the calf, the anterior cutaneous branches of the femoral nerve, the infrapatellar branches of the saphenous nerve and the arteriovenous network of the knee joint. In the deep layer, there is the cavity of the knee joint.

2. 3. 36 ST 36 Zúsānlǐ 足三裏

Skin---subcutaneous tissue---anterior tibial muscle---interosseous membrane of leg---posterior tibial muscle.

In the superficial layer, there is the lateral cutaneous nerve of the calf. In the deep layer, there are the branches or tributaries of the anterior tibial artery and vein.

2. 3. 37 ST 37 Shàngjùxū 上巨虛

Skin---subcutaneous tissue---anterior tibial muscle---interosseous membrane of leg---posterior tibial muscle.

In the superficial layer, there is the lateral cutaneous nerve of the calf. In the deep layer, there are the anterior tibia artery and vein and the deep peroneal nerve. If the needle is inserted too deep, it may injure the posterior tibial artery and vein and the tibial nerve.

2. 3. 38 ST 38 Tiáokǒu 條口

Skin---subcutaneous tissue---anterior tibial muscle---interosseous membrane of leg---posterior tibial muscle.

In the superficial layer, there is the lateral cutaneous nerve of the calf. In the deep layer, there are the anterior tibial artery and vein and the deep peroneal nerve. If the needle is inserted too deep, it may injure the posterior tibial artery and vein.

2. 3. 39 ST 39 Xiàjùxū 下巨虛

Skin---subcutaneous tissue---anterior tibial muscle---interosseous membrane of leg---posterior tibial muscle.

In the superficial layer, there is the lateral cutaneous nerve of the calf. In the deep layer, there are the anterior tibial artery and vein and the deep peroneal nerve.

2. 3. 40 ST 40 Fēnglóng 豐隆

Skin---subcutaneous tissue---long extensor muscle of toes---long extensor muscle of great toe---interosseous membrane of leg---posterior tibial muscle.

In the superficial layer, there is the lateral cutaneous nerve of the calf. In the deep layer, there are the branches or tributaries of the anterior tibial artery and vein and the branches of the deep peroneal nerve.

2. 3. 41 ST 41 Jiěxī 解谿

Skin---subcutaneous tissue---between tendons of long extensor muscle of great toe and long extensor muscle of toes---talus.

In the superficial layer, there are the medial dorsal cutaneous nerves and the subcutaneous veins. In the deep layer, there are the deep peroneal nerve and the anterior tibial artery and vein.

2. 3. 42 ST 42 Chōngyáng 衝陽

Skin---subcutaneous tissue---between tendons of long extensor muscle of great toe and long extensor muscle of toes---short extensor muscle of great toe---intermediate cuneiform bone.

In the superficial layer, there are the medial dorsal cutaneous nerve and the dorsal venous network of the foot. In the deep layer, there are the dorsal pedal artery and vein and the deep peroneal nerve.

2. 3. 43 ST 43 Xiāngǔ 陷谷

Skin---subcutaneous tissue---tendon of long extensor muscle of toes---medial side of tendon of short extensor muscle of toes---2nd dorsal interosseous muscle---oblique head of adductor of great toe.

In the superficial layer, there are the medial dorsal cutaneous nerve and the dorsal venous network of the foot. In the deep layer, there are the 2nd dorsal metatarsal artery and vein.

2. 3. 44 ST 44 Nèitíng 内庭

Skin---subcutaneous tissue---between tendons of long and short extensor muscles of 2nd and 3rd toes---between heads of 2nd and 3rd metatarsal bones.

In the superficial layer, there are the dorsal digital nerve of the medial dorsal pedal cutaneous nerve and the dorsal arteriovenous network of the foot. In the deep layer, there are the dorsal artery and vein.

2. 3. 45 ST 45 Lìduì 厲兑

Skin---subcutaneous tissue---root of nail.

There are the dorsal digital nerve of the medial dorsal pedal cutaneous nerve and the dorsal digital arteriovenous network in this area.

4. Points of the Spleen Meridian of Foot-Taiyin, SP

足太陰脾經穴

Zútàiyīn Píjīng Xué

2. 4. 1 SP 1 Yǐnbái 隱白

Skin---subcutaneous tissue---root of nail.

There are the branches of the medial dorsal cutaneous nerve of the foot, the dorsal digital nerve and the dorsal digital artery and vein in this area.

2. 4. 2 SP 2 Dàdū 大都

Skin---subcutaneous tissue---base of 1st phalanx.

There are the proper digital plantar nerve of the medial plantar nerve, the superficial venous network and the branches or tributaries of the medial plantar artery and vein.

2. 4. 3 SP 3 **Tàibái** 太白

Skin---subcutaneous tissue---abductor muscle of great toe---short flexor muscle of great toe.

In the superficial layer, there are the saphenous nerve and the superficial venous network. In the deep layer, there are the branches or tributaries of the medial plantar artery and vein and the branches of the medial plantar nerve.

2. 4. 4 SP 4 **Gōngsūn** 公孫

Skin---subcutaneous tissue---abductor muscle of great toe---short flexor muscle of great toe---tendon of long flexor muscle of great toe.

In the superficial layer, there are the medial branches of the foot from saphenous nerve and the tributaries of the dorsal venous arch of the foot. In the deep layer, there are the branches or tributaries of the medial plantar artery and vein and the branches of the medial plantar nerve.

2. 4. 5 SP 5 **Shāngqiū** 商丘

Skin---subcutaneous tissue---medial (triangular) ligament---medial malleolus of tibia.

In the superficial layer, there are the saphenous nerve and the great saphenous vein. In the deep layer, there are the branches or tributaries of the medial anterior malleolar artery and vein.

2. 4. 6 SP 6 **Sānyīnjiāo** 三陰交

Skin---subcutaneous tissue---long flexor muscle of toes---posterior tibial muscle---long flexor muscle of great toe.

In the superficial layer, there are the medial cutaneous branches of the leg from the saphenous nerve and the tributaries of the great saphenous vein. In the deep layer, there are the tibial nerve and the posterior tibial artery and vein.

2. 4. 7 SP 7 **Lòugǔ** 漏谷

Skin---subcutaneous tissue---triceps muscle of calf---long flexor muscle of toes---posterior tibial muscle.

In the superficial layer, there are the medial cutaneous branches of the leg from the saphenous nerve and the great saphenous vein. In the deep layer, there are the tibial nerve and the posterior tibial artery and vein.

2. 4. 8 SP 8 **Dìjī** 地機

Skin---subcutaneous tissue---gastrocnemius muscle---soleus muscle.

In the superficial layer, there are the medial cutaneous branches of the leg from the saphenous nerve and the great saphenous vein. In the deep layer, there are the tibial nerve and the posterior tibial artery and vein.

2. 4. 9 SP 9 **Yīnlíngquán** 陰陵泉

Skin---subcutaneous tissue---tendon of semitendinous muscle---medial head of gastrocnemius muscle.

In the superficial layer, there are the medial cutaneous branches of the leg from the saphenous nerve, the great saphenous vein and the branches of the descending genicular artery. In the deep layer, there are the medial inferior genicular artery and vein.

2. 4. 10 SP 10 **Xuèhǎi** 血海

Skin---subcutaneous tissue---medial vastus muscle of thigh.

In the superficial layer, there are the anterior cutaneous branches of the femoral nerve and the tributaries of the great saphenous vein. In the deep layer, there are the muscular branches of the femoral artery and vein and the muscular branches of the femoral nerve.

2. 4. 11 SP 11 **Jīmén** 箕門

Skin---subcutaneous tissue---medial vastus muscle of thigh.

In the superficial layer, there are the anterior cutaneous branches of the femoral nerve and the tributaries of the great saphenous vein. In the deep layer, there are the femoral artery and vein, the saphenous nerve and the muscular branches of the femoral nerve.

2. 4. 12 SP 12 Chōngmén 衝門

Skin---subcutaneous tissue---aponeurosis of external oblique muscle of abdomen---internal oblique muscle of the abdomen---transverse muscle of abdomen---iliopsoas muscle.

In the superficial layer, there are the branches or tributaries of the superficial circumflex iliac artery and vein, the lateral cutaneous branches of the anterior branches of the 11th and 12th thoracic nerves and the 1st lumbar nerve. In the deep layer, there are the muscular branches of the anterior branches of the 11th and 12th thoracic nerve and the 1st lumbar nerve, the femoral nerve, and the deep circumflex iliac artery and vein.

2. 4. 13 SP 13 Fǔshè 府舍

Skin---subcutaneous tissue---aponeurosis of external oblique muscle of abdomen---internal oblique muscle of abdomen---transverse muscle of abdomen.

In the superficial layer, there are the branches or tributaries of the superficial circumflex iliac artery and vein, the lateral cutaneous branches of the anterior branches of the 11th and 12th thoracic nerves and the 1st lumbar nerve. In the deep layer, there are the anterior branches of the 11th and 12th thoracic nerves and the 1st lumbar nerve and their accompanying arteries and veins.

2. 4. 14 SP 14 Fùjié 腹結

Skin---subcutaneous tissue---external oblique muscle of abdomen---internal oblique muscle of abdomen----transverse muscle of abdomen.

In the superficial layer, there are the lateral cutaneous branches of the anterior branches of the 10th to 12th thoracic nerves and the tributaries of the thoracoepigastric vein. In the deep layer, there are the muscular branches of the anterior branches of the 10th to 12th thoracic nerves and their accompanying arteries and veins.

2. 4. 15 SP 15 Dàhéng 大横

Skin---subcutaneous tissue---external oblique muscle of abdomen---internal oblique muscle of abdomen---transverse muscle of abdomen.

In the superficial layer, there are the lateral cutaneous branches of the anterior branches of the 9th to 11th thoracic nerves and the tributaries of the thoracoepigastric vein. In the deep layer, there are the muscular branches of the anterior branches of the 9th to 11th thoracic nerves and their accompanying arteries and veins.

2. 4. 16 SP 16 Fùāi 腹哀

Skin---subcutaneous tissue---external oblique muscle of abdomen---internal oblique muscle of abdomen---transverse muscle of abdomen.

In the superficial layer, there are the lateral cutaneous branches of the anterior branches of the 7th to 9th thoracic nerves and the tributaries of the thoracoepigastric vein. In the deep layer, there are the muscular branches of the anterior branches of the 7th to 9th thoracic nerves and their accompanying arteries and veins.

2. 4. 17 SP 17 Shìdòu 食竇

Skin---subcutaneous tissue---anterior serratus muscle---external intercostal muscle.

In the superficial layer, there are the lateral cutaneous branches of the 5th intercostal nerve and the thoracoepigastric vein. In the deep layer, there are the branches of the long thoracic nerve, the 5th intercostal nerve and the 5th posterior intercostal artery and vein.

2. 4. 18 SP 18 Tiānxī 天豁

Skin---subcutaneous tissue---greater pectoral muscle---smaller pectoral muscle.

In the superficial layer, there are the lateral cutaneous branches of the 4th intercostal nerve and the tributaries of the thoracoepigastric vein. In the deep layer, there are the branches of the medial pectoral nerve and the lateral pectoral nerve, the pectoral branches of the thoracoacromial artery and vein and the branches or tributaries of the lateral thoracic artery and vein.

2. 4. 19 SP 19 Xiōngxiāng 胸鄉

Skin---subcutaneous tissue---greater pectoral muscle---smaller pectoral muscle.

In the superficial layer, there are the lateral cutaneous branches of the 3rd intercostal nerve and the tributaries of the thoracoepigastric vein. In the deep layer, there are the branches of the medial pectoral nerve and the lateral pectoral nerve, the pectoral branches of the thoracoacromial artery vein and the branches or tributaries of the lateral thoracic artery and vein.

2. 4. 20 SP 20 Zhōuróng 周榮

Skin---subcutaneous tissue---great pectoral muscle---smaller pectoral muscle.

In the superficial layer, there are the lateral cutaneous branches of the 2nd intercostal nerve and the superficial vein. In the deep layer, there are the medial pectoral nerve, the lateral pectoral nerve and the pectoral branches of the thoracoacromial artery and vein.

2. 4. 21 SP 21 Dàbāo 大包

Skin---subcutaneous tissue---anterior serratus muscle.

In the superficial layer, there are the lateral cutaneous branches of the 6th intercostal nerve and the tributaries of the thoracoepigastric vein. In the deep layer, there are the branches of the long thoracic nerve and the branches or tributaries of the thoracodorsal artery and vein.

5. Points of the Heart Meridian of Hand-Shaoyin, HT
手少陰心經穴
Shǒushàoyīn Xīnjīng Xué

2. 5. 1 HT 1 Jíquán 極泉

Skin---subcutaneous tissue---brachial plexus and axillary artery and vein---tendon of latissimus muscle of back---teres major muscle.

In the superficial layer, there is the intercostobrachial nerve. In the deep layer, there are the radial nerve, the ulnar nerve, the median nerve, the medial cutaneous nerve of forearm, the medial cutaneous nerve of the arm and the axillary artery and vein.

2. 5. 2 HT 2 Qīnglíng 青靈

Skin---subcutaneous tissue---medial intermuscular septum of arm and brachial muscle.

In the superficial layer, there are the medial cutaneous nerve of the arm, the medial cutaneous nerve of the forearm and the basilic vein. In the deep layer, there are the brachial artery and vein, the median nerve, the ulnar nerve, the superior ulnar collateral artery and vein and the brachial triceps muscle.

2. 5. 3 HT 3 Shàohǎi 少海

Skin---subcutaneous tissue---round pronator muscle---brachial muscle.

In the superficial layer, there are the medial cutaneous nerve of the forearm and the basilic vein. In the deep layer, there are the median nerve, the anastomotic branches of the ulnar recurrent artery and vein and the inferior ulnar collateral artery and vein.

2. 5. 4 HT 4 Língdào 靈道

Skin---subcutaneous tissue---between ulnar flexor muscle of wrist and superficial flexor muscle of fingers---deep flexor muscle of fingers---quadrate pronator muscle.

In the superficial layer, there are the medial cutaneous nerve of the forearm and the tributaries of the basilic vein. In the deep layer, there are the ulnar artery and vein and the ulnar nerve.

2. 5. 5 HT 5 Tōnglǐ 通裏

Skin---subcutaneous tissue---between ulnar flexor muscle of wrist and superficial flexor muscle of fingers---deep flexor muscle of fingers---quadrate pronator muscle.

In the superficial layer, there are the medial cutaneous nerve of the forearm and the tributaries of the basilic vein. In the deep layer, there are the ulnar artery and vein and the ulnar nerve.

2. 5. 6 HT 6 Yīnxì 陰郄

Skin---subcutaneous tissue---radial border of tendon of ulnar flexor muscle of wrist---ulnar nerve.

In the superficial layer, there are the medial cutaneous nerve of the forearm and the tributaries of the basilic vein. In the deep layer, there are the ulnar artery and vein.

2. 5. 7 HT 7 Shénmén 神門

Skin---subcutaneous tissue---radial border of tendon of ulnar flexor muscle of wrist.

In the superficial layer, there are the medial cutaneous nerve of the forearm, the tributaries of the basilic vein and the palmar branches of the ulnar nerve. In the deep layer, there are the ulnar artery and vein and the ulnar nerve.

2. 5. 8 HT 8 Shàofǔ 少府

Skin---subcutaneous tissue---palmar aponeurosis---between tendons of superficial and deep flexor muscle of the 4th and 5th fingers---4th lumbrical muscle---4th dorsal interosseous muscle.

In the superficial layer, there are the palmar branches of the ulnar nerve. In the deep layer, there are the common palmar digital artery and vein and the proper palmar digital nerve from the ulnar nerve.

2. 5. 9 HT 9 Shàochōng 少衝

Skin---subcutaneous tissue---root of nail.

There are the dorsal digital branches of the proper palmar digital nerve of the ulnar nerve and the anteriovenous network formed by the dorsal digital branches of the proper palmar digital arteries and veins in this area.

6. Points of the Small Intestine Meridian of Hand-Taiyang, SI
手太陽小腸經穴
Shǒutàiyáng Xiǎochángjīng Xué

2. 6. 1 SI 1 Shàozé 少澤

Skin---subcutaneous tissue---root of nail.

There are the dorsal digital branches of the proper palmar digital nerve of the ulnar nerve and the anteriovenous network formed by the dorsal digital branches of the ulnar palmar arteries and veins of the little finger in this area.

2. 6. 2 SI 2 Qiángŭ 前谷

Skin---subcutaneous tissue---base of proximal phalanx of 5th finger.

There are the dorsal digital nerve and the proper palmar digital nerve of the ulnar nerve and the ulnar palmar artery and vein of the 5th finger in this area.

2. 6. 3 SI 3 Hòuxī 後谿

Skin---subcutaneous tissue---abductor muscle of 5th finger---short flexor muscle of 5th finger.

In the superficial layer, there are the dorsal branches of the ulnar nerve, the palmar branches of the ulnar nerve and the subcutaneous superficial vein. In the deep layer, there are the proper ulnar palmar artery and vein and the proper palmar digital nerve of the 5th finger.

2. 6. 4 SI 4 Wàngŭ 腕骨

Skin---subcutaneous tissue---abductor muscle of 5th finger---pisometacarpal ligament.

In the superficial layer, there are the medial cutaneous nerve of the forearm, the palmar branches of the ulnar nerve, the dorsal branches of the ulnar nerve and the superficial vein. In the deep layer, there are the branches or tributaries of the ulnar artery and vein.

2. 6. 5 SI 5 Yánggŭ 陽谷

Skin---subcutaneous tissue---anterior side of tendon of ulnar extensor muscle of wrist.

In the superficial layer, there are the dorsal branches of the ulnar nerve and the basilic vein. In the deep layer, there are the dorsal branches of the ulnar artery.

2. 6. 6 SI 6 Yănglăo 養老

Skin---subcutaneous tissue---tendon of ulnar extensor muscle of wrist.

In the superficial layer, there are the medial cutaneous nerve of the forearm, the posterior cutaneous nerve of the forearm, the dorsal branches of the ulnar nerve and the tributaries of the basilic vein. In the deep layer, there is the network of the dorsal carpal arteries and veins.

2. 6. 7 SI 7 Zhīzhèng 支正

Skin---subcutaneous tissue---ulnar flexor muscle of wrist---deep flexor muscle of fingers ---interosseous membrane of forearm.

In the superficial layer, there are the medial cutaneous nerve of the forearm and the tributaries of the basilic vein. In the deep layer, there are the ulnar artery and vein and the ulnar nerve.

2. 6. 8 SI 8 Xiăohăi 小海

Skin---subcutaneous tissue---groove of ulnar nerve.

In the superficial layer, there are the ulnar branches of the medial cutaneous nerve of the forearm, the medial cutaneous nerve of the arm and the tributaries of the basilic vein. In the deep layer, there are the ulnar nerve, the arteriovenous network formed by the superior ulnar collateral arteries and veins and the posterior branches of the ulnar recurrent artery and vein on the posterior lateral side of the ulnar nerve.

2. 6. 9 SI 9 Jiānzhēn 肩貞

Skin---subcutaneous tissue---posterior part of deltoid muscle---long head of brachial triceps muscle---teres major muscle---tendon of latissimus muscle of back.

In the superficial layer, there are the lateral cutaneous branch of the 2nd intercostal nerve and the superior lateral cutaneous nerve of the arm. In the deep layer, there is the radial nerve.

2. 6. 10 SI 10 Nàoshū 臑俞

Skin---subcutaneous tissue---deltoid muscle---infraspinous muscle.

In the superficial layer, there is the lateral supraclavicular nerve. In the deep layer, there are the branches or tributaries of the suprascapular artery and vein and posterior circumflex humeral artery and vein.

2. 6. 11 SI 11 Tiānzōng 天宗

Skin---subcutaneous tissue---trapezius muscle---infraspinous muscle.

In the superficial layer, there are the cutaneous branches of the posterior branches of the 4th thoracic nerve and their accompanying arteries and veins. In the deep layer, there are the branches of the suprascapular nerve and the branches or tributaries of the circumflex scapular artery and vein.

2. 6. 12 SI 12 Bǐngfēng 秉風

Skin---subcutaneous tissue---trapezius muscle---supraspinous muscle.

In the superficial layer, there are the cutaneous branches of the posterior branches of the 2nd thoracic nerve and their accompanying arteries and veins. In the deep layer, there are the branches of the suprascapular nerve and the branches or tributaries of the suprascapular artery and vein.

2. 6. 13 SI 13 Qūyuán 曲垣

Skin---subcutaneous tissue---trapezius muscle---supraspinous muscle.

In the superficial layer, there are the cutaneous branches of the posterior branches of the 2nd and 3rd thoracic nerves and their accompanying arteries and veins. In the deep layer, there are the muscular branches of the suprascapular nerve, the branches or tributaries of the suprascapular artery and vein and the dorsal scapular artery and vein.

2. 6. 14 SI 14 Jiānwàishū 肩外俞

Skin---subcutaneous tissue---trapezius muscle---rhomboid muscle.

In the superficial layer, there are the cutaneous branches of the posterior branches of the 1st and 2nd thoracic nerves and their accompanying arteries and veins. In the deep layer, there are the branches or tributaries of the transverse cervical artery and vein and muscular branches of the dorsal scapular nerve.

2. 6. 15 SI 15 Jiānzhōngshū 肩中俞

Skin---subcutaneous tissue---trapezius muscle---rhomboid muscle.

In the superficial layer, there are the posterior branches of the 8th cervical nerve and the cutaneous branches of the posterior branches of the 1st thoracic nerve. In the deep layer, there are the accessory nerve, the branches of the dorsal scapular nerve and the transverse cervical artery and vein.

2. 6. 16 SI 16 Tiānchuāng 天窗

Skin---subcutaneous tissue---posterior border of sternocleidomastoid muscle---levator muscle of scapula---splenius muscle of neck and head.

In the superficial layer, there are the greater auricular nerve, the lesser occipital nerve and the external jugular vein. In the deep layer, there are the branches or tributaries of the ascending cervical artery and jugular vein.

2. 6. 17 SI 17 Tiānróng 天容

Skin---subcutaneous tissue---posterior side of facial artery---tendons of digastric muscle and stylohyoid muscle.

In the superficial layer, there are the greater auricular nerve and the external jugular vein. In the deep layer, there are the facial artery and vein, the internal jugular vein, the accessory nerve, the vagus nerve, the hypoglossal nerve and the superior cervical ganglion.

2. 6. 18 SI 18 Quánliáo 顴髎

Skin---subcutaneous tissue---zygomatic muscle---masseter muscles---temporal muscle.

In the superficial layer, there are the branches of the infraorbital nerve from the maxillary nerve, the zygomatic and buccal branches of the facial nerve, and the branches or tributaries of the transverse facial artery and vein. In the deep layer, there are the branches of the mandibular nerve from the trigeminal nerve.

2. 6. 19 SI 19 Tīnggōng 聽宮

Skin---subcutaneous tissue---external meatal cartilage.

There are the auriculotemporal nerve and the branches or tributaries of the anterior auricular branches of the superficial temporal artery and vein in this area.

7. Points of Bladder Meridian of Foot-Taiyang, BL
足太陽膀胱經穴
Zútàiyáng Pángguāngjīng Xué

2. 7. 1 BL 1 Jīngmíng 睛明

Skin---subcutaneous tissue---orbicular muscle of eye---upper side of superior lacrimal duct ---between internus muscle of the eye and orbital lamina of ethmoid bone.

In the superficial layer, there are the supratrochlear nerve of the ophthalmic branches of the trigeminal nerve, and the branches or tributaries of the angular artery and vein. In the deep layer, there are the branches or tributaries of the ophthalmic artery and vein, the branches of the ophthalmic nerve and the branches of the oculomotor nerve.

2. 7. 2 BL 2 Cuánzhú 攢竹

Skin---subcutaneous tissue---orbicular muscle of eye.

In the superficial layer, there are the supratrochlear nerve of the frontal nerve, and the branches or tributaries of the superior orbital artery and vein. In the deep layer, there are the temporal and zygomatic branches of the facial nerve.

2. 7. 3 BL 3 Méichōng 眉衝

Skin---subcutaneous tissue---frontal belly of occipitofrontal muscle.

In the superficial layer, there are the supratrochlear nerve and the supratrochlear artery and vein. In the deep layer, there are the subaponeurotic loose connective tissue and the pericranium.

2. 7. 4 BL 4 Qūchāi 曲差

Skin---subcutaneous tissue---frontal belly of occipitofrontal muscle.

In the superficial layer, there are the supratrochlear nerve and the supratrochlear artery and vein. In the deep layer, there are the subaponeurotic loose connective tissue and the pericranium.

2. 7. 5 BL 5 Wǔchù 五處

Skin---subcutaneous tissue---frontal belly of occipitofrontal muscle.

In the superficial layer, there are the supratrochlear nerve and the supratrochlear artery and vein. In the deep layer, there are the subaponeurotic loose connective tissue and the pericranium.

2. 7. 6 BL 6 Chéngguāng 承光

Skin---subcutaneous tissue---epicranial aponeurosis.

In the superficial layer, there are the supraorbital nerve and the supraorbital artery and vein. In the deep layer, there are the subaponeurotic loose connective tissue and the pericranium.

2. 7. 7 BL 7 Tōngtiān 通天

Skin---subcutaneous tissue---epicranial aponeurosis.

In the superficial layer, there are the supraorbital nerve and the supraorbital artery and vein, the interneural and intervascular anastomotic network of the greater occipital nerve, the occipital artery and vein, the auriculotemporal nerve and the superficial temporal artery and vein. In the deep layer, there are the subaponeurotic loose connective tissue and the pericranium.

2. 7. 8 BL 8 Luòquè 絡郤

Skin---subcutaneous tissue---epicranial aponeurosis.

In the superficial layer, there are the greater occipital nerve and the occipital artery and vein. In the deep layer, there are the subaponeurotic loose connective tissue and the pericranium.

2. 7. 9 BL 9 Yùzhěn 玉枕

Skin---subcutaneous tissue---epicranial aponeurosis.

In the superficial layer, there are the greater occipital nerve and the occipital artery and vein. In the deep layer, there are the subaponeurotic loose connective tissue and the pericranium.

2. 7. 10 BL 10 Tiānzhù 天柱

Skin---subcutaneous tissue---trapezius muscle---medial border of splenius muscle of head ---semispinal muscle of head.

In the superficial layer, there are the medial branches of the posterior branches of the 3rd cervical nerve and the subcutaneous vein. In the deep layer, there is the greater occipital nerve.

2. 7. 11 BL 11 Dàzhù 大杼

Skin---subcutaneous tissue---trapezius muscle---rhomboid muscle---superior posterior serratus muscle---splenius muscle of neck---erector spinal muscle.

In the superficial layer, there are the medial cutaneous branches of the posterior branches of the 1st and 2nd thoracic nerves and the medial cutaneous branches of the accompanying posterior intercostal arteries and veins. In the deep layer, there are the muscular branches of the posterior branches of the 1st and 2nd thoracic nerves and the branches of the dorsal branches of the related posterior intercostal arteries and veins.

2. 7. 12 BL 12 Fēngmén 風門

Skin---subcutaneous tissue---trapezius muscle---rhomboid muscle---superior posterior serratus muscle----splenius muscle of neck---erector spinal muscle.

In the superficial layer, there are the medial cutaneous branches of the posterior branches of the 2nd and 3rd thoracic nerves and the medial cutaneous branches of the dorsal branches of the accompanying intercostal arteries and veins. In the deep layer, there are the muscular branches of the posterior branches of the 2nd and 3rd thoracic nerves and the branches of the dorsal branches of the related posterior intercostal arteries and veins.

2. 7. 13 BL 13 Fèishū 肺俞

Skin---subcutaneous tissue---trapezius muscle---rhomboid muscle---superior posterior serratus muscle---erector spinal muscle.

In the superficial layer, there are the medial cutaneous branches of the posterior branches of the 3rd and 4th thoracic nerves and the medial cutaneous branches of the dorsal branches of the accompanying posterior intercostal arteries and veins. In the deep layer, there are the muscular branches of the posterior branches of the 3rd and 4th thoracic nerves and the branches or tributaries of the dorsal branches of the related posterior intercostal arteries and veins.

2. 7. 14 BL 14 Juéyīnshū 厥陰俞

Skin---subcutaneous tissue---trapezius muscle---rhomboid muscle---erector spinal muscle.

In the superficial layer, there are the medial cutaneous branches of the posterior branches of the 4th and 5th thoracic nerves and the dorsal branches of the accompanying posterior intercostal arteries and veins. In the deep layer, there are the muscular branches of the posterior branches of the 4th and 5th thoracic nerves and the branches or tributaries of the dorsal branches of the related posterior intercostal arteries and veins.

2. 7. 15 BL 15 Xīnshū 心俞

Skin---subcutaneous tissue---trapezius muscle---inferior border of rhomboid muscle ---erector spinal muscle.

In the superficial layer, there are the medial cutaneous branches of the posterior branches of the 5th and 6th thoracic nerves and the accompanying arteries and veins. In the deep layer, there are the muscular branches of the posterior branches of the 5th and 6th thoracic nerves and the branches or tributaries of the dorsal branches of the related posterior intercostal arteries and veins.

2. 7. 16 BL 16 Dūshū 督俞

Skin---subcutaneous tissue---trapezius muscle---erector spinal muscle.

In the superficial layer, there are the medial cutaneous branches of the posterior branches of the 6th and 7th thoracic nerves and the accompanying arteries and veins. In the deep layer, there are the muscular branches of the posterior branches of the 6th and 7th thoracic nerves and the branches or tributaries of the dorsal branches of the related posterior intercostal arteries and veins.

2. 7. 17 BL 17 Géshū 膈俞

Skin---subcutaneous tissue---trapezius muscle---latissimus muscle of the back---erector spinal muscle.

In the superficial layer, there are the medial cutaneous branches of the posterior branches of the 7th and 8th thoracic nerves and the accompanying arteries and veins. In the deep layer, there are the muscular branches of the posterior branches of the 7th and 8th thoracic nerves and the branches or tributaries of the dorsal branches of the related posterior intercostal arteries and veins.

2. 7. 18 BL 18 Gānshū 肝俞

Skin---subcutaneous tissue---trapezius muscle---latissimus muscle of back---inferior posterior serratus muscle---erector spinal muscle.

In the superficial layer, there are the cutaneous branches of the posterior branches of the 9th and 10th thoracic nerves and the accompanying arteries and veins. In the deep layer, there are the muscular branches of the posterior branches of the 9th and 10th thoracic nerves and the branches or tributaries of the related posterior intercostal arteries and veins.

2. 7. 19 BL 19 Dǎnshū 膽俞

Skin---subcutaneous tissue---trapezius muscle---latissimus muscle of back---inferior posterior serratus muscle---erector spinal muscle.

In the superficial layer, there are the cutaneous branches of the posterior branches of the

10th and 11th thoracic nerves and the accompanying arteries and veins. In the deep layer, there are the muscular branches of the posterior branches of the 10th and 11th thoracic nerves and the branches or tributaries of the related posterior intercostal arteries and veins.

2. 7. 20 BL 20 Píshū 脾俞

Skin---subcutaneous tissue---latissimus muscle of back---inferior posterior serratus muscle ---erector spinal muscle.

In the superficial layer, there are the cutaneous branches of the posterior branches of the 11th and 12th thoracic nerves and the accompanying arteries and veins. In the deep layer, there are the muscular branches of the posterior branches or the 11th and 12th thoracic nerves and the branches or tributaries of the related intercostal and infracostal arteries and veins.

2. 7. 21 BL 21 Wèishū 胃俞

Skin---subcutaneous tissue---superficial layer of thoracolumbar fascia and aponeurosis of latissimus muscle of back---erector spinal muscle.

In the superficial layer, there are the cutaneous branches of the posterior branches of the 12th thoracic and 1st lumbar nerves and the accompanying arteries and veins. In the deep layer, there are the muscular branches of the posterior branches of the 12th thoracic and 1st lumbar nerves and the branches or tributaries of the related arteries and veins.

2. 7. 22 BL 22 Sānjiāoshū 三焦俞

Skin---subcutaneous tissue---aponeurosis of latissimus muscle of back and superficial layer of thoracolumbar fascia---erector spinal muscle.

In the superficial layer, there are the cutaneous branches of the posterior branches of the 1st and 2nd lumbar nerves and the accompanying arteries and veins. In the deep layer, there are the muscular branches of the posterior branches of the 1st and 2nd lumbar nerves and the branches or tributaries of the dorsal branches of the related lumbar arteries and veins.

2. 7. 23 BL 23 Shènshū 腎俞

Skin---subcutaneous tissue---aponeurosis of latissimus muscle of back and superficial layer of thoracolumbar fascia---erector spinal muscle.

In the superficial layer, there are the cutaneous branches of the posterior branches of the 2nd and 3rd lumbar nerves and the accompanying arteries and veins. In the deep layer, there are the muscular branches of the posterior branches of the 2nd and 3rd lumbar nerves and the branches or tributaries of the dorsal branches of the related lumbar arteries and veins.

2. 7. 24 BL 24 Qìhǎishū 氣海俞

Skin---subcutaneous tissue---aponeurosis of latissimus muscle of back and superficial layer of thoracolumbar fascia---erector spinal muscle.

In the superficial layer, there are the cutaneous branches of the posterior branches of the 3rd and 4th lumbar nerves and the accompanying arteries and veins. In the deep layer, there are the muscular branches of the posterior branches of the 3rd and 4th lumbar nerves and the branches or tributaries of the related lumbar arteries and veins.

2. 7. 25 BL 25 Dàchángshū 大腸俞

Skin---subcutaneous tissue---aponeurosis of latissimus muscle of back and superficial layer of thoracolumbar fascia---erector spinal muscle.

In the superficial layer, there are the cutaneous branches of the posterior branches of the 4th and 5th lumbar nerves and the accompanying arteries and veins. In the deep layer, there are the muscular branches of the posterior branches of the 4th and 5th lumbar nerves and the branches or tributaries of the related lumbar arteries and veins.

2. 7. 26 BL 26 Guānyuánshū 關元俞

Skin---subcutaneous tissue---superficial layer of thoracolumbar fascia---erector spinal muscle.

In the superficial layer, there are the cutaneous branches of the posterior branches of the 5th lumbar and 1st sacral nerves and the accompanying arteries and veins. In the deep layer, there are the muscular branches of the posterior branches of the 5th lumbar nerves.

2. 7. 27 BL 27 Xiǎochángshū 小腸俞

Skin---subcutaneous tissue---medial border of greatest gluteal muscle---tendon of erector spinal muscle.

In the superficial layer, there are the middle clunial nerves. In the deep layer, there are the branches of the inferior gluteal nerve and the muscular branches of the posterior branches of the related spinal nerves.

2. 7. 28 BL 28 Pángguāngshū 膀胱俞

Skin---subcutaneous tissue---greatest gluteal muscle---tendon of erector spinal muscle.

In the superficial layer, there are the middle clunial nerves. In the deep layer, there are the branches of the inferior gluteal nerve and the muscular branches of the posterior branches of the related spinal nerves.

2. 7. 29 BL 29 Zhonglǚshū 中膂俞

Skin---subcutaneous tissue---greatest gluteal muscle---sacrotuberous ligament.

In the superficial layer, there are the middle clunial nerves. In the deep layer, there are the branches or tributaries of the superior and inferior gluteal arteries and veins and the branches of the inferior gluteal nerve.

2. 7. 30 BL 30 Báihuānshū 白環俞

Skin---subcutaneous tissue---greatest gluteal muscle---sacrotuberous ligament---piriform muscle.

In the superficial layer, there are the middle and inferior clunial nerves. In the deep layer, there are the branches or tributaries of the superior and inferior gluteal arteries and veins and the sacral nervous plexus and sacral venous plexus.

2. 7. 31 BL 31 Shàngliáo 上髎

Skin---subcutaneous tissue---superficial layer of thoracolumbar fascia---erector spinal muscle ---1st posterior sacral foramen.

In the superficial layer, there is the middle clunial nerve. In the deep layer, there are the posterior branches of the 1st sacral nerve and the lateral sacral artery and vein.

2. 7. 32 BL 32 Cìliáo 次髎

Skin---subcutaneous tissue---erector spinal muscle---2nd posterior sacral foramen.

In the superficial layer, there is the middle clunial nerve. In the deep layer, there are the posterior branches of the 2nd sacral nerve and the lateral sacral artery and vein.

2. 7. 33 BL 33 Zhōngliáo 中髎

Skin---subcutaneous tissue---greatest gluteal muscle---erector spinal muscle.

In the superficial layer, there is the middle clunial nerve. In the deep layer, there are the posterior branches of the 3rd sacral nerve and the lateral sacral artery and vein.

2. 7. 34 BL 34 Xiàliáo 下髎

Skin---subcutaneous tissue---greatest gluteal muscle—erector spinal muscle.

In the superficial layer, there is the middle clunial nerve. In the deep layer, there are the branches or tributaries of the superior and inferior gluteal arteries and veins, the inferior gluteal nerve of the 4th sacral nerve and the posterior branches of the lateral sacral artery and vein.

2. 7. 35 BL 35 Hùiyáng 會陽

Skin---subcutaneous tissue---greatest gluteal muscle---tendon of levator ani muscle.

In the superficial layer, there is the middle clunial nerve. In the deep layer, there are the branches or tributaries of the inferior gluteal artery and vein and the inferior gluteal nerve.

2. 7. 36 BL 36 Chéngfú 承扶

Skin---subcutaneous tissue---greatest gluteal muscle---long head of biceps muscle of thigh and semitendinous muscle.

In the superficial layer, there are the branches of the posterior femoral cutaneous nerve and the inferior clunial nerve. It the deep layer, there are the trunk of the posterior femoral cutaneous nerve, the sciatic nerve and the accompanying arteries and veins.

2. 7. 37 BL 37 Yīnmén 殷門

Skin---subcutaneous tissue---long head of biceps muscle of thigh and semitendinous muscle.

In the superficial layer, there is the posterior femoral cutaneous nerve. In the deep layer, there are the sciatic nerve and the accompanying artery and vein and the perforating branches of the deep femoral artery.

2. 7. 38 BL 38 Fúxì 浮郄

Skin---subcutaneous tissue---medial border of tendon of biceps muscle of thigh---lateral head of gastrocnemius muscle.

In the superficial layer, there is the posterior femoral cutaneous nerve. In the deep layer, there are the common peroneal nerve, the lateral cutaneous nerve of the calf and the lateral superior genicular artery and vein.

2. 7. 39 BL 39 Wěiyáng 委陽

Skin---subcutaneous tissue---biceps muscle of thigh---lateral head of gastrocnemius muscle ---origin of popliteal muscle and plantar muscle.

In the superficial layer, there is the posterior femoral cutaneous nerve. In the deep layer, there are the common peroneal nerve and the lateral cutaneous nerve of the calf.

2. 7. 40 BL 40 Wěizhōng 委中

Skin---subcutaneous tissue---between lateral and medial heads of gastrocnemius muscle.

In the superficial layer, there are the posterior femoral cutaneous nerve and the small saphenous vein. In the deep layer, there are the tibial nerve, the popliteal artery and vein, and the peroneal artery.

2. 7. 41 BL 41 Fùfēn 附分

Skin---subcutaneous tissue---trapezius muscle---rhomboid muscle---superior posterior serratus muscle---erector spinal muscle.

In the superficial layer, there are the cutaneous branches of the posterior branches of the 2nd and 3rd thoracic nerves and the accompanying arteries and veins. In the deep layer, there are the dorsal scapular nerve, the dorsal scapular artery and vein, the muscular branches of the posterior branches of the 2nd and 3rd thoracic nerves and the branches or tributaries of the dorsal branches of the related posterior intercostal arteries and veins.

2. 7. 42 BL 42 Pòhù 魄户

Skin---subcutaneous tissue---trapezius muscle---rhomboid muscle---superior posterior serratus muscle---erector spinal muscle.

In the superficial layer, there are the cutaneous branches of the posterior branches of the 3rd and 4th thoracic nerves and the accompanying arteries and veins. In the deep layer, there are the dorsal scapular nerve, the dorsal scapular artery and vein, the muscular branches of the posterior branches of the 3rd and 4th thoracic nerves and the branches or tributaries of the dorsal branches of the related posterior intercostal arteries and veins.

2. 7. 43 BL 43 Gāohuāng 膏肓

Skin---subcutaneous tissue---trapezius muscle---rhomboid muscle---erector spinal muscle.

In the superficial layer, there are the cutaneous branches of the posterior branches of the 4th and 5th thoracic nerves and the accompanying arteries and veins. In the deep layer, there are the dorsal scapular nerve, the dorsal scapular artery and vein, the muscular branches of the posterior branches of the 4th and 5th thoracic nerves and the branches or tributaries of the dorsal branches of the related posterior intercostal arteries and veins.

2. 7. 44 BL 44 Shéntáng 神堂

Skin---subcutaneous tissue---trapezius muscle---rhomboid muscle---erector spinal muscle.

In the superficial layer, there are the cutaneous branches of the posterior branches of the 5th and 6th thoracic nerves and the accompanying arteries and veins. In the deep layer, there are the dorsal scapular nerve, the dorsal scapular artery and vein, the muscular branches of the posterior branches of the 5th and 6th thoracic nerves and the branches or tributaries of the dorsal branches of the related posterior intercostal arteries and veins.

2. 7. 45 BL 45 Yìxǐ 譩譆

Skin---subcutaneous tissue---trapezius muscle---rhomboid muscle---erector spinal muscle.

In the superficial layer, there are the cutaneous branches of the posterior branches of the 6th and 7th thoracic nerves and the accompanying arteries and veins. In the deep layer, there are the dorsal scapular nerve, the dorsal scapular artery and vein, the muscular branches of the posterior branches of the 6th thoracic nerve and the branches or tributaries of the dorsal branches of the related posterior intercostal arteries and veins.

2. 7. 46 BL 46 Géguān 膈關

Skin---subcutaneous tissue---trapezius muscle---rhomboid muscle---erector spinal muscle.

In the superficial layer, there are the cutaneous branches of the posterior branches of the 7th and 8th thoracic nerves and the accompanying arteries and veins. In the deep layer, there are the dorsal scapular nerve, the dorsal scapular artery and vein, the muscular branches of the posterior branches of the 7th and 8th thoracic nerves and the branches or tributaries of the dorsal branches of the related posterior intercostal arteries and veins.

2. 7. 47 BL 47 Húnmén 魂門

Skin---subcutaneous tissue---latissimus muscle of back---inferior posterior serratus muscle ---erector spinal muscle.

In the superficial layer, there are the lateral cutaneous branches of the posterior branches of the 9th and 10th thoracic nerves and the accompanying arteries and veins. In the deep layer, there are the muscular branches of the posterior branches of the 9th and 10th thoracic nerves and the branches or tributaries of the dorsal branches of the related posterior intercostal arteries and veins.

2. 7. 48 BL 48 Yánggāng 陽綱

Skin---subcutaneous tissue---latissimus muscle of back---inferior posterior serratus muscle ---erector spinal muscle.

In the superficial layer, there are the lateral cutaneous branches of the posterior branches of the 10th and 11th thoracic nerves and the accompanying arteries and veins. In the deep layer, there are the muscular branches of the posterior branches of the 10th and 11th thoracic nerves and the branches or tributaries of the dorsal branches of the related posterior intercostal arteries and veins.

2. 7. 49 BL 49 Yìshè 意舍

Skin---subcutaneous tissue---latissimus muscle of back---inferior posterior serratus muscle ---erector spinal muscle.

In the superficial layer, there are the lateral cutaneous branches of the posterior branches of the 11th and 12th thoracic nerves and the accompanying arteries and veins. In the deep layer, there are the muscular branches of the posterior branches of the 11th and 12th thoracic nerves and the branches or tributaries of the dorsal branches of the related posterior intercostal arteries and veins.

2. 7. 50 BL 50 Wèicāng 胃倉

Skin---subcutaneous tissue---latissimus muscle of back---inferior posterior serratus muscle ---erector spinal muscle---lumbar quadrate muscle.

In the superficial layer, there are the lateral cutaneous branches of the posterior branches of the 12th thoracic and 1st lumbar nerves and the accompanying arteries and veins. In the deep layer, there are the muscular branches of the posterior branches of the 12th thoracic and 1st lumbar nerve and the branches or tributaries of the dorsal branches of the related arteries and veins.

2. 7. 51 BL 51 Huāngmén 肓門

Skin---subcutaneous tissue---aponeurosis of latissimus muscle of back---erector spinal muscle ---lumbar quadrate muscle.

In the superficial layer, there are the lateral cutaneous branches of the posterior branches of the 1st and 2nd lumbar nerves and the accompanying arteries and veins. In the deep layer, there are the muscular branches of the posterior branches of the 1st and 2nd lumbar nerves and the branches or tributaries of the dorsal branches of the 1st lumbar artery and vein.

2. 7. 52 BL 52 Zhìshì 志室

Skin---subcutaneous tissue---aponeurosis of latissimus muscle of back---erector spinal muscle---lumbar quadrate muscle.

In the superficial layer, there are the lateral cutaneous branches of the posterior branches of the 1st and 2nd lumbar nerves and the accompanying arteries and veins. In the deep layer, there are the muscular branches of the posterior branches of the 1st and 2nd lumbar nerves and the branches or tributaries of the related lumbar arteries and veins.

2. 7. 53 BL 53 Bāohuāng 胞肓

Skin---subcutaneous tissue---greatest gluteal muscle---middle gluteal muscle.

In the superficial layer, there are the superior and middle clunial nerves. In the deep layer, there are the superior gluteal artery and vein and the superior gluteal nerve.

2. 7. 54 BL 54 Zhìbiān 秩邊

Skin---subcutaneous tissue---greatest gluteal muscle---middle gluteal muscle---least gluteal muscle.

In the superficial layer, there are the middle and inferior clunial nerves. In the deep layer, there are the superior and inferior gluteal arteries and veins, and the superior and inferior gluteal nerves.

2. 7. 55 BL 55 Héyáng 合陽

Skin---subcutaneous tissue---gastrocnemius muscle---plantar muscle.

In the superficial layer, there are the small saphenous vein, the posterior cutaneous nerve of the thigh and the medial cutaneous nerve of the calf. In the deep layer, there are the popliteal artery and vein and the tibial nerve.

2. 7. 56 BL 56 Chéngjīn 承筋

Skin---subcutaneous tissue---gastrocnemius muscle---soleus muscle.

In the superficial layer, there are the small saphenous vein and the medial cutaneous nerve of the calf. In the deep layer, there are the posterior tibial artery and vein, the peroneal artery and vein and the tibial nerve.

2. 7. 57 BL 57 Chéngshān 承山

Skin---subcutaneous tissue---gastrocnemius muscle---soleus muscle.

In the superficial layer, there are the small saphenous vein and the medial cutaneous nerve of the calf. In the deep layer, there are the tibial nerve and the posterior tibial artery and vein.

2. 7. 58 BL 58 Fēiyáng 飛揚

Skin---subcutaneous tissue---triceps muscle of calf---long flexor muscle of great toe.

In the superficial layer, there is the lateral cutaneous nerve of calf. In the deep layer, there are the tibial nerve and the posterior tibial artery and vein.

2. 7. 59 BL 59 Fūyáng 跗陽

Skin---subcutaneous tissue---short peroneal muscle---long flexor muscle of great toe.

In the superficial layer, there are the sural nerve and small saphenous vein. In the deep layer, there are the branches of the tibial nerve and the muscular branches of the posterior tibial artery and vein.

2. 7. 60 BL 60 Kūnlún 昆侖

Skin---subcutaneous tissue---loose connective tissue anterior to Archilles tendon.

In the superficial layer, there are the sural nerve and small saphenous vein. In the deep layer, there are the branches or tributaries of the peroneal artery and vein.

2. 7. 61 BL 61 Púcān 僕參

Skin---subcutaneous tissue---calcaneus.

There are the tributaries of the small saphenous vein, the lateral calcaneal branches of the sural nerve and the calcaneal branches of the peroneal artery and vein in this area.

2. 7. 62 BL 62 Shēnmài 申脈

Skin---subcutaneous tissue---tendon of long peroneal muscle---tendon of short peroneal muscle---lateral talocalcaneal ligament.

There are the branches of the small saphenous vein, the sural nerve and the lateral anterior malleolus artery and vein in this area.

2. 7. 63 BL 63 Jīnmén 金門

Skin---subcutaneous tissue---tendon of long peroneal muscle and abductor muscle of little toe.

There are the lateral dorsal cutaneous nerve of the foot and the lateral vein of the foot (the small saphenous vein) in this area.

2. 7. 64 BL 64 Jīnggǔ 京骨

Skin---subcutaneous tissue---abductor muscle of little toe.

There are the lateral dorsal cutaneous nerve of the foot and the lateral vein of the foot (the small saphenous vein) in this area.

2. 7. 65 BL 65 Shùgǔ 束骨

Skin---subcutaneous tissue---abductor muscle of little toe---tendon of opponens muscle of little toe---short flexor muscle of little toe.

In the superficial layer, there are the lateral dorsal cutaneous nerve of the foot and the tributaries of the arch of the dorsal veins of the foot. In the deep layer, there are the proper digital plantar nerve and the proper digital plantar arteries and veins.

2. 7. 66 BL 66 Zútōnggǔ 足通谷

Skin---subcutaneous tissue---plantar surface of proximal end of little toe.

There are the lateral dorsal cutaneous nerve of the foot, the tributaries of the arch of the dorsal veins of the foot, and the proper digital plantar arteries and veins in this area.

2. 7. 67 BL 67 Zhìyīn 至陰

Skin---subcutaneous tissue---root of nail.

There are the dorsal digital nerve of the lateral dorsal cutaneous nerve of the foot and the arteriovenous network of the dorsal digital arteries and veins in this area.

8. Points of the Kidney Meridian of Foot-Shaoyin, KI

足少陰腎經穴

Zúshàoyīn Shènjīng Xué

2. 8. 1 KI 1 Yǒngquán 涌泉

Skin---subcutaneous tissue---plantar aponeurosis---2nd common digital nerve of sole---2nd lumbrical muscle.

In the superficial layer, there are the branches of the medial plantar nerve. In the deep layer, there are the 2nd common digital nerve of the sole and the 2nd common digital artery and vein of the sole.

2. 8. 2 KI 2 Rángǔ 然谷

Skin---subcutaneous tissue---abductor muscle of great toe---tendon of long flexor muscle of toes.

In the superficial layer, there are the medial cutaneous branches of the saphenous nerve to the leg, the cutaneous branches of the medial plantar nerve and the tributaries of the dorsal venous network of the foot. In the deep layer, there are the medial planter nerve and the medial plantar artery and vein.

2. 8. 3 KI 3 Tàixī 太谿

Skin---subcutaneous tissue---between tendons of posterior tibial muscle and long flexor muscle of toes and tendon of plantar muscle and Achilles tendon---long flexor muscle of great toe.

In the superficial layer, there are the medial cutaneous branches of the saphenous nerve to the leg and the tributaries of the great saphenous vein. In the deep layer, there are the tibial nerve and the posterior tibial artery and vein.

2. 8. 4 KI 4 Dàzhōng 大鐘

Skin---subcutaneous tissue---anterior side of tendon of plantar muscle and Archilles tendon ---calcaneus.

In the superficial layer, there are the medial cutaneous branches of the saphenous nerve to the leg and the tributaries of the great saphenous vein. In the deep layer, there is the arterial network formed by the medial malleolus branches and the calcaneal branches of the posterior tibial artery.

2. 8. 5 KI 5 Shuǐquán 水泉

Skin---subcutaneous tissue---medial side of calcaneus.

In the superficial layer, there are the medial cutaneous branches of the saphenous nerve to the leg and the tributaries of the great saphenous vein. In the deep layer, there are the posterior tibial artery and vein, the medial and lateral plantar nerves and the medial calcaneal branches from the tibial nerve.

2. 8. 6 KI 6 Zhàohǎi 照海

Skin---subcutaneous tissue---tendon of posterior tibial muscle.

In the superficial layer, there are the medial cutaneous branches of the saphenous nerve to the leg and the tributaries of the great saphenous vein. In the deep layer, there are the branches or tributaries of the medial tarsal artery and vein.

2. 8. 7 KI 7 Fùliū 複溜

Skin---subcutaneous tissue---anterior side of tendon of plantar muscle and Archilles tendon ---long flexor of great toe.

In the superficial layer, there are the medial cutaneous branches of the saphenous nerve to the leg and the tributaries of the great saphenous vein. In the deep layer, there are the tibial nerve and the posterior tibial artery and vein.

2. 8. 8 KI 8 Jiāoxìn 交信

Skin---subcutaneous tissue---long flexor muscle of toes---posterior side of posterior tibial muscle---long flexor muscle of great toe.

In the superficial layer, there are the medial cutaneous branches of the saphenous nerve to the leg and the tributaries of the great saphenous vein. In the deep layer, there are the tibial nerve and the posterior tibial artery and vein.

2. 8. 9 KI 9 Zhùbīn 築賓

Skin---subcutaneous tissue---triceps muscle of calf.

In the superficial layer, there are the medial cutaneous branches of the saphenous nerve to the leg and the superficial veins. In the deep layer, there are the tibial nerve and the posterior tibial artery and vein.

2. 8. 10 KI 10 Yīngǔ 陰谷

Skin---subcutaneous tissue---between tendons of semimembranous muscle and semitendinous muscle---medial head of gastrocnemius muscle.

In the superficial layer, there are the posterior cutaneous nerve of the thigh and the subcutaneous vein. In the deep layer, there are the branches or tributaries of the superior medial genicular artery and vein.

2. 8. 11 KI 11 Hénggǔ 横骨

Skin---subcutaneous tissue---anterior sheath of rectus muscle of abdomen---pyramidal muscle---rectus muscle of abdomen.

In the superficial layer, there are the anterior cutaneous branches of the iliohypogastric nerve and the tributaries of the superficial epigastric vein. In the deep layer, there are the branches or tributaries of the inferior epigastric artery and vein and the branches of the anterior branches of the 11th and 12th thoracic nerves.

2. 8. 12 KI 12 Dàhè 大赫

Skin---subcutaneous tissue---anterior sheath of rectus muscle of abdomen----superior and lateral border of pyramidal muscle---rectus muscle of abdomen.

In the superficial layer, there are the branches or tributaries of the superficial epigastric artery and vein, the anterior cutaneous branches of the anterior branches of the 11th and 12th thoracic and 1st lumbar nerves and the accompanying arteries and veins. In the deep layer, there are the branches or tributaries of the inferior epigastric artery and vein, the muscular branches of the anterior branches of the 11th and 12th thoracic nerves and the related intercostal arteries and veins.

2. 8. 13 KI 13 Qìxué 氣穴

Skin---subcutaneous tissue---anterior sheath of rectus muscle of abdomen---rectus muscle of abdomen.

In the superficial layer, there are the branches or tributaries of the superficial epigastric artery and vein, the anterior cutaneous branches of the anterior branches of the 11th and 12th thoracic and 1st lumbar nerves and the accompanying arteries and veins. In the deep layer, there are the branches or tributaries of the inferior epigastric artery and vein, the muscular branches of the anterior branches of the 11th and 12th thoracic nerves and the related intercostal arteries and veins.

2. 8. 14 KI 14 Sìmǎn 四满

Skin---subcutaneous tissue---anterior sheath of rectus muscle of abdomen---rectus muscle of abdomen.

In the superficial layer, there are the branches or tributaries of the superficial epigastric artery and vein, the anterior cutaneous branches of the anterior branches of the 10th to 12th thoracic nerves and the accompanying arteries and veins. In the deep layer, there are the branches or tributaries of the inferior epigastric artery and vein, the muscular branches of the anterior branches of the 10th to 12th thoracic nerves and the related intercostal arteries and veins.

2. 8. 15 KI 15 Zhōngzhù 中注

Skin---subcutaneous tissue---anterior sheath of rectus muscle of abdomen---rectus muscle of abdomen.

In the superficial layer, there are the periumbilical subcutaneous venous network, the anterior cutaneous branches of the anterior branches of the 10th to 12th thoracic nerves and the accompanying arteries and veins. In the deep layer, there are the branches or tributaries of the inferior epigastric artery and vein, the muscular branches of the anterior branches of the 10th to 12th thoracic nerves and the related intercostal arteries and veins.

2. 8. 16 KI 16 Huāngshū 肓俞

Skin---subcutaneous tissue---anterior sheath of rectus muscle of abdomen---rectus muscle of abdomen.

In the superficial layer, there are the periumbilical subcutaneous venous network, the anterior cutaneous branches of the anterior branches of the 9th to 11th thoracic nerves and the accompanying arteries and veins. In the deep layer, there are the arteriovenous network formed by the anastomosis of the superior epigastric arteries and veins with the inferior epigastric arteries and veins, the muscular branches of the anterior branches of the 9th to 11th thoracic nerves and the related intercostal arteries and veins.

2. 8. 17 KI 17 Shāngqū 商曲

Skin---subcutaneous tissue---anterior sheath of rectus muscle of abdomen---rectus muscle of abdomen.

In the superficial layer, there are the superficial epigastric vein, the anterior cutaneous branches of the anterior branches of the 8th to 10th thoracic nerves and the accompanying arteries and veins. In the deep layer, there are the branches or tributaries of the superior epigastric artery and vein, the muscular branches of the anterior branches of the 8th to 10th thoracic nerves and the related intercostal arteries and veins.

2. 8. 18 KI 18 Shíguān 石關

Skin---subcutaneous tissue---anterior sheath of rectus muscle of abdomen---recuts muscle of abdomen.

In the superficial layer, there are the superficial epigastric vein, the anterior branches of the 7th to 9th thoracic nerves and the accompanying arteries and veins. In the deep layer, there are the branches or tributaries of the superior epigastric artery and vein, the muscular branches of the anterior branches of the 7th to 9th thoracic nerves and the related intercostal arteries and veins.

2. 8. 19 KI 19 Yīndū 陰都

Skin---subcutaneous tissue---anterior sheath of rectus muscle of abdomen---rectus muscle of abdomen.

In the superficial layer, there are the superficial epigastric vein, the anterior cutaneous branches of the anterior branches of the 7th to 9th thoracic nerves and the accompanying arteries and veins. In the deep layer, there are the branches or tributaries of the superior epigastric artery and vein, the muscular branches of the anterior branches of the 7th to 9th thoracic nerves and the related intercostal arteries and veins.

2. 8. 20 KI 20 Fùtōnggǔ 腹通谷

Skin---subcutaneous tissue---anterior sheath of rectus straight muscle of abdomen---rectus muscle of abdomen.

In the superficial layer, there are the superficial epigastric vein, the anterior cutaneous branches of the anterior branches of the 6th to 8th thoracic nerves and the accompanying arteries and veins. In the deep layer, there are the branches or tributaries of the superior epigastric artery and vein, the muscular branches of the anterior branches of the 6th to 8th thoracic nerves and the related intercostal arteries and veins.

2. 8. 21 KI 21 Yōumén 幽門

Skin---subcutaneous tissue---anterior sheath of rectus muscle of abdomen---rectus muscle of abdomen.

In the superficial layer, there are the anterior cutaneous branches of the anterior branches of the 6th to 8th thoracic nerves and the accompanying arteries and veins. In the deep layer, there are the branches or tributaries of the superior epigastric artery and vein, the muscular branches of the anterior branches of the 6th to 8th thoracic nerves and the related intercostal arteries and veins.

2. 8. 22 KI 22 Bùláng 步廊

Skin---subcutaneous tissue---greater pectoral muscle.

In the superficial layer, there are the anterior cutaneous branches of the 5th intercostal nerve and the perforating branches of the internal thoracic artery and vein. In the deep layer, there are the branches of the medial and lateral pectoral nerves.

2. 8. 23 KI 23 Shénfēng 神封

Skin---subcutaneous tissue---greater pectoral muscle.

In the superficial layer, there are the anterior cutaneous branches of the 4th intercostal nerve and the perforating branches of the internal thoracic artery and vein. In the deep layer, there are the branches of the medial and lateral pectoral nerves.

2. 8. 24 KI 24 Língxū 靈墟

Skin---subcutaneous tissue---greater pectoral muscle.

In the superficial layer, there are the anterior cutaneous branches of the 3rd intercostal nerves and the perforating branches of the internal thoracic artery and vein. In the deep layer, there are the branches of the medial and lateral pectoral nerves.

2. 8. 25 KI 25 Shéncáng 神藏

Skin---subcutaneous tissue---greater pectoral muscle.

In the superficial layer, there are the anterior cutaneous branches of the 2nd intercostal nerve and the perforating branches of the internal thoracic artery and vein. In the deep layer, there are the branches of the medial and lateral pectoral nerves.

2. 8. 26 KI 26 Yùzhōng 彧中

Skin---subcutaneous tissue---great pectoral muscle.

In the superficial layer, there are the anterior cutaneous branches of the 1st intercostal nerve, the medial supraclavicular nerve and the perforating branches of the internal thoracic artery and vein. In the deep layer, there are the branches of the medial and lateral pectoral nerves.

2. 8. 27 KI 27 Shūfǔ 俞府

Skin---subcutaneous tissue---great pectoral muscle.

In the superficial layer, there are the medial supraclavicular nerve. In the deep layer, there are the branches of the medial and lateral pectoral nerves.

9. Points of the Pericardium Meridian of Hand-Jueyin, PC

手厥陰心包經穴

Shǒujuéyīn Xīnbāojīng Xué

2. 9. 1 PC 1 Tiānchí 天池

Skin---subcutaneous tissue---greater pectoral muscle---smaller pectoral muscle.

In the superficial layer, there are the lateral cutaneous branches of the 4th intercostal nerve and the tributaries of the thoracoepigastric vein. In female, besides the above-mentioned vessel and nerve, there are also the glandular tissues in the subcutaneous layer. In the deep layer, there are the medial and lateral pectoral nerves and the branches or tributaries of the lateral thoracic artery and vein.

2. 9. 2 PC 2 Tiānquán 天泉

Skin---subcutaneous tissue---brachial biceps muscle---brachial muscle---tendon of coracobrachial muscle.

In the superficial layer, there are the branches of the medial brachial cutaneous nerve. In the deep layer, there are the musculocutaneous nerve and the muscular branches of the brachial artery and vein.

2. 9. 3 PC 3 Qūzé 曲澤

Skin---subcutaneous tissue---medial nerve---brachial muscle.

In the superficial layer, there are the medial vein of the elbow and the medial cutaneous nerve of the forearm. In the deep layer, there are the brachial artery and veins, the arteriovenous network formed by the palmar branches of the ulnar recurrent artery and vein with the anterior branches of the inferior ulnar collateral artery and vein, and the trunk of the median nerve.

2. 9. 4 PC 4 Xīmén 郄門

Skin---subcutaneous tissue---between tendons of radial flexor muscle of wrist and long palmar muscle---superficial flexor muscle of fingers---deep flexor muscle of fingers---interosseous membrane of forearm.

In the superficial layer, there are the branches of the lateral and medial cutaneous nerves of the forearm and the median vein of the forearm. In the deep layer, there are the median nerve and the accompanying arterv and vein and the anterior interosseous artery and nerve.

2. 9. 5 PC 5 Jiānshǐ 間使

Skin---subcutaneous tissue---between tendons of radial flexor muscle of wrist and long palmar muscle---superficial flexor muscle of fingers---deep flexor muscle of fingers---quadrate pronate muscle---interosseous membrane of forearm.

In the superficial layer, there are the branches of the lateral and medial cutaneous nerves and the median vein of the forearm. In the deep layer, there are the median nerve and the accompanying artery and vein and the anterior interosseous artery and nerve.

2. 9. 6 PC 6 Nèiguān 內關

Skin---subcutaneous tissue---between tendons of radial flexor muscle of wrist and long palmar muscle---superficial flexor muscle of fingers---deep flexor muscle of fingers---quadrate pronate muscle.

In the superficial layer, there are the branches of the medial and lateral cutaneous nerves and the median vein of the forearm. In the deep layer, there are the median nerve and the accompanying artery and vein in the superficial flexor muscle of the fingers, the long flexor muscle of the thumb and the deep flexor muscle of the fingers. There are the anterior interosseous artery, vein and nerve on the anterior side of the interosseous membrane of the forearm.

2. 9. 7 PC 7 Dàlíng 大陵

Skin---subcutaneous tissue---between tendons of long palmar muscle and radial flexor muscle of wrist---between tendons of flexor muscle of thumb and superficial flexor muscle of fingers and deep flexor muscle of fingers---distal side of radiocarpal joint.

In the superficial layer, there are the medial and lateral cutaneous nerves of the forearm, the palmar branches of the median nerve and the palmar venous network of the wrist. In the deep layer, the median nerve may be injured if the needle is inserted between and beyond the long palmar muscle and the radial flexor muscle of the wrist.

2. 9. 8 PC 8 Láogōng 勞宫

Skin---subcutaneous tissue---palmar aponeurosis---between tendons of superficial and deep flexor muscle of fingers on radial side---raidal side of second lumbrical muscle---first palmar interosseous muscle and second dorsal interosseous muscle.

In the superficial layer, there are the palmar branches of the median nerve and the venous network of the palmar side. In the deep layer, there are the common palmar digital artery and the proper palmar digital nerve of the median nerve.

2. 9. 9 PC 9 Zhōngchōng 中衝

Skin---subcutaneous tissue.

There are the terminal branches of the proper palmar digital nerve of the median nerve, and the arteriovenous network of the proper palmar digital arteries and veins in this area. Inside the subcutaneous tissue are the rich fiber bundles between the skin and the periosteum of the distal phalanx.

10. Points of the Sanjiao (Triple Energizer) Meridian of Hand-Shaoyang, SJ (TE)

手少陽三焦經穴

Shǒushàoyáng Sānjiāojīng Xué

2. 10. 1 SJ 1 Guānchōng 關衝

Skin---subcutaneous tissue---root of nail.

In the subcutaneous tissue, there are the branches of the dorsal digital branches of the proper palmar digital nerve from the ulnar nerve, and the arteriovenous network of the dorsal branches of the proper palmar digital arteries and veins.

2. 10. 2 SJ 2 Yèmén 液門

Skin---subcutaneous tissue---between bases of 4th and 5th proximal phalangeal bones ---4th dorsal interosseous muscle and 4th lumbrical muscle.

In the superficial layer, there are the dorsal digital nerve of the ulnar nerve and the dorsal venous network of the hand. In the deep layer, there are the dorsal digital artery and vein.

2. 10. 3 SJ 3 Zhōngzhǔ 中渚

Skin---subcutaneous tissue---4th dorsal interosseous muscle.

In the superficial layer, there are the dorsal digital nerve of the ulnar nerve and the ulnar part of the dorsal venous network of the hand. In the deep layer, there is the 4th dorsal metacarpal artery.

2. 10. 4 SJ 4 Yángchí 陽池

Skin---subcutaneous tissue---ligament of dorsum of wrist---between tendons of extensor muscle of fingers and extensor muscle of little finger---radiocarpal joint.

In the superficial layer, there are the dorsal branches of the ulnar nerve, the dorsal venous network of the wrist and the terminal branches of the posterior cutaneous nerve of the forearm. In the deep layer, there are the branches of the dorsal carpal branch of the ulnar artery.

2. 10. 5 SJ 5 Wàiguān 外關

Skin---subcutaneous tissue---extensor muscle of little finger and extensor muscle of fingers ---long extensor muscle of thumb and extensor muscle of index finger.

In the superficial layer, there are the posterior cutaneous nerve of the forearm and the tributaries of the cephalic and basilic veins. In the deep layer, there are the posterior interosseous artery and vein and the posterior interosseous nerve.

2. 10. 6 SJ 6 Zhīgōu 支溝

Skin---subcutaneous tissue---extensor muscle of little finger---long extensor muscle of thumb---interosseous membrane of forearm.

In the superficial layer, there are the posterior cutaneous nerve of the forearm and the tributaries of the cephalic and basilic veins. In the deep layer, there are posterior interosseous artery and vein and the posterior interosseous nerve.

2. 10. 7 SJ 7 Huìzōng 會宗

Skin---subcutaneous tissue---ulnar extensor muscle of wrist---extensor muscle of index finger---interosseous membrane of forearm.

In the superficial layer, there are the posterior cutaneous nerve of the forearm and the tributaries of the basilic vein. In the deep layer, there are the branches or the tributaries of the posterior interosseous artery and vein of the forearm and the branches of the posterior interosseous nerve of the forearm.

2. 10. 8 SJ 8 Sānyángluò 三陽絡

Skin---subcutaneous tissue---extensor muscle of fingers---long abductor muscle of thumb ---short extensor muscle of thumb---interosseous membrane of forearm.

In the superficial layer, there are the posterior cutaneous nerve of the forearm and the tributaries of the cephalic and basilic veins. In the deep layer, there are the branches or tributaries of the posterior interosseous artery and vein of the forearm and the branches of the posterior interosseous nerve of the forearm.

2. 10. 9 SJ 9 Sìdú 四瀆

Skin---subcutaneous tissue---extensor muscle of little finger and ulnar extensor muscle of wrist---long abductor and extensor muscle of thumb.

In the superficial layer, there are the posterior cutaneous nerve of the forearm and the tributaries of the cephalic and basilic veins. In the deep layer, there are the posterior interosseous artery and vein and the posterior interosseous nerve.

2. 10. 10 SJ 10 Tiānjǐng 天井

Skin---subcutaneous tissue---brachial triceps muscle.

In the superficial layer, there is the posterior brachial cutaneous nerve. In the deep layer, there are the arteriovenous network of the elbow joint and the muscular branches of the radial nerve.

2. 10. 11 SJ 11 Qīnglěngyuān 清冷淵

Skin---subcutaneous tissue---brachial triceps muscle.

In the superficial layer, there is the posterior brachial cutaneous nerve. In the deep layer, there are the median collateral arterv and vein and the muscular branches of the radial nerve.

2. 10. 12 SJ 12 Xiāoluò 消濼

Skin---subcutaneous tissue---long head of brachial triceps muscle---medial head of brachial triceps muscle.

In the superficial layer, there is the posterior brachial cutaneous nerve. In the deep layer, there are the median collateral artery and vein and the muscular branches of the radial nerve.

2. 10. 13 SJ 13 Nàohuì 臑會

Skin---subcutaneous tissue---long head and lateral head of brachial triceps muscle---radial nerve---medial head of brachial triceps muscle.

In the superficial layer, there is the posterior brachial cutaneous nerve. In the deep layer, there are the radial nerve and the deep brachial artery and vein.

2. 10. 14 SJ 14 Jiānliáo 肩髎

Skin---subcutaneous tissue---deltoid muscle---teres minor muscle---teres major muscle

---tendon of latissimus muscle of back.

In the superficial layer, there is the lateral supraclavicular nerve. In the deep layer, there are the axillary nerve and the posterior circumflex humeral artery and vein.

2. 10. 15 SJ 15 Tiānliáo 天髎

Skin---subcutaneous tissue---trapezius muscle---supraspinous muscle.

In the superficial layer, there are the supraclavicular nerve and the lateral cutaneous branches of the posterior branches of the 1st thoracic nerve. In the deep layer, there are the branches or tributaries of the dorsal scapular artery and vein, the branches or tributaries of the suprascapular artery and vein, and the suprascapular nerve.

2. 10. 16 SJ 16 Tiānyǒu 天牖

Skin---subcutaneous tissue---between sternocleidomastoid muscle and trapezius muscle ---splenius muscle of head and neck---semispinal muscles of head and neck.

In the superficial layer, there are the tributaries of the external jugular vein, the great auricular nerve and the lesser occipital nerve. In the deep layer, there are the branches or tributaries of the occipital artery and vein, and the ascending branches of the deep cervical artery and vein.

2. 10. 17 SJ 17 Yìfēng 翳風

Skin---subcutaneous tissue---parotid gland.

In the superficial layer, there are the great auricular nerve and the tributaries of the external jugular vein. In the deep layer, there are the posterior auricular artery of the external carotid artery and the facial nerve.

2. 10. 18 SJ 18 Chìmài 瘈脈

Skin---subcutaneous tissue---posterior auricular muscle.

There are the great auricular nerve, the posterior auricular branches of the facial nerve and the posterior auricular artery and vein in this area.

2. 10. 19 SJ 19 Lúxī 顱息

Skin---subcutaneous tissue---posterior auricular muscle.

There are the great auricular nerve, the lesser occipital nerve, the posterior auricular branches of the facial nerve, and the auricular branches of the posterior auricular artery and vein in this area.

2. 10. 20 SJ 20 Jiǎosūn 角孫

Skin---subcutaneous tissue---superior auricular muscle---superficial temporal fascia and temporal muscle.

There are the branches of the auriculotemporal nerve and the anterior auricular branches of the superficial temporal artery and vein in this area.

2. 10. 21 SJ 21 Ěrmén 耳門

Skin---subcutaneous tissue---parotid gland.

There are the auriculotemporal nerve, the anterior auricular branches of the superficial temporal artery and vein, and the temporal branches of the facial nerve in this area.

2. 10. 22 SJ 22 Ěrhéliáo 耳和髎

Skin---subcutaneous tissue---anterior auricular muscle---superficial temporal fascia and temporal muscle.

In the superficial layer, there are the auriculotemporal nerve, the temporal branches of the facial nerve, and the branches or tributaries of the superficial temporal artery and vein. In the deep layer, there are the anterior and posterior deep temporal nerves from the mandibular division of the trigeminal nerve.

2. 10. 23 SJ 23 Sīzhúkōng 絲竹空

Skin---subcutaneous tissue---orbicular muscle of eye.

There are the supraorbital nerve, the zygomaticofacial nerve, the temporal and zygomatic branches of the facial nerve, and the frontal branches of the superficial temporal artery and vein in this area.

11. Points of the Gallbladder Meridian of Foot-Shaoyang, GB

足少陽膽經穴

Zúshàoyáng Dǎnjīng Xué

2. 11. 1 GB 1 Tóngzǐliáo 瞳子髎

Skin---subcutaneous tissue---orbicular muscle of eye---temporal fascia---temporal muscle.

In the superficial layer, there are the zygomaticofacial and zygomaticotemporal branches of the zygomatic nerve. In the deep layer, there are the anterior and posterior deep temporal nerves and the branches of the anterior and posterior deep temporal arteries and veins.

2. 11. 2 GB 2 Tīnghuì 聽會

Skin---subcutaneous tissue--capsule of parotid gland---parotid gland.

In the superficial layer, there are the auriculotemporal nerve and the great auricular nerve. In the deep layer, there are the superficial temporal artery and vein and the plexus of the facial nerve.

2. 11. 3 GB 3 Shàngguān 上關

Skin---subcutaneous tissue---superficial temporal fascia---deep temporal fascia---loose connective tissue---temporal muscle.

In the superficial layer, there are the auriculotemporal nerve, the temporal branch of the facial nerve and the superficial temporal artery and vein. In the deep layer, there are the branches of the anterior and posterior deep temporal nerves.

2. 11. 4 GB 4 Hànyàn 頷厭

Skin---subcutaneous tissue---superior auricular muscle---temporal fascia---temporal muscle.

In the superficial layer, there are the auriculotemporal nerve and the parietal branches of the superficial temporal artery and vein. In the deep layer, there are the branches of the anterior and posterior deep temporal nerves.

2. 11. 5 GB 5 Xuánlú 懸盧

Same as Hànyàn (GB 4).

2. 11. 6 GB 6 Xuánlí 懸釐

Same as Hànyàn (GB 4).

2. 11. 7 GB 7 Qūbìn 曲鬢

Same as Hànyàn (GB 4).

2. 11. 8 GB 8 Shuàigǔ 率谷

Skin---subcutaneous tissue---superior auricular muscle---temporal fascia---temporal muscle.

There are the anastomotic branches of the auriculotemporal and greater occipital nerves and the parietal branches of the superficial temporal artery and vein in this area.

2. 11. 9 GB 9 Tiānchōng 天衝

Skin---subcutaneous tissue---superior auricular muscle---temporal fascia---temporal muscle.

There are the anastomotic branches of the auriculotemporal nerve and the lesser and greater occipital nerves, the parietal branches of the superficial temporal artery and vein, and the posterior auricular artery and vein in this area.

2. 11. 10 GB 10 Fúbái 浮白

Skin---subcutaneous tissue---epicranial aponeurosis.

There are the anastomotic branches of the lesser and greater occipital nerves and the posterior auricular artery and vein in this area.

2. 11. 11 GB 11 Tóuqiàoyīn 頭竅陰

Skin---subcutaneous tissue---epicranial aponeurosis.

There are the lesser occipital nerve and the branches of the posterior auricular artery and vein in this area.

2. 11. 12 GB 12 Wángŭ 完骨

Skin---subcutaneous tissue---sternocleidomastoid muscle---splenius muscle of head---longest muscle of head.

In the superficial layer, there are the lesser occipital nerve and the branches or tributaries of the posterior auricular artery and vein. In the deep layer, there are the deep cervical artery and vein. If the needle is inserted too deep, the vertebral artery may be injured.

2. 11. 13 GB 13 Běnshén 本神

Skin---subcutaneous tissue---frontal belly of occipitofrontal muscle.

There are the supraorbital artery and vein, the supraorbital nerve, and the frontal branches of the superficial temporal artery and vein in this area.

2. 11. 14 GB 14 Yángbái 陽白

Skin---subcutaneous tissue---frontal belly of occipitofrontal muscle.

There are the lateral branches of the supraorbital nerve and lateral branches of the supraorbital artery and vein in this area.

2. 11. 15 GB 15 Tóulínqì 頭臨泣

Skin---subcutaneous tissue---epicranial aponeurosis---loose connective tissue below aponeurosis.

There are the supraorbital nerve and the supraorbital artery and vein in this area.

2. 11. 16 GB 16 Mùchuāng 目窗

Skin---subcutaneous tissue---galea aponeurosis---loose connective tissue below aponeurosis.

There are the supraorbital nerve and the frontal branches of the superficial temporal artery and vein in this area.

2. 11. 17 GB 17 Zhèngyíng 正營

Skin---subcutaneous tissue---epicranial aponeurosis---loose connective tissue below aponeurosis.

There are the anatomotic branches of the supraorbital and greater occipital nerves and the parietal branches of the superficial temporal artery and vein in this area.

2. 11. 18 GB 18 Chénglíng 承靈

Skin---subcutaneous tissue---epicranial aponeurosis---loose connective tissue below aponeurosis.

There are the greater occipital nerve and the branches of the occipital artery and vein in this area.

2. 11. 19 GB 19 Nǎokōng 腦空

Skin---subcutaneous tissue---occipital belly of occipitofrontal muscle.

There are the greater occipital nerve, the occipital artery and vein, and the posterior auricular branches of the facial nerve in this area.

2. 11. 20 GB 20 Fēngchí 風池

Skin---subcutaneous tissue---between trapezius muscle and sternocleidomastoid muscle ---splenius muscle of head---semispinal muscle of head---between large posterior straight muscle of head and superior oblique muscle of head.

In the superficial layer, there are the lesser occipital nerve and the branches or tributaries of the occipital artery and vein. In the deep layer, there is the suboccipital nerve.

2. 11. 21 GB 21 Jiānjǐng 肩井

Skin---subcutaneous tissue---trapezius muscle---levator muscle of scapula.

In the superficial layer, there are the supraclavicular nerve and the branches or tributaries of the superficial cervical artery and vein. In the deep layer, there are the branches or tributaries of the transverse cervical artery and vein and the branches of the dorsal scapular nerve.

2. 11. 22 GB 22 Yuānyè 淵腋

Skin---subcutaneous tissue---anterior serratus muscle---external intercostal muscle

In the superficial layer, there are the lateral cutaneous branches of the 3rd to 5th intercostal nerves, the long thoracic nerve and the lateral thoracic artery and vein. In the deep layer, there are the 4th intercostal nerve and the 4th posterior intercostal artery and vein.

2. 11. 23 GB 23 Zhéjīn 輒筋

Skin---subcutaneous tissue---anterior serratus muscle---external intercostal muscle.

In the superficial layer, there are the lateral cutaneous branches of the 3rd to 5th intercostal nerves and the branches or tributaries of the lateral thoracic artery and vein. In the deep layer, there are the 4th intercostal nerve and 4th posterior intercostal artery and vein.

2. 11. 24 GB 24 Rìyuè 日月

Skin---subcutaneous tissue---external oblique muscle of abdomen---external intercostal muscle.

In the superficial layer, there are the lateral cutaneous branches of the 6th to 8th intercostal nerves and the accompanying arteries and veins. In the deep layer, there are the 7th intercostal nerve and the 7th posterior intercostal artery and vein.

2. 11. 25 GB 25 Jīngmén 京門

Skin---subcutaneous tissue---external oblique muscle of abdomen---internal oblique muscle of abdomen---transverse muscle of abdomen.

In the superficial layer, there are the lateral cutaneous branches of the anterior branches of the 11th and 12th thoracic nerves and the accompanying arteries and veins. In the deep layer, there are the muscular branches of the anterior branches of the 11th and 12th thoracic nerves and the related intercostal and subcostal arteries and veins.

2. 11. 26 GB 26 Dàimài 帶脈

Skin---subcutaneous tissue---external oblique muscle of abdomen---internal oblique muscle of abdomen---transverse muscle of abdomen.

In the superficial layer, there are the lateral cutaneous branches of the anterior branches of the 9th to 11th thoracic nerves and the accompanying arteries and veins. In the deep layer, there are the muscular branches of the anterior branches of the 9th to 11th thoracic nerves and the related arteries and veins.

2. 11. 27 GB 27 Wǔshū 五樞

Skin---subcutaneous tissue---external oblique muscle of abdomen---internal oblique muscle of abdomen---transverse muscle of abdomen.

In the superficial layer, there are the lateral cutaneous branches of the anterior branches of the 11th and 12th thoracic and 1st lumbar nerves and accompanying arteries and veins. In the deep layer, there are the deep circumflex iliac artery and vein, the muscular branches of the anterior branches of the 11th and 12th thoracic and 1st lumbar nerves and the related arteries and veins.

2. 11. 28 GB 28 Wéidào 維道

Skin---subcutaneous tissue---external oblique muscle of abdomen---internal oblique muscle of abdomen---transverse muscle of abdomen---iliopsoas muscle.

In the superficial layer, there are the superficial circumflex iliac artery and vein, the lateral cutaneous branches of the anterior branches of the 11th and 12th thoracic and 1st lumbar nerves and the accompanying arteries and veins. In the deep layer, there are the deep circumflex iliac artery and vein, the lateral cutaneous nerve of the thigh, the muscular branches of the anterior branches of the 11th and 12th thoracic and 1st lumbar nerves and the related arteries and veins.

2. 11. 29 GB 29 Jūliáo 居髎

Skin---subcutaneous tissue---fascia lata---middle gluteal muscle---least gluteal muscle.

In the superficial layer, there are the superior clunial nerve and the lateral cutaneous branches of the iliohypogastric nerve. In the deep layer, there are the branches or tributaries of the superior gluteal artery and vein and the superior gluteal nerve.

2. 11. 30 GB 30 Huántiào 環跳

Skin---subcutaneous tissue---greatest gluteal muscle---sciatic nerve---quadrate muscle of thigh.

In the superficial layer, there is the superior clunial nerve. In the deep layer, there are the sciatic nerve, the inferior gluteal nerve, the posterior cutaneous nerve of the thigh, and the inferior gluteal artery and vein.

2. 11. 31 GB 31 Fēngshì 風市

Skin---subcutaneous tissue---iliotibial tract---lateral muscle of thigh---intermediate vastus muscle of thigh.

In the superficial layer, there is the lateral cutaneous nerve of the thigh. In the deep layer, there are the muscular branches of the descending branches of the lateral circumflex femoral artery and the muscular branches of the femoral nerve.

2. 11. 32 GB 32 Zhōngdú 中瀆

Skin---subcutaneous tissue---iliotibial tract---lateral vastus muscle of thigh---intermediate vastus muscle of thigh.

In the superficial layer, there is the lateral cutaneous nerve of the thigh. In the deep layer, there are the muscular branches of the descending branches of the lateral circumflex femoral artery and vein and the muscular branches of the femoral nerve.

2. 11. 33 GB 33 Xīyángguān 膝陽關

Skin---subcutaneous tissue---posterior border of iliotibial tract---anterior side of lateral head of gastrocnemius muscle.

In the superficial layer, there is the lateral cutaneous nerve of the thigh. In the deep layer, there are the lateral superior genicular artery and vein.

2. 11. 34 GB 34 Yánglíngquán 陽陵泉

Skin---subcutaneous tissue---long peroneal muscle---long extensor muscle of toes.

In the superficial layer, there is the lateral sural cutaneous nerve. In the deep layer, there are the anterior recurrent tibial artery and vein, the branches or tributaries of the lateral inferior genicular artery and vein, and the branches of common peroneal nerve.

2. 11. 35 GB 35 Yángjiāo 陽交

Skin---subcutaneous tissue---triceps muscle of calf---long peroneal muscle---posterior intermuscular septum---long flexor muscle of great toe.

In the superficial layer, there is the lateral sural cutaneous nerve. In the deep layer, there are the peroneal artery and vein, the posterior tibial artery and vein, and the tibial nerve.

2. 11. 36 GB 36 Wàiqiū 外丘

Skin---subcutaneous tissue---long and short peroneal muscles---anterior intermuscular septum---long extensor muscle of toes---long extensor muscle of great toe.

In the superficial layer, there is the lateral sural cutaneous nerve. In the deep layer, there are the superficial and deep peroneal nerves and the anterior tibial artery and vein.

2. 11. 37 GB 37 Guāngmíng 光明

Skin---subcutaneous tissue---short peroneal muscle---anterior intermuscular septum---long extensor muscle of toes---long extensor muscle of great toe---interosseous membrane of leg ---posterior tibial muscle.

In the superficial layer, there are the superficial peroneal nerve and the lateral sural cutaneous nerve. In the deep layer, there are the deep peroneal nerve and the anterior tibial artery and vein.

2. 11. 38 GB 38 Yángfǔ 陽輔

Skin---subcutaneous tissue---long extensor muscle of toes---long extensor muscle of the great toe---interosseous membrane of leg---posterior tibial muscle.

In the superficial layer, there are the lateral sural cutaneous nerve and the superficial peroneal nerve. In the deep layer, there are the peroneal artery and vein.

2. 11. 39 GB 39 Xuánzhōng 懸鍾

Skin---subcutaneous tissue---long extensor muscle of toes---interosseous membrane of leg.

In the superficial layer, there is the lateral sural cutaneous nerve. In the deep layer, there are the branches of the deep peroneal nerve. If the needle penetrates through the interosseous membrane of the leg, the peroneal artery and vein may be injured.

2. 11. 40 GB 40 Qiūxū 丘墟

Skin---subcutaneous tissue---short extensor muscle of toes---lateral talocalcaneal ligament ---tarsal sinus.

There are the superficial vein of the dorsum of the foot, the lateral dorsal cutaneous nerve of the foot, the intermediate dorsal cutaneous nerve of the foot, and the lateral anterior malleolar artery and vein in this area.

2. 11. 41 GB 41 Zúlínqì 足臨泣

Skin---subcutaneous tissue---4th dorsal interosseous muscle and 3rd plantar interosseous muscle.

There are the venous network of the dorsum of the foot, the intermediate dorsal cutaneous nerve of the foot, the 4th dorsal metatarsal artery and vein, and the branches of the lateral plantar nerve in this area.

2. 11. 42 GB 42 Dìwǔhuì 地五會

Skin---subcutaneous tissue---tendon of long extensor muscle of toes---lateral side of tendon of short extensor muscle of toes---4th dorsal interosseous muscle---3rd plantar interosseous muscle.

In the superficial layer, there are the intermediate dorsal cutaneous nerve of the foot, the venous network of the dorsum of the foot and the dorsal metatarsal artery and vein. In the deep layer, there are the common digital plantar nerve and the common digital plantar artery and vein.

2. 11. 43 GB 43 Xiáxī 俠谿

Skin---subcutaneous tissue---between tendons of 4th long and short extensor muscles of toe and tendons of 5th long and short extensor muscle of toe---between bases of 4th and 5th proximal phalangeal bones.

There are the dorsal digital nerve of the intermediate dorsal cutaneous nerve of the foot and the dorsal digital artery and vein in this area.

2. 11. 44 GB 44 Zúqiàoyīn 足竅陰

Skin---subcutaneous tissue---root of nail.

There are the dorsal digital nerve of the intermediate dorsal cutaneous nerve of the foot, and the arteriovenous network formed by the dorsal digital arteries and veins of the foot with the proper plantar arteries and veins in this area.

12. Points of the Liver Meridian of Foot-Jueyin, LR

足厥陰肝經穴

Zújuéyīn Gānjīng Xué

2. 12. 1 LR 1 Dàdūn 大敦

Skin---subcutaneous tissue---root of nail.

There are the lateral dorsal nerve of the great toe from the deep peroneal nerve and the dorsal digital artery and vein in this area.

2. 12. 2 LR 2 Xíngjiān 行間

Skin---subcutaneous tissue---between base of proximal phalangeal bone of great toe and head of 2nd metatarsal bone.

There are the dorsal digital nerve of the deep peroneal nerve and the dorsal digital artery and vein in this area.

2. 12. 3 LR 3 Tàichōng 太衝

Skin---subcutaneous tissue---between tendons of long extensor muscle of great toe and long extensor muscle of toes---lateral side of short extensor muscle of great toe---1st dorsal interosseous muscle.

In the superficial layer, there are the venous network of the dorsum of the foot and the medial dorsal cutaneous nerve of the foot. In the deep layer, there are the deep peroneal nerve and the 1st dorsal metatarsal artery and vein.

2. 12. 4 LR 4 Zhōngfēng 中封

Skin---subcutaneous tissue---medial side of tendon of anterior tibial muscle---between talus and medial malleolus of tibia.

There are the branches of the medial dorsal cutaneous nerve of the foot, the medial anterior malleolar artery and the superficial dorsal vein of the foot in this area.

2. 12. 5 LR 5 Lígōu 蠡溝

Skin---subcutaneous tissue---medial surface of tibia.

There are the medial cutaneous branches of the leg from the saphenous nerve and the great saphenous vein in this area.

2. 12. 6 LR 6 Zhōngdū 中都

Skin---subcutaneous tissue---medial surface of tibia.

There are the medial cutaneous branches of the leg from the saphenous nerve and the great saphenous vein in this area.

2. 12. 7 LR 7 Xīguān 膝關

Skin---subcutaneous tissue---gastrocnemius muscle.

In the superficial layer, there are the medial cutaneous branches of the leg from the saphenous nerve and the tributaries of the great saphenous vein. In the deep layer, there are the popliteal artery and vein and the tibial nerve.

2. 12. 8 LR 8 Qūquán 曲泉

Skin---subcutaneous tissue---posterior border of sartorius muscle---posterior border of tendon of gracilis muscle---tendon of semimembranous muscle---medial head of gastrocnemius muscle.

In the superficial layer, there are the saphenous nerve and the great saphenous vein. In the deep layer, there are the branches or tributaries of the medial superior genicular artery and vein.

2. 12. 9 LR 9 Yīnbāo 陰包

Skin---subcutaneous tissue---between sartorius muscle and gracilis muscle---great adductor muscle.

In the superficial layer, there are the cutaneous branches of the obturator nerve and the tributaries of the great saphenous vein. In the deep layer, there are the muscular branches of the femoral nerve, the saphenous nerve and the femoral artery and vein.

2. 12. 10 LR 10 Zúwǔlǐ 足五裏

Skin---subcutaneous tissue---long adductor muscle---short adductor muscle---great adductor muscle.

In the superficial layer, there are the anterior cutaneous branches of the femoral nerve and the saphenous vein. In the deep layer, there are the anterior and posterior branches of the obturator nerve, the muscular branches of the deep femoral artery and vein, and the muscular branches of the medial femoral circumflex artery and vein.

2. 12. 11 LR 11 Yīnlián 陰廉

Skin---subcutaneous tissue---long adductor muscle---short adductor muscle---small adductor muscle.

In the superficial layer, there are the anterior cutaneous branches of the femoral nerve, the great saphenous vein and the superficial inguinal lymph nodes. In the deep layer, there are the anterior and posterior branches of the obturator nerve and the muscular branches of the medial femoral circumflex artery and vein.

2. 12. 12 LR 12 Jímài 急脈

Skin---subcutaneous tissue---pectineal muscle---lateral obturator muscle.

In the superficial layer, there are the anterior cutaneous branches of the femoral nerve, the great saphenous vein and the superficial inguinal lymph nodes. In the deep layer, there are the external pudendal artery and vein, the branches or tributaries of the medial femoral circumflex artery and vein, and the anterior branches of the obturator nerve.

2. 12. 13 LR 13 Zhāngmén 章門

Skin---subcutaneous tissue---external oblique muscle of abdomen---internal oblique muscle of abdomen---transverse muscle of abdomen.

In the superficial layer, there are the lateral cutaneous branches of the anterior branches of the 10th and 11th thoracic nerves and the tributaries of the superficial thoracoepigastric vein. In the deep layer, there are the 10th and 11th thoracic nerves and the branches or tributaries of the 10th and 11th posterior intercostal arteries and veins.

2. 12. 14 LR 14 Qīmén 期門

Skin---subcutaneous tissue---inferior border of greater pectoral muscle---external oblique muscle of abdomen---external intercostal muscle---internal intercostal muscle.

In the superficial layer, there are the lateral cutaneous branches of the 6th intercostal nerve and the tributaries of the thoracoepigastric vein. In the deep layer, there are the 6th intercostal nerve and the branches or tributaries of the 6th posterior intercostal artery and vein.

13. Points of the Du Meridian (Governor Vessel), DU (GV)

督脈穴

Dūmài Xué

2. 13. 1 DU 1 Chángqiáng 長強

Skin---subcutaneous tissue---anococcygeal ligament.

In the superficial layer, there are the posterior branches of the coccygeal nerve. In the deep layer, there are the anal nerve of the pudendal nerve and the anal artery and vein of the internal pudendal artery and vein.

2. 13. 2 DU 2 Yāoshū 腰俞

Skin---subcutaneous tissue---dorsal sacrococcgyeal ligament---sacral canal.

In the superficial layer, there are the posterior branches of the 5th sacral nerve. In the deep layer, there is the coccygeal plexus.

2. 13. 3 DU 3 Yāoyángguān 腰陽關

Skin---subcutaneous tissue---supraspinal ligament---interspinal ligament---interarcuate ligament.

In the superficial layer, there are the medial branches of the posterior branches of the 4th lumbar nerve and the accompanying artery and vein. In the deep layer, there are the external (posterior) vertebral venous plexus between the adjacent spinous processes, the branches of the posterior branches of the 4th lumbar nerve and the branches or tributaries of the dorsal branches of the 4th lumbar artery and vein.

2. 13. 4 DU 4 Mìngmén 命門

The layer structures of the needle insertion are the same as those in Yāoyángguān (DU 3).

In the superficial layer, there are the medial branches of the posterior branches of the 2nd lumbar nerve and the accompanying artery and vein. In the deep layer, there are the external (posterior) vertebral venous plexus between the adjacent spinous process, the branches of the posterior branches of the 2nd lumbar nerve and the branches or tributaries of the dorsal branches of the 2nd lumbar artery and vein.

2. 13. 5 DU 5 Xuánshū 懸樞

Skin---subcutaneous tissue---supraspinal ligament---interspinal ligament.

In the superficial layer, there are the medial branches of the posterior branches of the 1st lumbar nerve and the accompanying artery and vein. In the deep layer, there are the external (posterior) vertebral venous plexus between the adjacent spinous processes, the branches of the posterior branches of the 1st lumbar nerve and the branches or tributaries of the dorsal branches of the 1st lumbar artery and vein.

2. 13. 6 DU 6 Jǐzhōng 脊中

Skin---subcutaneous tissue---supraspinal ligament---interspinal ligament.

In the superficial layer, there are the medial cutaneous branches of the posterior branches of the 11th thoracic nerve and the accompanying artery and vein. In the deep layer, there are the external (posterior) vertebral venous plexus between the adjacent spinous processes, the branches of the posterior branches of the 11th thoracic nerve and the branches or tributaries of the dorsal branches of the 11th posterior intercostal artery and vein.

2. 13. 7 DU 7 Zhōngshū 中樞

The layer structures of the needle insertion are the same as those in Jǐzhōng (DU 6).

In the superficial layer, there are the medial cutaneous branches of the posterior branches of the 10th thoracic nerve and the accompanying artery and vein. In the deep layer, there are the external (posterior) vertebral venous plexus between the adjacent spinous processes, the branches of the posterior branches of the 10th thoracic nerve and the branches or tributaries of the dorsal branches of the 10th posterior intercostal artery and vein.

2. 13. 8 DU 8 Jīnsuō 筋縮

The layer structures of the needle insertion are the same as those in Jǐzhōng (DU 6).

In the superficial layer, there are the medial cutaneous branches of the posterior branches of the 9th thoracic nerve and the accompanying artery and vein. In the deep layer, there are the external (posterior) vertebral venous plexus between the adjacent spinous processes, the branches of the posterior branches of the 9th thoracic nerve and the branches or tributaries of the dorsal branches of the 9th posterior intercostal artery and vein.

2. 13. 9 DU 9 Zhìyáng 至陽

The layer structures of the needle insertion are the same as those in Jǐzhōng (Du 6).

In the superficial layer, there are the medial cutaneous branches of the posterior branches of the 7th thoracic nerve and the accompanying artery and vein. In the deep layer, there are the external (posterior) vertebral venous plexus between the adjacent spinous processes, the branches of the posterior branches of the 7th thoracic nerve and the branches or tributaries of the dorsal branches of the 7th posterior intercostal artery and vein.

2. 13. 10 DU 10 Língtái 靈台

The layer structures of the needle insertion are the same as those in Jǐzhōng (DU 6).

In the superficial layer, there are the medial cutaneous branches of the posterior branches of the 6th thoracic nerve and the accompanying artery and vein. In the deep layer, there are the external (posterior) vertebral venous plexus between the adjacent spinous processes, the branches of the posterior branches of the 6th thoracic nerve and the branches or tributaries of the dorsal branches of the 6th posterior intercostal artery and vein.

2. 13. 11 DU 11 **Shéndào** 神道

The layer structures of the needle insertion are the same as those in Jǐzhōng (DU 6).

In the superficial layer, there are the medial cutaneous branches of the posterior branches of the 5th thoracic nerve and the accompanying artery and vein. In the deep layer, there are the external (posterior) vertebral venous plexus between the adjacent spinous processes, the branches of the posterior branches of the 5th thoracic nerve and the branches or tributaries of the dorsal branches of the 5th posterior intercostal artery and vein.

2. 13. 12 DU 12 **Shēnzhù** 身柱

The layer structures of the needle insertion are the same as those in Jǐzhōng (DU 6).

In the superficial layer, there are the medial cutaneous branches of the posterior branches of the 3rd thoracic nerve and the accompanying artery and vein. In the deep layer, there are the external (posterior) vertebral venous plexus between the adjacent spinous processes, the branches of the posterior branches of the 3rd thoracic nerve and the branches or tributaries of the dorsal branches of the 3rd posterior intercostal artery and vein.

2. 13. 13 DU 13 **Táodào** 陶道

The layer structures of the needle insertion are the same as those in Jǐzhōng (DU 6).

In the superficial layer, there are the medial cutaneous branches of the posterior branches of the 1st thoracic nerve and the accompanying artery and vein. In the deep layer, there are the external (posterior) vertebral venous plexus between the adjacent spinous processes, the branches of the posterior branches of the 1st thoracic nerve and the branches or tributaries of the dorsal branches of the 1st posterior intercostal artery and vein.

2. 13. 14 DU 14 **Dàzhuī** 大椎

The layer structures of the needle insertion are the same as those in Jǐzhōng (DU 6).

In the superficial layer, there are the medial branches of the posterior branches of the 8th cervical nerve and the subcutaneous venous plexus between the adjacent spinous processes. In the deep layer, there are the external (posterior) vertebral venous plexus between the adjacent spinous processes and the branches of the posterior branches of the 7th cervical nerve.

2. 13. 15 DU 15 **Yǎmén** 啞門

Skin---subcutaneous tissue---between left and right trapezius muscles---nuchal ligament (between left and right splenius muscles of head)---between left and right semispinal muscles of head.

In the superficial layer, there are the 3rd occipital nerve and the subcutaneous vein. In the deep layer, there are the branches of the posterior branches of the 2nd and 3rd cervical nerves, the external (posterior) vertebral venous plexus and the branches or tributaries of the occipital artery and vein.

2. 13. 16 DU 16 **Fēngfǔ** 風府

Skin---subcutaneous tissue---between left and right tendons of trapezius muscles---nuchal ligament (between left and right semispinal muscles of head)---between left and right larger and lesser posterior straight muscles of head.

In the superficial layer, there are the branches of the greater occipital nerve and the 3rd occipital nerve and the branches or tributaries of the occipital artery and vein. In the deep layer, there are the branches of the suboccipital nerve.

2. 13. 17 DU 17 **Nǎohù** 腦户

Skin---subcutaneous tissue---between occipital belly of left and right occipitofrontal muscles ---subaponeurotic loose tissue.

There are the branches of the greater occipital nerve and the branches or tributaries of the occipital artery and vein in this area.

2. 13. 18 DU 18 Qiángjiān 强間

Skin---subcutaneous tissue---epicranial aponeurosis---subaponeurotic loose tissue.

There are the greater occipital nerve and anastomotic network of the left and right occipital arteries and veins in this area.

2. 13. 19 DU 19 Hòudǐng 後頂

Skin---subcutaneous tissue---epicranial aponeurosis---subaponeurotic loose tissue.

There are the great occipital nerve and the anastomotic network of the occipital arteries and veins with the superficial temporal arteries and veins in this area.

2. 13. 20 DU 20 Bǎihuì 百會

Skin---subcutaneous tissue---epicranial aponeurosis---subaponeurotic loose tissue.

There are the branches of the greater occipital and frontal nerves, and the anastomotic network of the left and right superficial temporal arteries and veins with the left and right occipital arteries and veins in this area.

2. 13. 21 DU 21 Qiándǐng 前頂

Skin---subcutaneous tissue---epicranial aponeurosis---subaponeurotic loose tissue.

There are the frontal nerve, the anastomotic network of the left and right superficial temporal arteries and veins with the left and right frontal arteries and veins in this area.

2. 13. 22 DU 22 Xìnhuì 顖會

Skin---subcutaneous tissue---epicranial aponeurosis---subaponeurotic loose tissue.

There are the frontal nerve and the anastomotic network of the left and right superficial temporal arteries and veins with the left and right frontal arteries and veins in this area.

2. 13. 23 DU 23 Shàngxīng 上星

Skin---subcutaneous tissue---epicranial aponeurosis---subaponeurotic loose tissue.

There are the branches of the frontal nerve and the branches or tributaries of the frontal artery and vein in this area.

2. 13. 24 DU 24 Shéntíng 神庭

Skin---subcutaneous tissue---between frontal belly of left and right occipitofrontal muscles ---subaponeurotic loose tissue.

There are the supratrochlear nerve from the frontal nerve and the branches or tributaries of the frontal artery and vein in this area.

2. 13. 25 DU 25 Sùliáo 素髎

Skin---subcutaneous tissue---septal cartilage of nose and lateral nasal cartilage. There are the lateral nasal branches of the anterior ethmoidal nerve and the dorsal nasal branches of the facial artery and vein in this area.

2. 13. 26 DU 26 Shuǐgōu 水溝

Skin---subcutaneous tissue---orbicular muscle of mouth.

There are the branches of the infraorbital nerve and the superior labial artery and vein in this area.

2. 13. 27 DU 27 Duìduān 兑端

Same as Shuǐgōu (DU 26).

2. 13. 28 DU 28 Yínjiāo 齦交

Transitional border of superior labial frenulum and upper gum---between deep surface of orbicular muscle of mouth and alveolar arch of maxillary bone.

There are the superior labial branches of the maxillary nerve, the infraorbital plexus formed by the branches of the infraorbital and facial nerves, and the superior labial artery and vein in this area.

14. Points of the Ren Meridian (Conception Vessel), RN (CA)

任脈穴

Rènmài Xué

2. 14. 1 RN 1 Huìyīn 會陰

Skin---subcutaneous tissue---central tendon of perineum.

In the superficial layer, there are the perineal branches of the posterior femoral cutaneous nerve and the perineal nervous branches of the pudendal nerve. In the deep layer, there are the branches of the pudendal nerve and the branches or tributaries of the internal pudendal artery and vein.

2. 14. 2 RN 2 Qūgǔ 曲骨

Skin---subcutaneous tissue---linea alba---transverse fascia---extraperitoneal fat tissue---parietal peritoneum.

In the superficial layer, there are the anterior cutaneous branches of the iliohypogastric nerve and the tributaries of the superficial epigastric vein. In the deep layer, there are the branches of the iliohypogastric nerve.

2. 14. 3 RN 3 Zhōngjí 中極

Skin---subcutaneous tissue---linea alba---transverse fascia---extraperitoneal fat tissue---parietal peritoneum.

In the superficial layer, there are the anterior cutaneous branches of the iliohypogastric nerve and the branches or tributaries of the superficial epigastric artery and vein. In the deep layer, there are the branches of the iliohypogastric nerve.

2. 14. 4 RN 4 Guānyuán 關元

Skin---subcutaneous tissue---linea alba---transverse fascia---extraperitoneal fat tissue---parietal peritoneum.

In the superficial layer, there are the anterior cutaneous branches of the anterior branch of the 12th thoracic nerve and the branches or tributaries of the superficial epigastric artery and vein. In the deep layer, there are the branches of the anterior branch of the 12th thoracic nerve.

2. 14. 5 RN 5 Shímén 石門

Skin---subcutaneous tissue---linea alba---transverse fascia---extraperitoneal fat tissue---parietal peritoneum.

In the superficial layer, there are the anterior cutaneous branches of the anterior branches of the 11th thoracic nerve and the tributaries of the superficial epigastric vein. In the deep layer, there are the branches of the anterior branches of the 11th thoracic nerve.

2. 14. 6 RN 6 Qìhǎi 氣海

Skin---subcutaneous tissue---linea alba---transverse fascia---extraperitoneal fat tissue---parietal peritoneum.

In the superficial layer, there are the anterior cutaneous branches of the anterior branch of the 11th thoracic nerve and the periumbilical venous network. In the deep layer, there are the branches of the anterior branch of the 11th thoracic nerve.

2. 14. 7 RN 7 Yīnjiāo 陰交

Skin---subcutaneous tissue---linea alba---transverse fascia---extraperitoneal fat tissue---parietal peritoneum.

In the superficial layer, there are the anterior cutaneous branches of the anterior branch of the 11th thoracic nerve and the periumbilical venous network. In the deep layer, there are the branches of the anterior branch of the 11th thoracic nerve.

2. 14. 8 RN 8 Shénquè 神闕

Skin---connective tissue---parietal peritoneum.

In the superficial layer, there are the anterior cutaneous branches of the anterior branch of the 10th thoracic nerve and the periumbilical venous network on the abdominal wall. In the deep layer, there are the branches of the anterior branch of the 10th thoracic nerve.

2. 14. 9 RN 9 Shuǐfēn 水分

Skin---subcutaneous tissue---linea alba---transverse fascia---extraperitoneal fat tissue---parietal peritoneum.

In the superficial layer, there are the anterior cutaneous branches of the anterior branch of the 9th thoracic nerve and the tributaries of the superficial epigastric vein. In the deep layer, there are the branches of the anterior branch of the 9th thoracic nerve.

2. 14. 10 RN 10 Xiàwǎn 下脘

Skin---subcutaneous tissue---linea alba---transverse fascia---extraperitoneal fat tissue---parietal peritoneum.

In the superficial layer, there are the anterior cutaneous branches of the anterior branch of the 9th thoracic nerve and the tributaries of the superficial epigastric vein. In the deep layer, there are the branches of the anterior branch of the 9th thoracic nerve.

2. 14. 11 RN 11 Jiànlǐ 建裏

Skin---subcutaneous tissue---linea alba---transverse fascia---extraperitoneal fat tissue---parietal peritoneum.

In the superficial layer, there are the anterior cutaneous branches of the anterior branch of the 8th thoracic nerve and the tributaries of the superficial epigastric vein. In the deep layer, there are the branches of the anterior branch of the 8th thoracic nerve.

2. 14. 12 RN 12 Zhōngwǎn 中脘

Skin---subcutaneous tissue---linea alba---transverse fascia---extraperitoneal fat tissue---parietal peritoneum.

In the superficial layer, there are the anterior cutaneous branches of the anterior branch of the 8th thoracic nerve and the tributaries of the superficial epigastric vein. In the deep layer, there are the branches of the anterior branch of the 8th thoracic nerve.

2. 14. 13 RN 13 Shàngwǎn 上脘

Skin---subcutaneous tissue---linea alba---transverse fascia---extraperitoneal fat tissue---parietal peritoneum.

In the superficial layer, there are the anterior cutaneous branches of the anterior branch of the 7th thoracic nerve and the tributaries of the superficial epigastric vein. In the deep layer, there are the branches of the anterior branch of the 7th thoracic nerve.

2. 14. 14 RN 14 Jùquè 巨闕

Skin---subcutaneous tissue---linea alba---transverse fascia---extraperitoneal fat tissue---parietal peritoneum.

In the superficial layer, there are the anterior cutaneous branches of the anterior branch of the 7th thoracic nerve and the superficial epigastric vein. In the deep layer, there are the branches of the anterior branch of the 7th thoracic nerve.

2. 14. 15 RN 15 Jiūwěi 鳩尾

Skin---subcutaneous tissue---linea alba---transverse fascia---extraperitoneal fat tissue---parietal peritoneum.

In the superficial layer, there are the anterior cutaneous branches of the anterior branch of the 7th thoracic nerve. In the deep layer, there are the branches of the anterior branch of the 7th thoracic nerve.

2. 14. 16 RN 16 Zhōngtíng 中庭

Skin---subcutaneous tissue---radiate sternocostal ligament and costoxiphoid ligament---xiphosternal synchondrosis.

There are the anterior cutaneous branches of the 6th intercostal nerve and the perforating branches of the internal thoracic artery and vein in this area.

2. 14. 17 RN 17 Dánzhōng 膻中

Skin---subcutaneous tissue---sternal body.

There are the anterior cutaneous branches of the 4th intercostal nerve and the perforating branches of the internal thoracic artery and vein in this area.

2. 14. 18 RN 18 Yùtáng 玉堂

Skin---subcutaneous tissue---sternal body.

There are the anterior cutaneous branches of the 3rd intercostal nerve and the perforating branches of the internal thoracic artery and vein in this area.

2. 14. 19 RN 19 Zǐgōng 紫宫

Skin---subcutaneous tissue---origin of greater pectoral muscle---sternal body.

There are the anterior cutaneous branches of the 2nd intercostal nerve and the perforating branches of the internal thoracic artery and vein in this area.

2. 14. 20 RN 20 Huágài 華蓋

Skin---subcutaneous tissue---origin of greater pectoral muscle---between manubrium of sternum and sternal body (sternal angle).

There are the anterior cutaneous branches of the 1st intercostal nerve and the perforating branches of the internal thoracic artery and vein in this area.

2. 14. 21 RN 21 Xuánjī 璇璣

Skin---subcutaneous tissue---origin of greater pectoral muscle---manubrium of sternum.

There are the medial supraclavicular nerve and the perforating branches of the internal thoracic artery and vein in this area.

2. 14. 22 RN 22 Tiāntū 天突

Skin---subcutaneous tissue---between two sternal heads of sternocleidomastoid muscles ---superior side of suprasternal notch---between bilateral sternothyroid muscles---anterior space of trachea.

In the superficial layer, there are the medial supraclavicular nerve, the platysma and the jugular arch of veins in the subcutaneous tissues. In the deep layer, there are the important structures, including the brachiocephalic trunk, the left common carotid artery, the aortic arch and the brachiocephalic vein.

2. 14. 23 RN 23 Liánquán 廉泉

Skin---subcutaneous tissue (including platysma)---between bilateral anterior bellies of digastric muscles---mylohyoid muscle---geniohyoid muscle---genioglossus muscle.

In the superficial layer, there are the cervical branches of the facial nerve and the branches of the superior branch of the transverse nerve of the neck. In the deep layer, there are the branches or tributaries of the lingual artery and vein and the branches of the hypoglossal and mylohyoid nerves.

2. 14. 24 RN 24 Chéngjiāng 承漿

Skin---subcutaneous tissue---orbicular muscle of mouth---depressor muscle of lower lip ---mental muscle.

There are the mental nerve of the inferior alveolar nerve and the mental artery and vein in this area.

EXTRA POINTS, EX
經外穴
JĪNGWÀI XUÈ

3. 1 Points of the Head and Neck, EX-HN
頭頸部穴
Tóujǐngbù Xué

3. 1. 1 EX-HN 1 Sìshéncōng 四神聰

Skin---subcutaneous tissue---epicranial aponeurosis---subaponeurotic loose connective tissue.

There are the network anastomosed by the occipital artery and vein, the parietal branches of the superficial temporal artery and vein with the supraorbital artery and vein, and the branches of the greater occipital, auriculotemporal and supraorbital nerves in this area.

3. 1. 2 EX-HN 2 Dāngyáng 當陽

Skin---subcutaneous tissue---frontal belly of occipitofrontal muscle or epicranial aponeurosis---subaponeurotic loose connective tissue.

There are the supraorbital nerve and the branches or tributaries of the supraorbital artery and vein in this area.

3. 1. 3 EX-HN 3 Yìntáng 印堂

Skin---subcutaneous tissue---procerus muscle.

There are the supratrochlear branch of the frontal nerve and the frontal artery from the ophthalmic artery and the accompanving vein in this area.

3. 1. 4 EX-HN 4 Yúyāo 魚腰

Skin---subcutaneous tissue---orbicular muscle of eye---frontal belly of occipitofrontal muscle.

There are the lateral branches of the supraorbital nerve, the branches of the facial nerve and the lateral branches of the supraorbital artery and vein in this area.

3. 1. 5 EX-HN 5 Tàiyáng 太陽

Skin---subcutaneous tissue---orbicular muscle of eye---temporal fascia---temporal muscle.

There are the zygomaticofacial branch of the zygomatic nerve, the temporal and zygomatic branches of the facial nerve, the temporal nerve of the mandibular nerve and the branches or tributaries of the superficial temporal artery and vein in this area.

3. 1. 6 EX-HN 6 Ěrjiān 耳尖

Skin---subcutaneous tissue---auricular cartilage.

There are the anterior auricular branches of the superficial temporal artery and vein, the posterior auricular branches of the posterior auricular artery and vein, the anterior auricular branches of the auriculotemporal nerve, the posterior auricular branches of the lesser occipital nerve, and the auricular branches of the facial nerve in this area.

3. 1. 7 EX-HN 7 Qiúhòu 球後

Skin---subcutaneous tissue---orbicular muscle of eye---adipose body of orbit---between inferior oblique muscle and inferior wall of orbit.

In the superficial layer, there are the branches of the infraorbital and facial nerves and the branches or tributaries of the infraorbital artery and vein. In the deep layer, there are the inferior branches of the oculomotor nerve, the branches or tributaries of the ophthalmic artery and vein, and the infraorbital artery and vein.

3. 1. 8 EX-HN 8 Shàngyíngxiāng 上迎香

Skin---subcutaneous tissue---levator muscle of upper lip and nasal ala.

There are the branches of the infraorbital and infratrochlear nerves, the buccal branches of the facial nerve, and the angular artery and vein in this area.

3. 1. 9 EX-HN 9 Nèiyíngxiāng 内迎香

Nasal mucosa---submucous loose connective tissue.

There are the arteriovenous network of the dorsal nasal branches of the facial artery and vein and the lateral nasal branches of the anterior ethmoidal nerve in this area.

3. 1. 10 EX-HN 10 Jùquán 聚泉

Tongue mucosa---submucous loose connective tissue---lingual muscle.

There are the lingual nerve from the mandibular nerve, the hypoglossal nerve, the nervous fibers of the tympanic cord, and the arteriovenous network of the lingual artery and vein in this area.

3. 1. 11 EX-HN 11 Hǎiqúan 海泉

Mucosa---submucous tissue---lingual muscle.

There are the lingual nerve from the mandibular nerve, the hypoglossal nerve, the nervous fibres of the tympanic cord from the facial nerve, the deep lingual artery from the lingual artery, and the deep lingual veins to the lingual vein in this area.

3. 1. 12 EX-HN 12 Jīnjīn 金津

Mucosa---submucous tissue---genioglossus muscle.

There are the gnathic nerve from the mandibular nerve, the hypoglossal nerve, the nervous fibres of the tympanic cord from the facial nerve, the deep lingual artery of the lingual artery and the deep lingual veins to the lingual vein in this area.

3. 1. 13 EX-HN 13 Yùyè 玉液

Same as Jīnjīn (EX-HN 12).

3. 1. 14 EX-HN 14 Yìmíng 翳明

Skin---subcutaneous tissue---sternocleidomastoid muscle---splenius muscle of head---longest muscle of head.

In the superficial layer, there are the branches of the great auricular nerve. In the deep layer, there are the deep cervical artery and vein.

3. 1. 15 EX-HN 15 Jǐngbǎiláo 頸百勞

Skin---subcutaneous tissue---trapezius muscle---superior posterior serratus muscle---splenius muscles of head and neck---semispinal muscle of head---multifidus muscle.

In the superficial layer, there are the cutaneous branches of the posterior branches of the 4th and 5th cervical nerves. In the deep layer, there are the branches of the posterior branches of the 4th and 5th cervical nerve.

3. 2 Points of the Chest and Abdomen, EX-CA

胸腹部穴

Xiōngfùbù Xué

3. 2. 1 EX-CA 1 Zǐgōng 子宫

Skin---subcutaneous tissue---aponeurosis of external oblique muscle of abdomen---internal oblique muscle of abdomen---transverse muscle of abdomen---transverse fascia of abdomen.

In the superficial layer, there are the lateral cutaneous branches of the iliohypogastric nerve and the superficial epigastric vein. In the deep layer, there are the branches of the iliohypogastric nerve and the branches or tributaries of the inferior epigastric artery and vein.

3. 3 Points of the Back, EX-B

背部穴

Bèibù Xué

3. 3. 1 EX-B 1 Dìngchuǎn 定喘

Skin---subcutaneous tissue---trapezius muscle---rhomboid muscle---superior posterior serratus muscle---splenius muscle of neck---erector spinal muscle.

In the superficial layer, there are the medial cutaneous branches of the posterior branch of the 8th cervical nerve. In the deep layer, there are the branches or tributaries of the deep cervical artery and vein and the transverse cervical artery and vein and the muscular branches of the posterior branches of the 8th cervical and 1st thoracic nerves.

3. 3. 2 EX-B 2 Jiájǐ 夾脊

The related muscles, blood vessels and nerves are not totally alike because the location of each point is different. The layer structures are usually: Skin---subcutaneous tissue---superficial muscles (trapezius muscle, latissimus muscle of back, rhomboid muscle, superior posterior serratus muscle, inferior posterior serratus muscle)---deep muscles (erector spinal muscle, transversospinal muscle).

In the superficial layer, there are the medial cutaneous branches of the posterior branches of the 1st thoracic nerve to the 5th lumbar nerve and the accompanying arteries and veins. In the deep layer, there are the muscular branches of the posterior branches of the 1st thoracic nerve to the 5th lumbar nerve, the branches or tributaries of the dorsal branches of the posterior intercostal arteries and veins or lumbar arteries and veins respectively.

3. 3. 3 EX-B 3 Wèiwǎnxiàshū 胃脘下俞

Skin---subcutaneous tissue---trapezius muscle---latissimus muscle of back---erector spinal muscle.

In the superficial layer, there are the cutaneous branches of the posterior branch of the 8th thoracic nerve and the accompanying artery and vein. In the deep layer, there are the muscular branches of the posterior branch of the 8th thoracic nerve and the branches or tributaries of the dorsal branches of the 8th posterior intercostal artery and vein.

3. 3. 4 EX-B 4 Pǐgēn 痞根

Skin---subcutaneous tissue---latissimus muscle of back---inferior posterior serratus muscle ---iliocostal muscle.

In the superficial layer, there are the lateral cutaneous branches of the posterior branch of the 12th thoracic nerve and the accompanying artery and vein. In the deep layer, there are the muscular branches of the posterior branch of the 12th thoracic nerve.

3. 3. 5 EX-B 5 Xiajíshū 下極俞

Skin---subcutaneous tissue---supraspinal ligament---interspinal ligament.

In the superficial layer, there are the medial branches of the posterior branch of the fourth lumbar nerve and the accompanying artery and vein. In the deep layer, there are the external (posterior) vertebral venous plexus of the spinous process, the posterior branch of the 4th lumbar nerve and the branch of the dorsal branch of the 4th lumbar artery and vein.

3. 3. 6 EX-B 6 Yāoyí 腰宜

Skin---subcutaneous tissue---superficial layer of thoracolumbar fascia---erector spinal muscle (or medial and superior border of greatest gluteal muscle).

In the superficial layer, there is the superior clunial nerve. In the deep layer, there are the muscular branches of the posterior branch of the 4th lumbar nerve and the branches or tributaries of the dorsal branches of the 4th lumbar artery and vein.

3. 3. 7 EX-B 7 Yāoyǎn 腰眼

Skin---subcutaneous tissue---superficial layer of thoracolumbar fascia and aponeurosis of latissimus muscle of back---iliocostal muscle---deep layer of thoracolumbar fascia---quadrate muscle of loins.

In the superficial layer, there are the superior clunial nerve and the cutaneous branches of the posterior branch of the 4th lumbar nerve. In the deep layer, there are the muscular branches of the posterior branch of the 4th lumbar nerve and the branches or tributaries of the 4th lumbar artery and vein.

3. 3. 8 EX-B 8 Shíqīzhūi 十七椎

Skin---subcutaneous tissue---supraspinal ligament---interspinal ligament.

In the superficial layer, there are the cutaneous branches of the posterior branch of the 5th lumbar nerve and the accompanying artery and vein. In the deep layer, there are the branches of the posterior branch of the 5th lumbar nerve and the external (posterior) vertebral venous plexus between the adjacent spinous processes.

3. 3. 9 EX-B 9 Yāoqí 腰奇

Skin---subcutaneous tissue---supraspinal ligament.

There are the branches of the posterior branches of the 2nd and 3rd sacral nerves and the accompanying artery and vein in this area.

3. 4. Points of the Upper Extremities, EX-UE
上肢穴
Shàngzhī Xué

3. 4. 1 EX-UE 1 Zhǒujiān 肘尖

Skin---subcutaneous tissue---subcutaneous bursa of olecranon---tendon of brachial triceps muscle.

There are the posterior cutaneous nerve of the forearm and the arteriovenous network around the elbow joint in this area.

3. 4. 2 EX-UE 2 Èrbái 二白

The medial point: Skin---subcutaneous tissue---between tendons of long palmar muscle and radial flexor muscle of wrist---superficial digital flexor muscle---median nerve---long flexor muscle of thumb---interosseous membrane of forearm.

In the superficial layer, there are the lateral cutaneous nerve of the forearm and the tributaries of the median brachial vein. In the deep layer, there are the median nerve and the median artery.

The lateral point: Skin---subcutaneous tissue---between radial flexor muscle of wrist and tendon of brachioradial muscle---superficial flexor muscle of fingers---long flexor muscle of thumb.

In the superficial layer, there are the lateral cutaneous nerve of the forearm and the tributaries of the cephalic vein. In the deep layer, there are the radial artery and vein.

3. 4. 3 EX-UE 3 Zhōngqúan 中泉

Skin---subcutaneous tissue---between tendons of extensor muscle and short radial extensor muscle of wrist.

There are posterior cutaneous nerve of the forearm, the branches of the superficial branch of the radial nerve, the dorsal venous network of the hand and the branches of the dorsal carpal branch of the radial artery in this area.

3. 4. 4 EX-UE 4 Zhōngkúi 中魁

Skin---subcutaneous tissue---dorsal digital aponeurosis.

There is the dorsal digital nerve in this area. Its radial branch originates from the radial nerve, and its ulnar branch originates from the ulnar nerve. There are the dorsal digital artery from the dorsal palmar artery and the dorsal digital vein to the dorsal venous network of the palm.

3. 4. 5 EX-UE 5 Dàgǔkōng 大骨空

Skin---subcutaneous tissue---tendon of long extensor muscle of thumb.

There are the dorsal digital nerve of the radial nerve and the dorsal digital artery and vein in this area.

3. 4. 6 EX-UE 6 Xiǎogǔkōng 小骨空

Skin---subcutaneous tissue---dorsal digital aponeurosis.

There are the branches or tributaries of the dorsal digital artery and vein and the branches of the dorsal digital nerve of the ulnar nerve in this area.

3. 4. 7 EX-UE 7 Yāotòngdiǎn 腰痛點

First point: Skin---subcutaneous tissue---tendons of digital extensor muscle and short radial extensor muscle of wrist.

Another point: Skin---subcutaneous tissue---between tendons of extensor muscle of little finger and extensor muscle of the 4th finger.

There are the dorsal venous network of the hand, the dorsal palmar artery, the superficial branches of the radial nerve and the dorsal branches of the hand from the ulnar nerve in the area of these two points.

3. 4. 8 EX-UE 8 Wàiláogōng 外勞宮

Skin---subcutaneous tissue---2nd dorsal interosseous muscle---1st palmar interosseous muscle.

There are the dorsal digital nerve from the superficial branch of the radial nerve, the dorsal venous network of the hand, and the dorsal palmar artery in this area.

3. 4. 9 EX-UE 9 Bāxié 八邪

Skin---subcutaneous tissue---dorsal interosseous muscle---palmar interosseous muscle---lumbrical muscle.

In the superficial layer, there are the dorsal metacarpal artery and vein or the dorsal digital artery and vein and the dorsal digital nerve. In the deep layer, there are the common digital palmar artery and vein or the proper palmar digital artery and vein and the proper palmar digital nerve.

3. 4. 10 EX-UE 10 Sìfèng 四縫

Skin---subcutaneous tissue---tendon of deep digital flexor muscle.

The blood vessels in the area of each point are the branches or tributaries of the proper palmar digital artery and vein and the subcutaneous digital vein. The nerve in the area of the point between the thumb and index or between the index and middle fingers is the proper palmar digital nerve from the median nerve; between the middle and ring fingers is the proper palmar digital nerve from the median nerve for the radial side and from the ulnar nerve for the ulnar side; between the index and little fingers is the proper palmar digital nerve from the ulnar nerve.

3. 4. 11 EX-UE 11 Shíxuān 十宣

Skin---subcutaneous tissue.

The nerves innervating the areas of the points on the thumb, index and middle finger are from the median nerve; on the ring finger is from both the median and ulnar nerves; on the little finger is from the ulnar nerve.

3. 5 Points of the Lower Extremities, EX-LE
下肢穴
Xiàzhī Xué

3. 5. 1 EX-LE 1 Kuāngǔ 髖骨

Kuāngǔ (EX-LE 1) on the lateral side: Skin---subcutaneous tissue---lateral muscle of thigh.

In the superficial layer, there are the anterior cutaneous branches of the femoral nerve and the lateral cutaneous nerve of the thigh. In the deep layer, there are the branches or tributaries of the descending branches of the lateral circumflex femoral artery and vein.

Kuāngǔ (EX-LE 1) on the medial side: Skin---subcutaneous tissue---medial of thigh.

In the superficial layer, there are the anterior cutaneous branches of the femoral nerve. In the deep layer, there are the muscular branches of the deep femoral artery and vein.

3. 5. 2 EX-LE 2 Hèdǐng 鶴頂

Skin---subcutaneous tissue---tendon of quadriceps muscle of thigh.

In the superficial layer, there are the anterior cutaneous branches of the femoral nerve and the tributaries of the great saphenous vein. In the deep layer, there is the arteriovenous network of the knee joint.

3. 5. 3 EX-LE 3 Bǎichóngwō 百蟲窩

Skin---subcutaneous tissue---medial intermuscle of thigh.

In the superficial layer, there are the anterior cutaneous branch of the femoral nerve and great saphenous vein. In the deep layer, there are the muscular branch of the femoral artery and vein and the femoral nerve.

3. 5. 4 EX-LE 4 Nèixīyǎn 内膝眼

Skin---subcutaneous tissue---between patellar ligament and medial patellar retinaculum ---articular capsule of knee joint and alar folds.

In the superficial layer, there are the infrapatellar branches of the saphenous nerve and the anterior cutaneous branches of the femoral nerve. In the deep layer, there is the arteriovenous network of the knee joint.

3. 5. 5 EX-LE 5 Xīyǎn 膝眼

The medial point of Xīyǎn (EX-LE 5) is also called Nèixīyǎn (EX-LE 4). For its layer anatomy, refer to Nèixīyǎn (EX-LE 4). The lateral point of Xīyǎn (EX-LE 5) is exactly the Dúbí (ST 35) of the Stomach Meridian of Foot-Yangming. For its layer anatomy, refer to Dúbí (ST 35).

3. 5. 6 EX-LE 6 Dǎnnáng 膽囊

Skin---subcutaneous tissue---long peroneal muscle.

In the superficial layer, there is the lateral sural cutaneous nerve. In the deep layer, there are the superficial peroneal nerve, the deep peroneal nerve and the anterior tibial artery and vein.

3. 5. 7 EX-LE 7 Lánwěi 闌尾

Skin---subcutaneous tissue---anterior tibial muscle---interosseous membrane of leg---posterior tibial muscle.

In the superficial layer, there are the lateral sural cutaneous nerve and the superficial veins. In the deep layer, there are the deep peroneal nerve and the anterior tibial artery and vein.

3. 5. 8 EX-LE 8 Nèihuáijiān 内踝尖

Skin---subcutaneous tissue---medial malleolus.

There are the branches of the medial cutaneous branch of the leg from the saphenous nerve, the medial melleolar network of the anterior tibial artery, the branches of the medial anterior malleolar artery and the medial malleolar branches of the posterior tibial artery in this area.

3. 5. 9 EX-LE 9 Wàihuáijiān 外踝尖

Skin---subcutaneous tissue---lateral malleolus.

There are the lateral malleolar network of the anterior tibial artery, the lateral malleolar branches of the peroneal artery, the branches of the sural nerve and the superficial peroneal nerve in this area.

3. 5. 10 EX-LE 10 Bāfēng 八風

The layer anatomy of Bāfēng (EX-LE 10) between the great and 2nd toes is the same as that in Xíngjiān (LR 2). The layer anatomy of Bāfēng (EX-LE 10) between the 2nd and 3rd toes is the same as that in Nèitíng (ST 44). The layer anatomy of Bāfēng (EX-LE 10) between the 4th and little toes is the same as that in Xiaxi (GB 43). The layer anatomy of Bāfēng (EX-LE 10) between the 3rd and 4th toes is: skin---subcutaneous tissue---between tendons of long and short extensor muscles of 3rd and 4th toes---between heads of 3rd and 4th metatarsal bones.

In the superficial layer, there are the dorsal digital nerve of the intermediate dorsal cutaneous nerve of the foot and the superficial venous network of the foot. In the deep layer, there are the dorsal digital artery from the dorsal metatarsal artery, and the dorsal digital veins to the dorsal metatarsal vein.

3. 5. 11 EX-LE 11 Dúyīn 獨陰

Skin---subcutaneous tissue---tendons of short and long flexor muscles of toes.

There are the proper digital plantar nerve and the branches or tributaries of the proper digital plantar artery and vein in this area.

3. 5. 12 EX-LE 12 Qìduān 氣端

Skin---subcutaneous tissue.

Innervation: The point on the great and 2nd toes is innervated by the dorsal digital nerves from the superficial peroneal and deep peroneal nerves, and the proper digital plantar nerve from the tibial nerve. The point on the 3rd and 4th toes is innervated by the dorsal digital nerve from the superficial peroneal nerve and the proper digital plantar nerve from the tibial nerve. The point on the little toe is innervated by the dorsal digital nerve from the sural nerve and from the superficial peroneal nerve, and the proper digital plantar nerve from the tibial nerve.

Vasculature: The points are supplied by the proper digital plantar artery from the medial and lateral plantar arteries of the foot and the dorsal digital artery from the dorsal artery of the foot.

APPENDICES

Appendices

1. Bibliography

Abbreviation Full Title

Bei Ji (備急) *Moxibustion for Emergencies* 備急灸法

Bian Lan (便覽) *Guide to Acupoints and Acupuncture Therapeutics* 針灸孔穴及其療法便覽

Ci Ding (刺疔) *Simple Acupuncture Method for Boils* 刺疔捷法

Da Cheng (大成) *A Great Compendium of Acupuncture and Moxibustion* 針灸大成

Da Quan (大全) *A Complete Work of Acupuncture and Moxibustion* 針灸大全

Fang An (方案) *The Standard Project of Acupoints* 穴位標準化方案

Fa Hui (發揮) *An Elaboration of the Fourteen Meridians* 十四經發揮

Feng Yuan (逢源) *The Origin of Acupuncture and Moxibustion* 針灸逢源

Gai Lun (概論) *An Outline of Acupoints* 腧穴學概論

Gang Mu (綱目) *An Outline of Medicine* 醫學綱目

Hui Bian (匯編) *An Expository Manual of Extra Acupoints* 經外奇穴匯編

Ji Cheng (集成) *Mian Xue Tang Compendium of Acupuncture and Moxibustion* 勉學堂針灸集成

Jia Yi (甲乙) *A-B Classic of Acupuncture and Moxibustion* 針灸甲乙經

Jian Bian (簡編) *Concise Book of Acupuncture and Moxibustion* 針灸學簡編

Jin Jian (金鑒) *Gold Mirror of Orthodox Medical Lineage* 醫宗金鑒

Ju Ying (聚英) *Essentials of Acupuncture and Moxibustion* 針灸聚英

Ling Shu (靈樞) *Miraculous Pivot* 靈樞經

Liu Ji (六集) *Six Collections of Acupuncture Prescriptions* 針方六集

Mai Jing (脈經) *The Classic of Sphygmology* 脈經

Mi Zhi (秘旨) *A Complete Work of Infantile Massotherapy* 小兒推拿方脈活嬰秘旨全書

Nan Jing (難經) *The Classic of Questions* 難經

Qi Xiao (奇效) *Prescriptions of Wonderful Efficacy* 奇效良方

Qian Jin (千金) *Essential Treasured Prescriptions for Emergencies* 備急千金要方

Qian Jin Yi (千金翼) *Supplement to Essential Treasured Prescriptions* 千金翼方

Ru Men (入門) *An Introduction to Medicine* 醫學入門

Shang Han Lun (傷寒論) *Treatise on Cold Diseases* 傷寒論

Shen Ying (神應) *Classic of God Merit* 神應經

Sheng Hui (聖惠) *Imperial Benevolent Prescriptions* 太平聖惠方

Sheng Ji (聖濟) *Imperial Medical Encyclopedia* 聖濟總録

Shi Ji (實際) *Practice of Clinical Studies* (in Japanese) 臨牀研究的實際（日文）

Su Wen (素問) *The Yellow Emperor's Canon of Internal Medicine: Plain Questions* 黄帝内經素問
Tong Ren (銅人) *Illustrated Manual of Points for Acupuncture and Moxibustion on a Bronze Statue with Acupoints* 銅人腧穴針灸圖經
Tu Pu (圖譜) *An Atlas of Extra Points for Acupuncture and Moxibustion* 針灸經外奇穴圖譜
Tu Yi (圖翼) *Supplements to Illustrated Classified Canon of Internal Medicine of the Yellow Emperor* 類經圖翼
Wai Tai (外台) *Clandestine Essentials from the Imperial Library* 外台秘要方
Wen Dui (問對) *Catechism of Acupuncture and Moxibustion* 針灸問對
Xiao Xue (小學) *Elementary Collections of Medical Classics* 醫經小學
Xin Shu (心書) *Bian Que's Medical Experiences* 扁鵲心書
Xun Jing (循經) *Studies on Acupoints Along Meridians* 循經考穴編
Yin Jing (銀精) *Essentials of Ophthalmology* 銀海精微
Yi Xin Fang (醫心方) *The Heart of Medical Prescriptions* 醫心方
Yu Long Jing (玉龍經) *Bian Que's Jade Dragon Classics of Acupuncture and Moxibustion* 扁鵲神應針灸玉龍經
Zhen Jiu Xue (針灸學) *Chinese Acupuncture and Moxibustion* 中國針灸學
Zhen Jiu Zhen Sui (針灸真髓) *Quintessence of Acupuncture and Moxibustion* (in Japanese) 針灸真髓 (日文)
Zhou Hou (肘後) *A Handbook of Prescriptions for Emergencies* 肘後備急方
Zi Sheng (資生) *Acupuncture-Moxibustion Classic for Saving Life* 針灸資生經
Zhejiang Journal of Traditional Chinese Medicine, No. 8, 1957
China Medical Journal, No. 6, 1956
Draft for Standard Acupuncture Nomenclature, WHO, 1988
Beijing Journal of Traditional Chinese Medicine, No. 11, 1954
Journal of Traditional Chinese Medicine, 1955
China Journal of Surgery, No. 8, 1959
New Materia Medica, No. 2, Vol. 8, 1957

2. Index of the Regular Points

3. Index of the Extra Points

Q

S

T

W

X

Y

Z

中医针灸经穴部位标准化
中国中医研究院针灸研究所编撰
国家中医药管理局审定
*
外文出版社出版
（中国北京百万庄路24号）
邮政编码100037
中国科学院印刷厂印刷
中国国际图书贸易总公司发行
（中国北京车公庄西路 21号）
北京邮政信箱第399号　邮政编码100044
1990年（16开）第一版
（英）
ISBN 0-8351-2749-4
ISBN 7-119-01368-8/R·62(外)
06000
14—E—2610S